Challenges and Innovative Solutions in Nasal Drug Delivery: From Formulation Development to Mode of Administration

Challenges and Innovative Solutions in Nasal Drug Delivery: From Formulation Development to Mode of Administration

Guest Editor

Anita Hafner

MDPI

Basel • Beijing • Wuhan • Barcelona • Belgrade • Novi Sad • Cluj • Manchester

Guest Editor
Anita Hafner
Faculty of Pharmacy
and Biochemistry
University of Zagreb
Zagreb
Croatia

Editorial Office
MDPI AG
Grosspeteranlage 5
4052 Basel, Switzerland

This is a reprint of the Special Issue, published open access by the journal *Pharmaceutics* (ISSN 1999-4923), freely accessible at: https://www.mdpi.com/journal/pharmaceutics/special_issues/87BUC5739Q.

For citation purposes, cite each article independently as indicated on the article page online and as indicated below:

Lastname, A.A.; Lastname, B.B. Article Title. *Journal Name* **Year**, *Volume Number*, Page Range.

ISBN 978-3-7258-7400-2 (Hbk)
ISBN 978-3-7258-7401-9 (PDF)
https://doi.org/10.3390/books978-3-7258-7401-9

Contents

About the Editor

Anita Hafner

Anita Hafner is a Full Professor with tenure at the University of Zagreb, Faculty of Pharmacy and Biochemistry, Department of Pharmaceutical Technology. Her primary research focuses on the development of nasal drug delivery systems through the simultaneous optimization of their biopharmaceutical properties and nasal deposition profiles. Her current work is particularly directed toward nasal drug delivery systems for pediatric and adolescent populations, with an emphasis on individualized administration approaches.

In 2008, she received the "For Women in Science" national award, granted by L'Oréal–UNESCO and the Ministry of Culture of the Republic of Croatia. In 2024 and 2025, she was included in the World's Top 2% Scientists list.

Preface

Nasal drug delivery is being continuously explored as a versatile and non-invasive route for local, systemic, and central nervous system (CNS) therapies. The possibility of direct nose-to-brain delivery offers a distinctive strategy to circumvent the limitations of the blood–brain barrier, challenging researchers to harness the untapped potential of this route. This Reprint brings together original studies and reviews that capture recent progress in this dynamic field.

The contributions span device innovation, formulation development, nasal deposition and bioavailability. Emphasis is placed on targeted delivery to the olfactory region, presenting advances in spray technologies and in vitro modeling. Novel formulation approaches, including nanoemulsions, thermogelling systems, and nanoparticulate carriers, highlight the role of delivery platforms in enhancing drug solubility, permeation, stability, mucosal retention, and targeted delivery. The use of permeation enhancers, as well as the importance of safety and translational considerations, are also addressed.

Beyond CNS delivery, the reprint includes the examples of broader applications such as systemic delivery, mucosal vaccination, and the prevention of airborne infections.

This Reprint is intended for researchers, clinicians and industry professionals engaged in the development of innovative nasal drug delivery strategies, offering a concise overview of current advances, along with insights into future perspectives in this rapidly evolving field.

Anita Hafner
Guest Editor

pharmaceutics

MDPI

Review

Lipid and Polymeric Nanoparticles: Successful Strategies for Nose-to-Brain Drug Delivery in the Treatment of Depression and Anxiety Disorders

Margarida Alberto [1], Ana Cláudia Paiva-Santos [1,2,*], Francisco Veiga [1,2] and Patrícia C. Pires [1,2,3,*]

1 Faculty of Pharmacy, University of Coimbra (FFUC), Azinhaga de Santa Comba, 3000-548 Coimbra, Portugal
2 Rede de Química e Tecnologia/Laboratório Associado para a Química Verde (REQUIMTE/LAQV), Group of Pharmaceutical Technology, Faculty of Pharmacy, University of Coimbra, 3000-548 Coimbra, Portugal
3 Health Sciences Research Centre, University of Beira Interior (CICS-UBI), Av. Infante D. Henrique, 6200-506 Covilhã, Portugal
* Correspondence: acsantos@ff.uc.pt (A.C.P.-S.); patriciapires@ff.uc.pt (P.C.P.)

Abstract: Intranasal administration has gained an increasing interest for brain drug delivery since it allows direct transport through neuronal pathways, which can be quite advantageous for central nervous system disorders, such as depression and anxiety. Nanoparticles have been studied as possible alternatives to conventional formulations, with the objective of improving drug bioavailability. The present work aimed to analyze the potential of intranasal nanoparticle administration for the treatment of depression and anxiety, using the analysis of several studies already performed. From the carried-out analysis, it was concluded that the use of nanoparticles allows the drug's protection from enzymatic degradation, and the modulation of its components allows controlled drug release and enhanced drug permeation. Furthermore, the results of in vivo studies further verified these systems' potential, with the drug reaching the brain faster and leading to increased bioavailability and, consequently, therapeutic effect. Hence, in general, the intranasal administration of nanoparticles leads to a faster onset of action, with increased and prolonged brain drug concentrations and, consequently, therapeutic effects, presenting high potential as an alternative to the currently available therapies for the treatment of depression and anxiety.

Keywords: anxiety; depression; intranasal; nose-to-brain; nanoparticles

1. Introduction

Mental health plays an extremely important role in society, and additional investment is needed in order to not only facilitate access to effective and existing treatments but also to strengthen the research and development of new treatments [1,2].

Depression is one of the leading causes of disability worldwide, contributing to the development of other diseases, which include neuropsychiatric, metabolic, and cardiovascular conditions. It is characterized by disinterest in day-to-day activities, sadness, irritability, fatigue, feelings of guilt, low self-esteem, sleep disorders, and suicidal thoughts, among others, which is associated with a decreased quality of life. Depression can be classified into two main groups: major depression, when symptoms are more intense, and there is a greater emotional burden, or minor depression, when there are fewer symptoms, allowing daily activities to be done properly. The most accepted theory regarding the pathogenesis of depression is based on a monoaminergic transmission disorder, in other words, a disruption in the transmission of serotonin, norepinephrine and dopamine in the brain due to the complex interaction of several social (e.g., traumatic life), psychological (e.g., personality) and biological (e.g., hereditary predisposition) factors. Most drugs used in the treatment of depression increase the availability of these neurotransmitters in the synaptic cleft, using several mechanisms of action, and include: selective serotonin reuptake inhibitors, such as fluoxetine, sertraline, and escitalopram; serotonin and norepinephrine reuptake inhibitors, such as venlafaxine; tricyclic antidepressants, such as amitriptyline; non-tricyclic antidepressants, such as trazodone and mirtazapine; monoamine oxidase inhibitors (MAOIs), such as moclobemide; among others, such as agomelatine, which acts as a melatonin receptor agonist and as a selective antagonist of serotonin reuptake [3–8].

On the other hand, anxiety is a type of central nervous system (CNS) disorder that frequently interferes with day-to-day activities and decreases performance in the workplace or in school. It can also be associated with increased cardiovascular morbidity and mortality. The most frequent symptoms of anxiety include feelings such as worry, helplessness, or fear that manifest physically through increased heart and respiratory rate, sweating, and tremors. There are different types of anxiety, such as obsessive-compulsive disorder, post-traumatic stress disorder, generalized anxiety disorder, social anxiety disorder, or separation anxiety disorder. Neuronal excitability is downregulated by the synaptic transmission of γ-aminobutyric acid (GABA); thus, when this system is inhibited, symptoms associated with anxiety arise. Pharmacological treatment of anxiety includes mostly anxiolytic drugs such as benzodiazepines (e.g., diazepam or alprazolam) that bind to the $GABA_A$ receptor, increasing GABAs affinity for the receptor and enhancing its action [9–11].

Depression and anxiety are two pathologies that are often associated; thus, a patient with depression tends to develop anxiety, and similarly, a patient with anxiety can progress to a depressive state. The presence of the two pathologies simultaneously intensifies the symptoms of both, making their treatment even more important [12,13].

Currently, the oral route of administration is the preferred route for drug administration in the treatment of depression and anxiety. However, this route has several disadvantages since drugs administered orally are exposed to first-pass hepatic metabolism and require regular administrations to ensure the constant presence of the drug at the site of action, the amount of drug that reaches the site of action (the brain) is restricted by the low permeability of the blood-brain barrier, and fluctuations in plasma concentrations can lead to side effects and loss of efficacy [7,8,14,15].

Therefore, since the prevalence of depression and anxiety has been increasing over the last few years, a growing number of studies have been developed in order to discover alternatives to the current treatments of these pathologies. One of these alternatives is the intranasal route of administration.

1.1. Intranasal Administration for Brain Drug Delivery

The intranasal route of administration is an alternative to the administration of drugs in the treatment of CNS pathologies which has several advantages over other routes, allowing to overcome the blood-brain barrier; transport of molecules of larger dimensions (up to about 1000 Da); avoid the first pass hepatic metabolism; minimize the side effects caused by drugs administered through the systemic circulation, reducing toxicity; reduce the drug dose that is necessary to achieve a therapeutically effective concentration at the site of action, and thus reach the therapeutic threshold. Additionally, in general, as a route of administration, it is simple, practical, and convenient since it does not require administration techniques involving coordination or swallowing (such as the oral route) or the aid of a health professional (such as the intravenous route), and noninvasive, which can contribute to increasing patient compliance [16–18].

These advantages are connected to the unique anatomy of the nasal cavity, which includes a direct connection to the CNS, allowing the drug to be transported to the brain. This makes the nasal cavity the only place in the human body where the nervous system is in direct contact with the surrounding environment. More specifically, the nasal cavity is divided into two parts by the nasal septum, and each part consists of three distinct regions: the vestibule, the olfactory region, and the respiratory region. The vestibule is located at the entrance of the nasal cavity and is responsible for the filtration of inhaled particles. It is the region that least contributes to the absorption of drugs. The respiratory region consists of turbinates, which are responsible for humidification and regulation of the temperature of inhaled air, contributing to the formation of an airflow that improves the contact between inhaled air and the nasal mucosa. The epithelium cells of this region are covered by microvilli and long cilia, which contribute to improved absorption. It is the main responsible region for systemic drug absorption, having a surface area of about 160 cm^2 and high vascularization, which provides a high blood flow. From systemic circulation, the drug can be transported to the brain, but in that case, it needs to cross the blood-brain barrier in order to reach the CNS. It can also contribute to the direct absorption of drugs into the CNS through the trigeminal nerve. The olfactory region occupies a surface area of approximately 10 cm^2, playing a crucial role in the absorption and transport of drugs to the brain. The olfactory epithelium consists of olfactory nerves, responsible for the direct transport of the drug from the nasal cavity to the brain, using the olfactory nerve. Hence, in short, intranasally administered drugs can reach the site of action in the brain directly, using the olfactory or trigeminal nerves (direct transport), or indirectly, being absorbed into the systemic circulation and then crossing the blood-brain barrier (indirect transport) (Figure 1) [16,17,19,20].

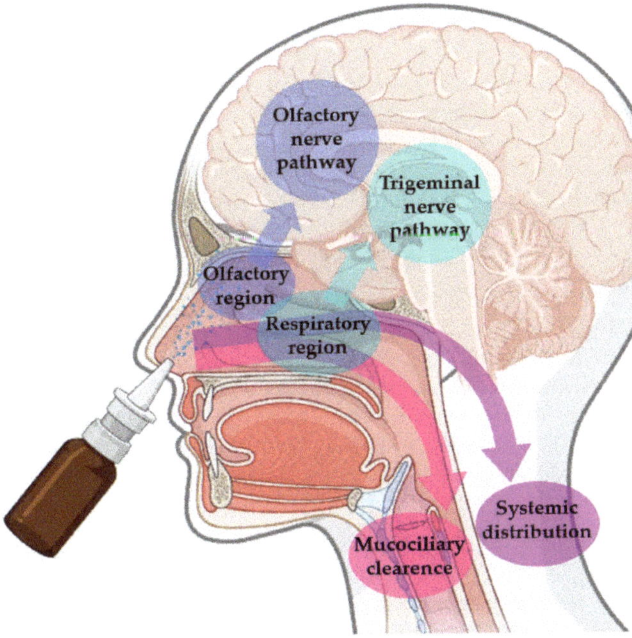

Figure 1. Pathways of brain drug transport after intranasal administration: direct transport (neuronal transport—olfactory nerve and trigeminal nerves) and indirect transport (systemic distribution).

Nevertheless, in spite of the many important advantages that intranasal administration presents, it is necessary to consider some limiting factors that hinder drug absorption, namely: the physical removal of the drug from the nasal cavity by mucociliary clearance mechanisms; enzymatic degradation in the mucus and nasal epithelium layer; and the volume of formulation that can be administered, that is limited to 25–200 µL, which turns this route of administration more appropriate for potent drugs. Mucociliary clearance has the function of protecting the respiratory system against bacteria and inhaled particles as a result of the combined effect of mucus and cilia that transport the particles from the anterior to the posterior region of the nasal cavity, being eliminated to the bottom of the throat. Hence, drug bioavailability is diminished by the high flow of nasal secretions and ciliary movement since these decrease the time of residence of the drugs in the nasal cavity, affecting the permeability through the mucosa. The enzymatic activity in the nasal cavity also constitutes a barrier to the absorption of drugs since several enzymes, such as the various isoforms of cytochrome P450, are present in the nasal mucosa and perform enzymatic degradation of various drugs [17,19–21]. The many strategies that have been developed to overcome these obstacles, as well as the factors that influence nasal drug absorption, are addressed in the following Sections 1.1.1 and 1.1.2.

1.1.1. Physicochemical and Formulation Factors That Influence Nasal Drug Absorption

Nasal absorption is influenced by several factors, namely anatomical and physiological factors (mucociliary clearance, enzymatic degradation, membrane transport, mucosal irritation, and deposition), physicochemical factors (molecular drug weight, lipophilicity and ionization state), and formulation factors (type and characteristics of the formulation, volume of administration, drug strength, viscosity, pH, osmolarity). When the drug is administered intranasally, it comes into direct contact with the nasal mucosa. The passage through the mucus layer is the first step to its absorption. Mucin, the main protein of the mucus, binds to drugs, hampering their diffusion. Additionally, alterations in pH or temperature may alter the structure of the mucus, making the diffusion of the drug more difficult. Moreover, the mucus has elastic and viscous properties that influence the transport of drugs; hence, if the mucus is more viscous, mucociliary clearance is reduced, and, therefore, the contact time between the drug and the mucosa is increased, which may contribute to improved drug absorption [17,20,21].

After passing through the mucus layer, the transport of the drug can be performed by different mechanisms that include: transcellular diffusion, in which transport is carried out through the membrane by passive diffusion or active transport; and paracellular diffusion, a passive process, in which the drug moves through the intercellular space. The lipophilicity of the drug is one of the most important factors that determines whether the transport will be performed by transcellular diffusion or paracellular diffusion. Lipophilic drugs are preferably transported through transcellular diffusion, showing fast and efficient absorption when administered intranasally. Hydrophilic drugs are mainly transported via paracellular diffusion, resulting in low absorption. The rate of a drug's diffusion through the nasal mucosa is also influenced by the state of ionization and molecular weight of the drug. Consequently, lipophilic and uncharged (neutral) drugs with low molecular weight are more easily absorbed when compared to hydrophilic, charged and/or high molecular weight molecules. Absorption also depends on the pKa of the drug and the pH at the absorption site, which presents values between 5.0 and 6.5 in the nasal mucosa. It is also influenced by the solubility of the drug since nose secretions have a more watery nature; therefore, the drug should present an appropriate aqueous solubility for better dissolution in the mucus itself [16,17,21,22].

In order to optimize drug transport to the action site after an intranasal administration, it is necessary to take into account certain characteristics of the formulation, for example, factors such as its capability to adhere to the mucosa, nasal permeability, and drug deposition in the olfactory epithelium. These characteristics should be elevated and should also allow a controlled and constant release of the drug. The excipients of the formulation should be selected, taking into account their functions, with the purpose of assigning properties to the formulation that allow to protect the drug and favor its administration and arrival of the drug at the action site. The excipients must also be compatible with the active substance and non-toxic or irritating to the nasal mucosa [17]. The concentration of the drug in the formulation and the volume of administration should also be taken into account since it is only possible to administer approximately 200 μL of formulation in the nasal cavity, which makes this route of administration suitable for potent drugs but challenging to drugs that require high doses or that have reduced solubility [17,18,23].

The pH of the formulation is also important and should be close to the pH of the nasal cavity to avoid mucosal irritation. Lysozyme found in nose secretions contributes to the dissolution of certain bacteria and helps to maintain acidic pH. Additionally, the pH of the formulation should be selected considering the stability of the drug and should also contribute to the existence of a higher fraction of non-ionized drug, while maintaining the functionality of the excipients. Another very important factor is the viscosity of the formulation, which should ensure contact with the nasal mucosa for an adequate period of time. Higher viscosity increases the time of contact of the drug with the mucosa and may contribute to increased absorption. However, formulations that are excessively viscous can decrease the diffusion of the drug from the formulation itself, reducing its absorption. Gel formulations can be used to increase the time of permanence of the drug in the nasal cavity and, consequently, improve its bioavailability. The most used gelling agents include cellulose derivatives (methylcellulose or carboxymethylcellulose) and carbopol. Also, considering that isotonic solutions are better tolerated, the osmolarity of the formulations should be between 285 and 310 mOsmol/L to avoid mucosal irritation. However, hypertonic solutions can be used since they transiently reduce ciliary activity, which can increase the retention time of the drug in the nasal cavity, promoting its absorption. Nevertheless, caution is required when hypertonic solutions are used in order to ensure that no damage is caused to the nasal mucosa [17,18,24–29].

1.1.2. Strategies Used to Improve Drug Absorption

Many different strategies have been developed in order to improve drug solubilization and absorption, such as the use of prodrugs, absorption enhancers, enzymatic inhibitors, mucoadhesive agents, and nanometric drug transport systems [30].

Structural changes in the drug molecule can help improve their characteristics by changing physicochemical properties such as molecular weight, partition coefficient, and solubility. These can be used to improve formulation drug strength, absorption through biological barriers, or premature metabolism. The grand majority of prodrugs are administered in their inactive form, requiring biotransformation to become their active form, which produces a pharmacological effect [17,28,29,31–33].

Absorption enhancers are excipients that can improve drug permeability, which is especially important for hydrophilic drugs. They act by altering the phospholipid bilayer and membrane fluidity or by alternately opening tight junctions between epithelial cells, improving paracellular transport. The most commonly used are surfactants (e.g., polysorbate, poloxamers), bile salts (e.g., sodium cholate), fatty acids (e.g., stearic acid, palmitic acid), chelators (e.g., ethylenediaminetetraacetic acid (EDTA), salicylates) and polymers (e.g., chitosan, poly(D,L–lacitde co– glycolide) (PLGA)) [17,22,34–36].

Enzymatic inhibitors can also be used to protect drugs against the enzymatic degradation that occurs in the nasal cavity, thereby increasing the available fraction of the drug for absorption and, consequently, bioavailability. Peptidase inhibitors and proteases, such as amastatin, boroleucine, bacitracin, and puromycin may be used [22,33,37,38].

Mucoadhesive agents increase the contact time between the formulation and the nasal mucosa, also favoring the paracellular transport of hydrophilic drugs and reducing mucociliary clearance by establishing a connection between mucin and a polymer. One of the possible mechanisms adopted by the mucoadhesive systems is the absorption of water from the nasal mucosa, which leads to the swelling of the polymer, and consequent penetration into the mucus with fixation of the formulation to the nasal cavity, improving the absorption of the drug. An example is chitosan, a biocompatible and biodegradable polymer, is widely used not only for its mucoadhesive properties but also for increasing permeability and paracellular transport, through interaction with the tight junctions [17,30,39–41].

Finally, another very promising and widely used strategy to improve drug absorption and bioavailability is the incorporation of drugs into nanometric transport systems, discussed in detail in the next Section 1.2.

1.2. Nanometric Drug Transport Systems

Nanometric drug transport systems are formulations that help transport the drug to the respective action site, allowing it to modulate the time and quantity of drug released. For the fraction that does not undergo transport via the direct route (neuronal transport), nanoparticles can be transported to the brain by interaction with the blood-brain barrier, mostly via receptor-mediated transcytosis, transporter-mediated transcytosis, absorption-mediated transcytosis, and transient opening of the blood-brain barrier itself [42–47]. These systems must be biocompatible, non-toxic, and easily eliminated or biodegradable. The main categories of nanometric systems are liposomes, nanoemulsions, and polymeric or lipid nanoparticles (Figure 2) [48].

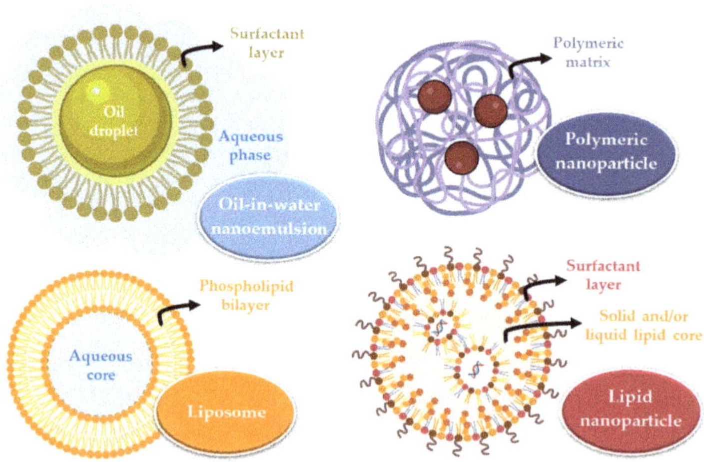

Figure 2. Main types of nanometric systems: liposomes, nanoemulsions, polymeric nanoparticles, and lipid nanoparticles.

Liposomes are vesicles composed of one or more phospholipid bilayers that surround an aqueous core and are variable in size (between 20 and 1000 nm). Their composition allows the incorporation of hydrophilic (in the core) or hydrophobic (in the phospholipid bilayers) drugs that will be transported to the site of action. Nevertheless, they have some disadvantages, which include system instability, the unwanted release of the encapsulated substance, irreproducibility between batches, difficulty controlling liposome size, and low encapsulation efficiency [49,50]. Nanoemulsions are thermodynamically stable systems, consisting of two immiscible liquids (oil and water) that, when mixed, form a single phase through the action of an emulsifying agent. These systems are usually smaller than 500 nm, and can either be oil-in-water or water-in-oil in nature. They are biodegradable and allow quick drug uptake to the brain. However, they also have some disadvantages, including their inability to solubilize substances with a high melting point, many times requiring large quantities of surfactants to stabilize the system (which may compromise their safe use), and a high production price [48,51,52].

On the other hand, nanoparticles are solid substances with a size that can vary between 10 and 1000 nm that allow to dissolve, encapsulate, absorb, or attach hydrophilic or lipophilic drugs (depending on the characteristics and composition of the nanoparticle). These systems have several advantages, such as: making it possible to avoid drug degradation, consequently increasing its concentration at the action site; having a reduced particle size, which results in higher surface area, allowing to overcome biological and physiological barriers; allowing drug targeting according to the nanoparticle's surface functionalization, directing it to the site of action. In intranasal administration, a particle size between 10 and 300 nm is advantageous since nanoparticles that are this size can be transported directly by the olfactory nerve to the brain. There are two major groups of nanoparticles: polymeric and lipid [33,46,48].

Polymeric nanoparticles can be divided into two groups, depending on the preparation method that is used and on the characteristics of the resulting system: nanocapsules, in which there is a reservoir system, which means the drug is confined to a cavity surrounded by a single polymer membrane that is present on the surface of the nanoparticle, coating it; or nanospheres, which are homogeneous matrix systems, in which the drug is uniformly dispersed or dissolved in. By modulating the polymer, it is possible to control the release of the drug to reach the desired therapeutic concentrations at the action site for the required period of time [33,48].

Lipid nanoparticles are subdivided into solid lipid nanoparticles (SLNs) and nanostructured lipid carriers (NLCs). SLNs are constituted by a solid lipid matrix, that is, by lipids that remain solid at room temperature and body temperature. The lipophilic drug is dissolved or dispersed in this matrix, which is surrounded by a surfactant layer in an aqueous dispersion that contributes to the stability of the nanoparticle. When compared to polymeric nanoparticles, lipid nanoparticles are considered more biocompatible and biodegradable, have low toxicity, are easy to produce on a large scale, have better physical stability, and good control of drug release. SLNs, however, have some disadvantages, namely the structural reorganization they undergo over time (such as recrystallization), because they only have one type of lipid, which creates a tighter internal structure with less space to incorporate drug molecules. In order to overcome this problem, the NLCs emerged, which have a matrix formed by a solid lipid and a liquid lipid. The addition of liquid lipids prevents crystallization and allows structural disorganization in the lipid matrix, creating larger spaces to incorporate the drug molecules in. Yet, despite the advantages of the NLC, SLN remains an effective system. Since the mucosa has a lipid nature, lipid nanoparticles can be transported by passive diffusion to the site of action [42,48,50].

Thus, nanometric drug transport systems, and specifically nanoparticles, present advantages for intranasal drug administration since they allow to protect the drug from mucociliary clearance and the enzymatic degradation that occurs in the nasal cavity, improve its absorption, and allow to modulate the time and quantity of drug available at the site of action, favoring transport through the biological membranes [30,53]. A summary of the ideal nanoparticle formulation characteristics for intranasal administration is depicted in Figure 3.

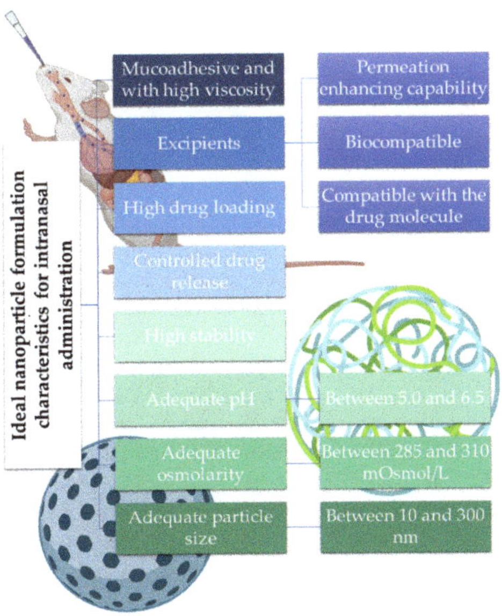

Figure 3. Summary of the ideal nanoparticle formulation characteristics for intranasal administration.

Taking into account the increased incidence of mental illness, and in particular depression and anxiety, an increasing need for safer, faster, and more effective treatments has been identified. Analyzing the advantages of intranasal administration together with the advantages of nanoparticles, the development of new formulations using nanoparticles for intranasal administration seems to have great potential as an alternative to existing treatments. The following sections will summarize and do a critical analysis of the already existing studies regarding the development and evaluation of nanoparticles for intranasal administration of antidepressant and anxiolytic drugs that may contribute to a more effective future treatment of these pathologies.

2. Nanoparticles as Efficient Strategies to Deliver Antidepressant and Anxiolytic Drugs to the Brain

2.1. Icariin

Icariin is a component of the aerial parts of the plant *Epimedium brevicornum* Maxim (Berberidaceae), which presents antidepressant-like effects. After oral administration, the reached plasma concentrations are very low, with the drug being weakly absorbed by this route, limiting its use in the treatment of depression.

A study conducted by Xu et al. [54] aimed to develop a nano thermoresponsive hydrogel (nanogel) to allow the encapsulation of icariin for intranasal administration in order to increase the amount of drug that reaches the brain, and to verify its antidepressant-like activity. Nanogel was obtained using alginate, an ionic polysaccharide with hydrophilic characteristics that allows the increase in the weak solubility of icariin in water, and divalent cations, which, when in contact with alginate, will enable the formation of reversible hydrogels (Figure 4A). Additionally, poloxamer 407 and poloxamer 188 were added to the developed hydrogel, due to their thermosensitive characteristics, with the objective of improving the bioavailability of icariin and stabilizing the nanosystem. Therefore, polymeric alginate nanoparticles were formulated, being placed in a matrix of poloxamers right after. Due to the presence of alginate, a mucoadhesive polymer, the developed semisolid formulation also had the ability to adhere to the nasal mucosa. The particle size of the icariin nanogel (73.80 nm) was smaller than the particle size of the drug-free vehicle (87.28 nm), which may be due to the fact that icariin is encapsulated in the nanogel through hydrogen bonds, with superior intermolecular forces. The polydispersity index (PDI, a particle size homogeneity index ranging from 0 to 1) and zeta potential (particle surface charge) of the optimized formulation were 0.15 and −19.2 mV, respectively, which means that the formulated nanogel presented homogeneous particle size and was potentially stable due to electrostatic repulsion between the charged nanoparticles.

In vitro drug release studies showed that the nanogel had a controlled release, allowing the drug to be fully released after 36 h. The antidepressant-like effects of the formulated nanogel were studied by conducting in vivo pharmacodynamic studies in mice, such as the forced swim test (Figure 4B), tail suspension test (Figure 4C), and open field test (Figure 4D). The results showed that the formulated nanogel allowed to reduce the immobility time of the mice after only one intranasal administration when compared with the oral administration of a drug solution that required administration for seven consecutive days. The results support that the antidepressant effect is the fastest with the intranasal administration of the nanogel. In vivo studies were also conducted in rats, using the CUMS (chronic unpredictable mild stress) model, which, when applied, leads to a reduction in body weight and decreases the preference for sucrose in depressed animals. The treatment with the formulated intranasal nanogel allowed to reverse these effects, overall increasing the rat's body weight (Figure 4E) and restoring their sucrose intake more significantly than any other treatment group (Figure 4F).

This study allowed us to conclude that the formulated icariin nanogel, when administered intranasally, presents relevant potential as a possible alternative for the treatment of depression.

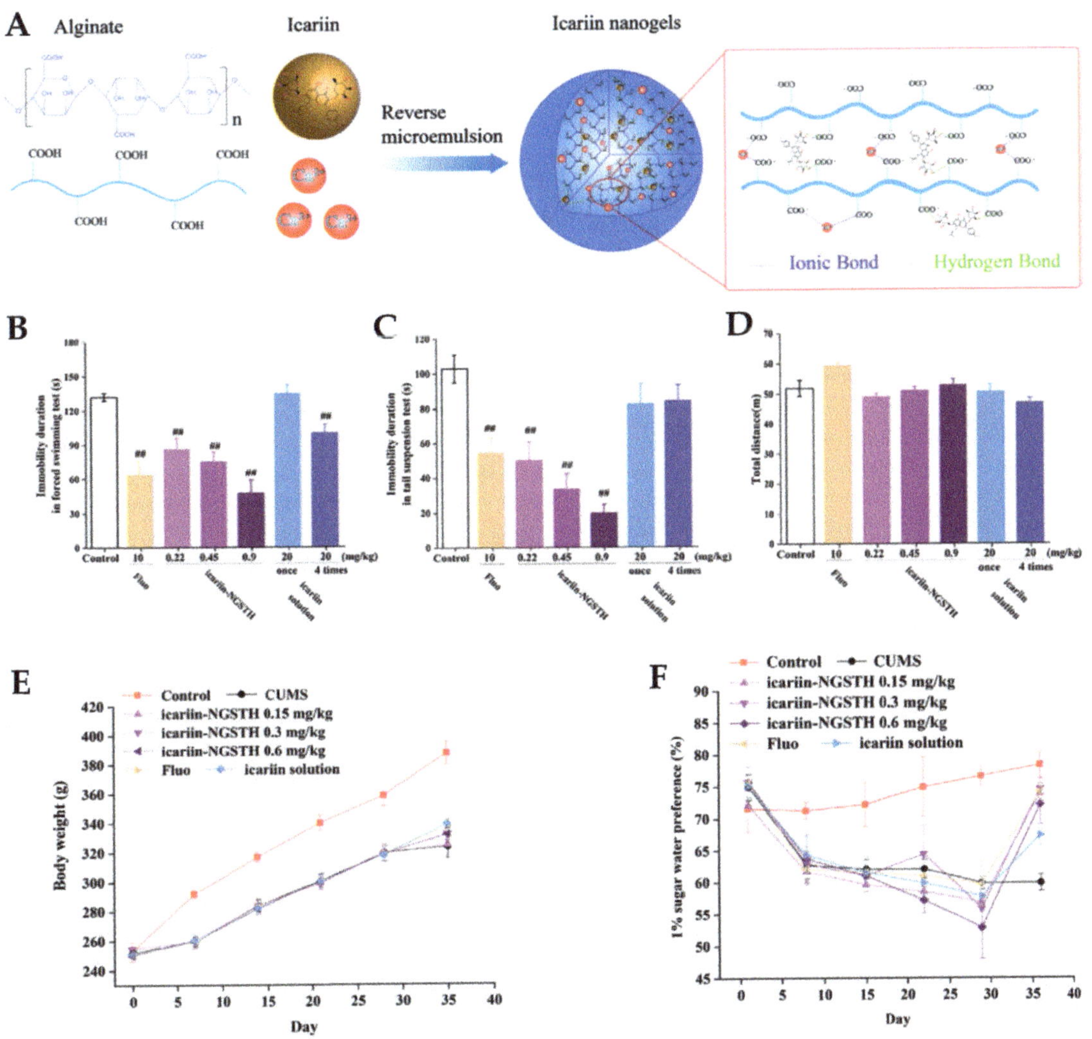

Figure 4. (**A**)—Schematic representation of the making of icariin nanogels; (**B**)—Immobility duration in a forced swimming test, (**C**)—Immobility duration in tail suspension test, and (**D**)—Total distance travelled in open field test, in mice, after intranasal administration of saline buffer (negative control), oral administration of a fluoxetine solution (Fluo, positive control), intranasal administration of the icariin nanogel (NGSTH), or oral administration of an icariin solution; (**E**)—Changes in body weight, and (**F**)—Changes in 1% sucrose preference, in rats, after no administration (CUMS) or intranasal administration of saline buffer (negative controls), oral administration of a fluoxetine solution (Fluo, positive control), intranasal administration of the icariin nanogel (NGSTH), or oral administration of an icariin solution; ## $p < 0.01$, compared with the negative control group; adapted from Xu et al. [54], reproduced with permission from Elsevier [License Number 5426000092048].

2.2. *Albiflorin*

Albiflorin is the main component of the root of *Radix Paeoniae Alba* (Ranunculaceae), presenting antioxidant, anti-inflammatory, and neuroprotective properties and antidepressant-like effects. Nevertheless, when administered orally, it has low bioavailability, not reaching effective brain concentrations to evidence a significant antidepressant-like effect.

To tackle these issues, a study conducted by Xu et al. [55] aimed to develop an intranasal albiflorin nanogel. Once again, the interaction of alginate with divalent cations was used for the formulation of the nanoparticles, with the subsequent addition of poloxamer 407 and poloxamer 188 to form the nanogel and in order to stabilize the system and allow a controlled release of the drug. The particle size of the nanogel was small (45.6 nm), as was the PDI (0.20), making it quite a homogeneous system. The obtained zeta potential was negative (−19.8 mV) due to the presence of alginate, a polyanion, in the composition of the nanoparticle.

In-vitro drug release studies showed a controlled release of the drug from the nanogel, being extended in time for about 12 h. Moreover, in vivo pharmacokinetic studies in rats, the drug was not only rapidly quantified in the brain, but also allowed the maintenance of prolonged concentrations over time, which indicated a rapid transport and a potential prolonged therapeutic effect. In-vivo pharmacodynamic studies were also conducted, in mice, with the purpose of evaluating the antidepressant activity of the formulation. The tail suspension test demonstrated that the intranasal administration of the nanogel significantly reduced the immobility time in mice when compared with intragastric or intravenous administration of fluoxetine (antidepressant drug of known efficacy) or albiflorin solutions. The CUMS model was applied in rats, causing a decrease in body weight as well as in sucrose intake, but these effects were once again reversed by intranasal administration of the albiflorin nanogel.

In conclusion, the formulated nanogel was able to encapsulate albiflorin and, when administered intranasally, provide a continuous and controlled release of the drug that made it possible to evidence its antidepressant-like effect, presenting potential as an alternative for the treatment of depression.

2.3. Fluoxetine

Fluoxetine is a selective serotonin reuptake inhibitor. The main problem associated with this drug is that it is prone to drug-drug interactions when administered orally since it is a CYP2D6 inhibitor and a substrate and inhibitor of the P-glycoprotein efflux transporter.

To tackle these issues, Vitorino et al. [56] aimed to develop a formulation based on lipid nanoparticles for intranasal administration of fluoxetine in order to find the optimal conditions to combine a rapid onset of action with a prolonged therapeutic effect. Initially, the components were screened, taking into account the relative solubility of fluoxetine in them. As a solid lipid, glyceryl palmitostearate (Precirol™ ATO 5), a biocompatible glyceride, was used. The selected liquid lipid was propylene glycol monocaprylate (type I) (Lauroglycol™ 90). Polysorbate 80 (Tween® 80) was used as a surfactant due to its good emulsifying capacity, biocompatibility, and ability to stabilize the nanosystem. In the optimization stage of the right component proportions (liquid lipid: solid lipid ratio and amount of surfactant), the main conclusions were: that formulations with higher surfactant concentration decreased permeability and extended drug release; that an increase in the amount of liquid lipid resulted in increased release and decreased permeability; that the increase in the concentration of liquid lipid and surfactant allowed to have smaller particles and a more homogeneous size; and that the formulation with the highest concentration of solid lipid and the lowest amount of surfactant achieved the best permeability. Thus, the optimized formulation had similar percentages of solid lipid and liquid lipid and low surfactant concentration, presenting a particle size of 154 nm, PDI of 0.514, and zeta potential of +19.7 mV. Although the particle size was small, and the zeta potential had a moderately high absolute value (which could contribute to particle stability), the PDI value was high, making this a reasonably heterogeneous formulation. The encapsulation efficiency (EE%) (amount of drug that is possible to incorporate in the lipid matrix) and drug loading (percentage of encapsulated drug divided by the total mass of the lipid matrix) were also determined, being around 74% and 13%, respectively.

In-vivo pharmacodynamic studies were conducted in mice, namely the forced swim test, applied one hour after the administration of the formulations. This allowed us to verify that both the intranasal nanoparticles and an oral fluoxetine solution (positive control) led to an increase in the mobility time when compared to the group of untreated animals. However, the immobility time was shorter after oral administration of the fluoxetine solution. These results may be related to the time elapsed between the administration of the drug and the performance of the test, since, in general, the drugs administered intranasally can take about 15 min to reach the brain

Based on the obtained results, since no comparative superiority was demonstrated in this study it is possible to conclude that the formulation of lipid nanoparticles administered intranasally presents potential as an alternative to oral administration when the oral route is not accessible.

2.4. Agomelatine

Agomelatine is a synthetic compound derived from melatonin used in the treatment of depression. It is an agonist of the melatonin MT1 and MT2 receptors and an antagonist of 5-HT2C serotonin receptors. This drug undergoes a substantial hepatic first-pass metabolism when administered orally, leading to an extremely low bioavailability. The study conducted by Jani et al. [57] aimed to solve these issues by analyzing the efficacy of the intranasal administration of agomelatine polymeric nanoparticles for the treatment of depression.

The formulated polymeric nanoparticles were obtained using the polymer PLGA, due to its low toxicity and poloxamer 407 as a surfactant to stabilize the nanoparticles. The optimization of the formulation considered the drug: polymer ratio and surfactant concentrations since they affect the particle size and the EE%. A statistical study allowed us to verify that by increasing the amount of PLGA the EE% also increases; however, after a certain amount of PLGA the EE% begins to decrease. The same was verified for the relation between surfactant concentration and EE%. Regarding particle size, it was concluded that it increases with the increase in the amount of PLGA, and decreases with the increase in the amount of surfactant. Thus, the optimized formulation aimed at the highest EE% value (98.3%) and the lowest particle size (116.06 nm). The zeta potential of the optimized formulation was −22.7 mV, and the PDI was less than 0.3, indicating that the formulated system was stable and the particle size distribution was homogeneous. Drug loading (49.2%) was also calculated.

In vitro drug release studies showed that the release of drug from the nanoparticles was more prolonged than the free drug, indicating an extended drug release, which can be seen as an advantage. Ex vivo permeation studies were performed using goat nasal mucosa, and the results allowed us to conclude that the permeability of the formulation was also superior to the permeability of a free drug suspension.

The forced swim test (in vivo pharmacodynamic study) was performed in rats and allowed to verify that, although the two analyzed formulations (PLGA nanoparticles and simple drug suspension) were able to reduce immobility time, the PLGA nanoparticles demonstrated the most significant reduction when compared to a group of untreated animals.

Thus, given the results of in vitro drug release, ex vivo drug permeation, and in-vivo pharmacodynamic studies, it is possible to conclude that the formulated nanoparticles have the potential for the treatment of depression when administered intranasally.

2.5. Venlafaxine

Venlafaxine is a serotonin and norepinephrine reuptake inhibitor. The oral administration of this drug is associated with several adverse effects, such as headaches and dizziness, among others, with low bioavailability and a short half-life time. Additionally, frequent administrations are necessary to produce the desired effect [37–39].

A study done by Haque et al. [58] aimed to tackle these issues by verifying the potential of chitosan nanoparticles to improve the transport of venlafaxine to the brain, using intranasal administration. The formulated polymeric nanoparticles were composed of chitosan, a polycation, and sodium tripolyphosphate (TPP), a polyanion. The optimized formulation considered a drug: polymer ratio of 1:1, and also took into account the proportion between chitosan and TPP concentrations since it affects the formulation of nanoparticles. The obtained nanoparticles presented a particle size of 167 nm, a PDI of 0.367, a zeta potential of +23.83 mV, and a pH of 5.12, thus concluding that the formulated system had a surface charge that increased its stability, with particle size and pH adequate for intranasal administration, although not being very homogeneous. It also presented an EE% of 79.3% and drug loading of 32.3%. In vitro drug release studies allowed us to conclude that the formulated nanoparticles presented a biphasic release profile, for which in the first 2 h there was a rapid release, followed by an extended release over 24 h. Drug permeation was analyzed in ex-vivo studies using pig nasal mucosa, and the use of chitosan nanoparticles allowed us to increase the permeability of venlafaxine 3-fold when compared with a venlafaxine solution. In vivo pharmacodynamic studies in rats (forced swim test) allowed us to conclude that the intranasal administration of the developed chitosan nanoparticles, when compared with the control group (saline solution), increased swimming time and locomotor activity and reduced immobility time. Pharmacokinetic parameters were also evaluated, such as the maximum concentration of venlafaxine in the brain and brain AUC, and the results were better for the intranasal nanoparticles (when compared with an intravenous or intranasal venlafaxine solution), and the intranasal route in general (when compared with the intravenous drug solution). These results could be attributed to the action of chitosan in paracellular transport enhancement and alternate opening of the tight junctions, and also its contribution to the reduction of mucociliary clearance. Brain targeting ratios, such as direct transport percentage (DTP%) and drug targeting efficiency (DTE%), were also calculated, presenting high values for the formulated nanoparticles (80.34% and 508.59%, respectively), supporting their capacity for brain targeting. Thus, the formulated nanoparticles, administered intranasally, were successful in increasing the transport of the drug from the nasal cavity to the brain, thus demonstrating potential as an alternative to the oral administration of venlafaxine.

Another study made by Haque et al. [59] aimed to analyze the potential of the intranasal administration of venlafaxine alginate and chitosan nanoparticles for the treatment of depression. To obtain the formulation, firstly, alginate was added to calcium chloride, which allowed the occurrence of inotropic pre-gelation, obtaining a pre-gelified nanonucleus, within which the drug was encapsulated. Then chitosan (positively charged) was added, which interacted with the negative charge of alginate, originating the nanogel. The optimization of the formulation took into account the concentrations of alginate, calcium chloride, and chitosan, and the drug: alginate ratio was set at 0.75:1. The pH was maintained between 5.7 and 6.1, being carefully optimized, since a higher pH results in chitosan precipitation, making it less available for the formation of the nanoparticles. Additionally, the addition of an alginate solution at neutral pH results in the non-protonation of the chitosan amine groups, stopping its ionic interaction with alginate. Particle size (173.7 nm), zeta potential (+37.4 mV), and PDI (0.391) allowed to confirm the reduced size and potential stability of the nanosystem, albeit being slightly heterogeneous. Drug loading (26.74%) and EE% (85.6%) were also determined. In-vitro drug release studies showed that the formulated nanoparticles had a biphasic release profile, with an initial faster release, followed by an extended release. Ex vivo permeation studies (pig nasal mucosa) showed that the formulated nanoparticles had an improved permeability when compared to a drug solution. In vivo pharmacodynamic studies (in rats), namely the forced swimming and locomotor activity tests, showed that, when compared with the control group (intranasal administration of a saline solution), the intranasal nanoparticles allowed to increase swimming time and locomotor activity and reduce immobility time. The pharmacokinetic parameters were also evaluated, and the brain concentrations and AUC of venlafaxine were significantly higher after intranasal administration of the nanoparticles when compared with intravenous administration and intranasal administration of a venlafaxine solution. DTE% (425.77%) and DTP% (76.52%) allowed us to conclude that intranasal administration of formulated nanoparticles also allowed a better brain targeting of the drug when compared with all other groups. Therefore, the study revealed that the formulated nanoparticles, administered intranasally, allowed us to achieve prolonged venlafaxine concentrations in the brain, probably due to an improvement in paracellular transport through the modulation of tight junctions between cells, presenting potential in the treatment of depression.

A third study, conducted by Cayero-Otero et al. [60], also aimed to find an intranasal nanosystem that would enable the controlled release of venlafaxine, maintaining therapeutic levels for a prolonged period of time. PLGA polymeric nanoparticles were developed, having two distinct ligands: transferrin (Tf) and a specific peptide against Tf receptor (TfRp). Ligands allow for the modification of the surface of nanoparticles, improving absorption and increasing permeability due to a better interaction between the cells and the nanosystems, allowing a targeted delivery. The non-functionalized nanoparticles (without ligand) originated with a particle size of 206.3 nm, PDI of 0.190, and zeta potential of −26.5 mV. The nanoparticles with Tf and the nanoparticles with TfRp originated a particle size of 218.6 nm and 216.3 nm, PDI of 0.078 and 0.067, and zeta potential of −19.5 mV and −19.6 mV, respectively. Hence, it is evident that although the ligands slightly increase the particle size, they also reduce the PDI, leading to more stable and homogeneous nanoparticles. EE% ranged from 48 to 50%, and drug loading from 10 to 12% for all formulations. The three formulations demonstrated a biphasic drug release profile. Initially, there was a fast release, and after that, there was a prolonged release for 10 days. It was possible to observe that the non-functionalized nanoparticles presented an overall higher cumulative drug release when compared to the functionalized nanoparticles. Hence, the ligands led to a decrease in drug release, probably due to the forming of an additional barrier on the surface of the nanoparticle. In-vivo pharmacokinetic studies, it was observed that the mice brain drug concentration 30 min after intranasal administration was much higher for the non-functionalized nanoparticles. This was justified by the authors as being due to the type of transport adopted by the different nanoparticles since the non-functionalized nanoparticles were preferably transported by the olfactory route, through facilitated transport or extracellular transport, taking only a few minutes to reach the brain; and the functionalized nanoparticles were preferably transported by endocytosis, which is a slower type of transport. Hence, compared to non-functionalized nanoparticles, functionalized nanoparticles take longer to reach the therapeutic action site, which can be a disadvantage if a rapid onset of action is desired. However, they have a more controlled release and may allow more prolonged therapeutic action. Hence, it was concluded that both the non-functionalized and functionalized developed nanoparticles had the potential to provide a controlled release of venlafaxine when administered intranasally and may be candidates as an alternative to the oral administration of this drug.

Comparing the three aforementioned studies, it is possible to observe that all of them formulated polymeric nanoparticles for venlafaxine encapsulation. The first two studies [58,59] had a particle size lower than 200 nm, but a PDI value higher than 0.3, which indicates that the particle size is small but not very homogeneous (considering an optimal value of < 0.3). The Zeta potential of both studies was positive. The third study [60] had an additional evaluation of the effect of surface ligands, and both functionalized and non-functionalized nanoparticles had a particle size higher than 200 nm, PDI less than 0.3 (which is indicative of homogeneity), and a negative zeta potential value. In vitro release studies of all the developed nanoparticles indicated a biphasic drug release, with an initial faster onset, followed by a prolonged release. In vivo pharmacodynamic studies also showed favorable results, supporting that the formulations allowed to potentiate the antidepressant action of venlafaxine. All the formulations developed in the three mentioned studies showed potential in the treatment of depression.

2.6. Desvenlafaxine

Desvenlafaxine is an active metabolite of venlafaxine, a second-generation serotonin and norepinephrine reuptake inhibitor. It has an oral bioavailability of about 80% and a half-life time of about 11 h; however, it is associated with several adverse symptoms such as increased blood pressure, nausea, and headaches, among others. In order to tackle these issues, a study conducted by Tong et al. [61] aimed to develop biodegradable and biocompatible polymeric nanoparticles for intranasal administration of desvenlafaxine for depression treatment.

The formulated polymeric nanoparticles were composed of: the polymer PLGA; chitosan, which was used due to its mucoadhesive properties; and polyvinyl alcohol (PVA), which in addition to chitosan, has the ability to stabilize the formulation. Particle size, PDI, zeta potential, EE%, and drug loading were, respectively, 172.5 nm, 0.254, +35.63 mV, 98.3%, and 49.15%. In-vitro drug release studies showed an initially fast drug release, probably of a drug present at the surface of the nanoparticles, followed by an extended release during 24 h, which probably corresponded to the fraction of the drug that was inside the nanoparticle, in its nucleus, by hydration and swelling of the nanoparticle matrix. A pH of 7.4 was considered for optimized nanoparticles. Also, there were no differences in drug release at pH 7.4 (physiological pH) when compared to pH 6.0 (pH within the range of nasal mucosa values).

In vivo pharmacokinetic studies in rats (Figure 5A), with intranasal and intravenous nanoparticle administration, and intranasal administration of a desvenlafaxine solution, showed that desvenlafaxine brain concentrations, half-life time ($t_{1/2}$) and AUC were higher when the administration was intranasal, regardless of the formulation that was used. Furthermore, these parameters were superior for the intranasal desvenlafaxine nanoparticles when compared to the drug solution. These results support intranasal administration for better pharmacokinetic parameters in the brain, as well as the use of nanoparticles for the incorporation of the drug. Additionally, the values of DTE% and DTP% were calculated and were higher for the formulated nanoparticles administered intranasally (544.23% and 81.62%, respectively), which indicates better efficiency in brain targeting when compared to the other comparative groups.

In-vivo pharmacodynamic studies (Figure 5B), such as the reserpine reversal test and the forced swim test, were conducted, administering the optimized nanoparticles intranasally or a desvenlafaxine solution intranasally or orally. The results were compared with the ones from a control group (intranasal administration of a saline solution). It was observed that only the intranasally administered formulations had a significant effect on the ability to reduce reserpine-induced immobility. Furthermore, the Forced Swim Test allowed to conclude that the intranasal nanoparticles had a more significantly reduced immobility and increased swimming, climbing, and locomotion time than all other groups.

Monoamine levels in the brain, and their association with antidepressant activity in different groups of rats subjected to the forced swim test, were also studied (Figure 5C). The results showed that the intranasal nanoparticles significantly improved serotonin and norepinephrine levels in the brain, supporting the theory that the levels of these two neurotransmitters decrease in stressful situations, particularly in depression.

In conclusion, the formulated nanoparticles, administered intranasally, allowed us to improve the pharmacokinetic and pharmacodynamic profile of desvenlafaxine, helping with the transport of the drug to the site of action in the brain, and showing promise as an alternative for depression treatment.

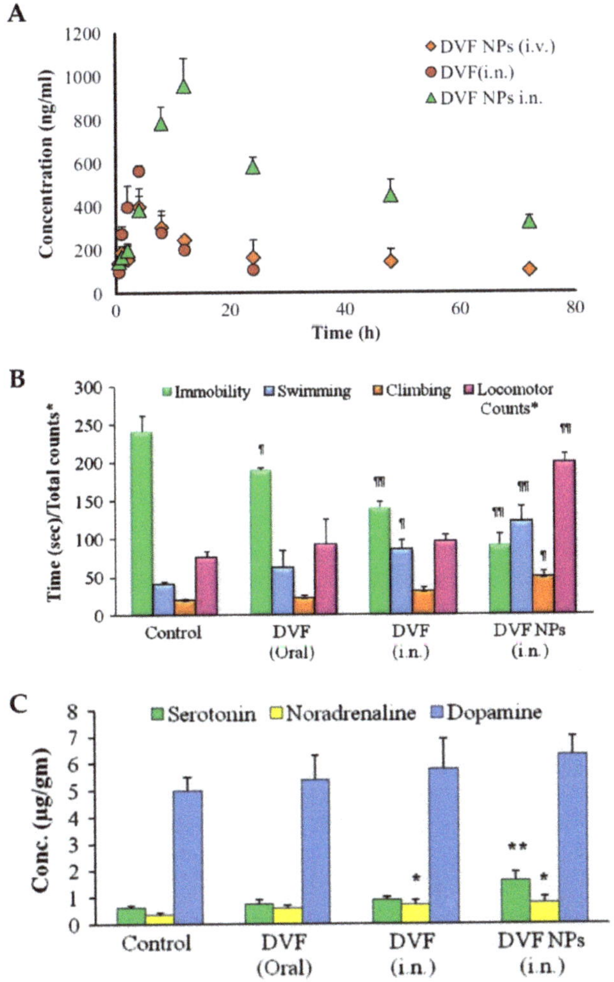

Figure 5. (**A**)—Desvenlafaxine brain concentration after intranasal administration of a drug solution (DVF (i.n.)) or the developed nanoparticles (DVF NPs i.n.), or the intravenous administration of the nanoparticles (DVF NPs (i.v.)); (**B**)—Evaluation of the antidepressant activity of intranasal desvenlafaxine nanoparticles (DVF NPs (i.n.)), intranasal desvenlafaxine solution (DVF (i.n.)) and oral desvenlafaxine solution (DVF (Oral)), in chronically depressed rats; (**C**)—Effect of intranasal desvenlafaxine nanoparticles (DVF NPs (i.n.)), intranasal desvenlafaxine solution (DVF (i.n.)) and oral desvenlafaxine solution (DVF (Oral)) on neurotransmitter levels in rat brain; ¶ and * represent $p < 0.05$, ¶¶ and ** represent $p < 0.01$; Conc.—concentration; DVF—desvenlafaxine; NPs—nanoparticles; adapted from Tong et al. [61], reproduced with permission from Elsevier [License Number 5426000412295].

2.7. Selegiline

Selegiline is a MAOi, with a dose-dependent therapeutic action and also presents neuroprotective effects. When administered orally, this drug undergoes extensive hepatic metabolism, having reduced bioavailability and also several associated adverse effects. A study conducted by Singh et al. [62] aimed to increase the efficacy of selegiline (hydrochloride form) through intranasal administration of thiolated chitosan nanoparticles in order to obtain an extended and controlled release of the encapsulated drug.

The formulated nanoparticles contained thiolated chitosan, which is obtained by coupling the primary amine groups of chitosan with thiol groups. This structural change improves the mucoadhesiveness and permeability enhancement capability of this polymer. TPP was also used as a polyanion that interacts with chitosan through electrostatic forces, causing chitosan to precipitate, forming spherical particles. The optimization of the formulation considered the thiolated chitosan: TPP ratio since it directly affects the particle size and its distribution. The optimized ratio was 5:1. The pH was also considered, being ideal between 5.0 and 5.5 (values in the range of the nasal mucosa). Also, with a pH above 5.5, there was the formation of unwanted white aggregates that disappeared when a reduction of pH was verified.

In vitro drug release was analyzed and compared between thiolated chitosan nanoparticles and unmodified chitosan nanoparticles. It was concluded that the unmodified nanoparticles showed a faster release profile in the first 2 h, due to the presence of a drug on the surface of the nanoparticles that is released faster when compared with thiolated chitosan nanoparticles, for which there was a formation of an in situ gel. This means that there is a high-density gel network that restricts the penetration of water at the site where the diffusion of the drug occurs, delaying the release. Nevertheless, after about 3 h, it was found that the release of the drug from thiolated chitosan nanoparticles was constant and extended, becoming higher than the release of unmodified chitosan after 13 h.

In-vivo pharmacodynamic studies in rats (stress-induced immobility, sucrose preference test, and locomotor activity), the intranasal administration of the thiolated chitosan nanoparticles was compared to the also intranasal administration of unmodified chitosan nanoparticles or a drug solution. The drug solution only showed significant effects on increased locomotor activity. Both nanoparticle types allowed reduced immobility time, restored sucrose intake, and increased locomotor activity, with better results being obtained after the administration of thiolated chitosan nanoparticles.

Additionally, another evaluated parameter was the formation of free radicals, namely nitrite, since oxidative stress has been associated with mood disorders. Its concentration was more significantly reduced when thiolated chitosan nanoparticles were administered, compared to the administration of the drug solution or the unmodified chitosan nanoparticles.

In conclusion, the formation of an in situ gel allows the improvement of the permeability and transport of the drug from the nasal cavity to the action site in the brain, and there was a significant advantage when using thiolated chitosan when compared to unmodified chitosan.

2.8. Tramadol

Tramadol is a synthetic opioid drug with central analgesic action. Aside from its affinity for opioid receptors, it is also able to inhibit the reuptake of the neurotransmitters serotonin and norepinephrine, thus presenting an antidepressant effect. Nevertheless, it is quite prone to metabolism; hence, the incorporation of tramadol in nanoparticles could allow protecting the drug from its labile nature. A study conducted by Kaur et al. [63] aimed to study the efficacy of the transport of tramadol to the brain using the intranasal administration of nanoparticles incorporated in an in situ gel for the treatment of depression.

The polymeric nanoparticles were composed of chitosan and TPP, and incorporated in a thermosensitive in situ gel made of poloxamer 407 and hydroxypropylmethylcellulose (HPMC) K15M. Benzalkonium chloride was also used as a cationic surfactant and as a stabilizer of the system. Chitosan and TPP were used in an optimized ratio of 1:1, and the optimized nanoparticles presented a particle size of 152.0 nm, PDI of 0.143, the zeta potential of +31 mV, and EE% of 85%. In-vitro drug release studies demonstrated a biphasic release of the drug, and the nanoparticles incorporated into the in situ gel presented a longer drug release when compared to a saline solution.

The forced swim test (in vivo pharmacodynamic study) was performed in rats, and it was possible to observe that the intranasal administration of the nanoparticles incorporated in the in situ gel allowed to reduce the immobility time and increase the locomotor activity. Body weight was also assessed before and after the treatment, and a significant improvement was observed after the administration of the nanoparticles when compared to the control group (no treatment). Furthermore, the sucrose preference test allowed us to verify that the intranasal nanoparticles in situ gel increased the intake of sucrose. Nitrite concentration was also evaluated, being significantly reduced after the treatment with the nanoparticles. It should also be noted that, in all these studies, the intranasal administration of a tramadol saline solution obtained unsatisfactory results.

Hence, in general, the developed tramadol nanoparticles in situ gel was able to ensure a controlled release of the drug, improving transport to the brain, and proving itself to be a possible alternative to oral administration of the drug.

2.9. Buspirone

Buspirone is an anxiolytic drug used in the treatment of generalized anxiety disorder. It acts as an agonist of pre-synaptic serotoninergic receptors in the hippocampal region of the brain, and as a partial agonist of post-synaptic serotoninergic receptors, in the raphe nucleus. It undergoes an extensive first-pass hepatic metabolism when administered orally, presenting reduced bioavailability. The study by Bari et al. [64] aimed to tackle this problem by assessing the efficacy of the brain transport of polymeric nanoparticles with the encapsulated drug, after intranasal administration, for the treatment of anxiety.

The formulated nanoparticles were either composed of thiolated chitosan or plain chitosan and also a mixture of TPP and alginate, which was used as a cross-linker. The optimization of the formulation considered the relationship between chitosan and cross-linker concentrations since it affects particle size and PDI values. The optimized chitosan and thiolated chitosan nanoparticles presented, respectively, a particle size of 195.7 nm and 208.3 nm and a PDI of 0.367 and 0.253. The decrease in PDI value indicates greater homogeneity of the system due to the presence of thiolated chitosan. It was also verified, by scanning electron microscopy (Figure 6A), that both formulations presented pores on the surface, which suggests the possibility of drug release by these same pores.

In vitro drug release was compared between the two formulations, and it was observed that the thiolation of chitosan did not affect it. Both formulations showed a biphasic release, with an initial fast release, followed by an extended release for 24 h, with more than 90% of the drug being released after that time. Nevertheless, ex vivo permeation studies (Figure 6B) showed that thiolated chitosan nanoparticles had better permeability when compared to unmodified chitosan nanoparticles. These results can be explained by the increased mucoadhesion since a strong ionic bond is formed between the thiolated chitosan amine group and the cell membrane sites, which results in the opening of the tight junctions.

Pharmacokinetic parameters were determined in vivo studies (Figure 6C) after intranasal administration of the thiolated chitosan nanoparticles or a buspirone solution or intravenous administration of the same drug solution. The brain concentration and AUC for the intranasal nanoparticles were higher than for all other groups at all points in time. It should also be noted that the concentration of buspirone in the brain that was obtained 30 min after administration was about three times higher for the intranasal nanoparticles, which indicates that this route of administration allows a faster reaching of the CNS bypassing the blood-brain barrier. DTP% (95.97%) and DTE% (78.94%) values were also higher after intranasal administration of the formulated nanoparticles (compared with the drug solution, also administered intranasally), further showing their superiority.

Therefore, it can be concluded that the developed polymeric nanoparticles are a possible noninvasive alternative to buspirone administration for the treatment of generalized anxiety disorder.

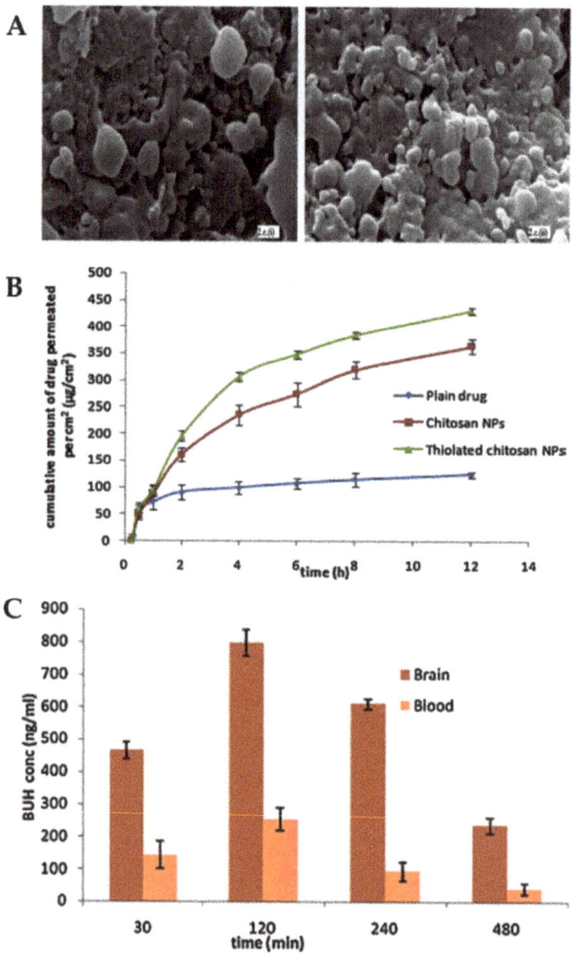

Figure 6. (**A**)—Scanning electron microscope images of the buspirone chitosan nanoparticles (on the left (2.c.(i))) and thiolated chitosan nanoparticles (on the right (2.c.(ii))); (**B**)—Ex vivo permeation study of buspirone chitosan nanoparticles (Chitosan NPs), thiolated chitosan nanoparticles (Thiolated chitosan NPs), and drug solution (Plain drug); (**C**)—Buspirone brain and blood concentrations after intranasal administration of the thiolated chitosan nanoparticles; BUH—buspirone; conc—concentration; NPs—nanoparticles; adapted from Bari et al. [64], reproduced with permission from Elsevier [License Number 5426000697685].

2.10. Riluzole

The mechanism of action of riluzole is not completely defined. It is assumed that it acts as an inhibitor of glutamate release and that it is associated with decreased oxidative stress, presenting the potential for the treatment of anxiety. This substance is subjected to an extensive first-pass effect metabolism when administered orally, which results in the reduction of its bioavailability. The study conducted by Nabi et al. [65] aimed to find a solution for this issue by developing polymeric nanoparticles for intranasal administration containing encapsulated riluzole in order to increase the concentration of the drug in the brain and to enhance its action in reducing oxidative stress.

Chitosan was used as a polymer in the formulation of the nanoparticles due to its mucoadhesive properties, and TPP was used as a polyanion. For comparative purposes, chitosan nanoparticles were formulated with and without Tf. Tf was added as a ligand in order to facilitate the transcytosis of the nanoparticles through the blood-brain barrier (for a fraction of the drug that will undergo indirect transport). The optimized formulations considered the drug:polymer: Tf ratio. The particle size and PDI for chitosan nanoparticles were 173.6 nm and 0.264, and for chitosan nanoparticles with Tf were 207.0 nm and 0.406, respectively. It was possible to observe an increase in particle size and PDI with the addition of Tf; therefore, nanoparticles without the ligand presented a more homogeneous system. The optimal pH value chosen for the formation of nanoparticles with Tf was 5.0, a value that is considered to be compatible with the nasal mucosa. In vitro drug release was shown to be initially fast, followed by an extended release. The cumulative release after 24 h was higher for the nanoparticles in which the ligand was used, followed by the nanoparticles without the ligand, and then a drug suspension. The same conclusions were reached in ex vivo permeation studies, with the nanoparticles with the ligand having higher permeation, followed by the nanoparticles without ligand, and with drug suspension permeating the least.

Intravenous or intranasal administration of a riluzole suspension and intranasal administration of the nanoparticles with Tf was done in rats to assess their pharmacokinetics. It was possible to observe higher brain drug concentrations for intranasal administration, in general, with it being more significant for the nanoparticles. The results also supported the hypothesis that the nanoparticles administered intranasally have an extended drug release, as seen in prolonged brain drug levels. DTE% (1138.46%) and DTP% (91.21%) values showed better results for the nanoparticles that contained the ligand, so it was concluded that the ligand allowed improved efficiency of brain drug transport. Pharmacodynamic studies conducted in rats (elevated plus maze model and Morris water maze test), showed that riluzole has substantial anxiolytic activity and that nanoparticles with and without ligands were able to improve learning capacity and memory in the animals subjected to the study. It was also possible to conclude that the treatment with both formulated nanoparticles (with and without ligand) was able to significantly reduce oxidative stress (although for this test, no significant difference was observed between the two types of nanoparticles).

Therefore, the formulated nanoparticles demonstrated potential for the treatment of anxiety through intranasal administration, with the use of Tf as a ligand being an additional advantage throughout the study, improving brain drug targeting.

3. Final Remarks

The current treatments for depression and anxiety disorders have several disadvantages that compromise drug bioavailability, with the amount of drug that reaches the intended site of action, the brain, being quite low. This can consequently compromise the therapeutic response. These treatments are also associated with several systemic adverse effects. Therefore, the intranasal route has been studied throughout these past years due to its great potential for improving the current therapies for these pathologies, bypassing their disadvantages. The administration through the intranasal route establishes direct contact between the surrounding environment of the nasal cavity and the CNS, allowing it to overcome the blood-brain barrier and also avoiding the metabolism of the first hepatic passage. This creates a decrease in adverse effects caused by the most prevalent route of administration, the oral route, which brings another major benefit for the patients.

Intranasal drug absorption depends on several anatomical, physiological, physicochemical, and formulation factors, which influence the extent of drug absorption and, consequently, the efficacy of the formulation administered in the nasal cavity. There are several strategies used to improve drug absorption. The analyzed studies show that the incorporation of drugs into nanoparticles is a way to protect the drug and transport it, also allowing a controlled release, which increases and prolongs its concentration in the therapeutical target site. The analyzed studies formulated different types of nanoparticles with different drugs in order to verify the potential of using these formulations, administered intranasally, for the treatment of depression and anxiety.

All studies that reported values of particle size, zeta potential, and PDI, demonstrated that they are, in general, adequate, conferring stability and homogeneity to the system. Moreover, these parameters can highly influence drug absorption and pharmacokinetics since, as already mentioned, nanoparticles with sizes between 10 and 300 nm can undergo direct brain transport (olfactory nerve), and lower PDI values are usually connected with lower variability in drug absorption and distribution. The reported values of EE%, DTE%, and DTP% were also promising, allowing for the achievement of an effective encapsulation of drugs and high brain targeting. The pharmacokinetic and pharmacodynamic studies presented promising results in the application of this type of formulation to produce the desired therapeutic effect. A more detailed comparison between the studies is hampered by the use of different animal models, sample collection times, administered doses, quantification methods, and of course, drugs.

For depression treatment, drugs such as icariin, albiflorin, fluoxetine, agomelatine, desvenlafaxine, venlafaxine, selegiline, and tramadol and, for anxiety, drugs such as buspirone and riluzole were studied. Hence, most studies focused on the treatment of depression. Although both pathologies interfere with the quality of life, depression is considered one of the main causes of disability in the world and can lead to suicide. Therefore, the treatment of this pathology can prevent death, and therefore this could be the reason for a higher focus on this pathology when compared to anxiety disorders.

Polymeric nanoparticles were the chosen nanoparticle type in most studies. This type of nanoparticle allows the control of the release of the drug, and in the majority of studies analyzed, it was reported that a biphasic release occurred: first, a faster release, followed by an extended release, that was maintained for a long period of time. Chitosan and alginate, two mucoadhesive polymers that allow to increase in the residence time of the drug in the nasal cavity and enhance its absorption and arrival at the site of action, were the most used polymers.

Moreover, the functionalization of nanoparticles with ligands, such as Tf or TfRp, as done in the studies conducted by Cayero-Otero et al. [60] and Nabi et al. [65], can allow improving drug absorption and permeability due to facilitated transcytosis of the nanosystems through the blood-brain barrier, which can be quite relevant for a fraction of the drug that will undergo indirect transport. For these functionalized nanoparticles, controlled drug release and permeation was observed, which can allow a more prolonged therapeutic action. In what concerns ligands that could facilitate nose-to-brain drug transport (direct transport), some reports have pointed out that the functionalization of nanoparticles with ligands that have highly expressed receptors in the olfactory region (such as lactoferrin) or glycoproteins (such as lectins) can increase drug transport by facilitated transcytosis and other related mechanisms [66].

Furthermore, the possible clinical application should not be considered until the biocompatibility of the developed nanosystems is assured. Most studies included in this review did not perform any safety studies. Yet, some studies chose their formulation's composition having in mind the biocompatibility of the used excipients, having searched for safety information priorly (especially from international health authorities, such as EMA and FDA). Although this information could make it more likely that the developed nanoparticles could be potentially safe, one should assess this by actually performing safety studies, for example, in animal nasal mucosa tissues (with the most common models being from pig or sheep) or cells, in order to assess if the developed formulations are actually safe for intranasal administration (no signs of toxicity/irritation/damage). Moreover, in order to increase patient safety, nanotherapeutics should be tailored according to the administration route and disease characteristics (composition compatible with administration site and site of action, adequate particle size, viscosity, pH, etc.). Here it is paramount to make use of adequate analytical tools and thorough prior formulation development planning [67].

Although this review focuses on small molecular weight drugs, intranasally administered biopharmaceuticals have also proven to be effective in the treatment of depression and anxiety disorders. Proteins and peptides such as brain-derived neurotrophic factor, nerve growth factor, neuropeptide Y, insulin, and oxytocin have proven to have potential therapeutic efficacy when administered through the intranasal route, which further shows the potential of intranasal administration [68]. Some of these high molecular weight drugs have also been formulated into nanosystems for intranasal delivery, but, to the best of our knowledge, not for the treatment of depression or anxiety disorders, which leaves scope for further research and development of new macromolecular therapies for these diseases [69–73].

In addition to in-vitro and in-vivo results, recent clinical evidence has surfaced on the effectiveness of the intranasal route for the treatment of major and treatment-resistant depression, with esketamine having proven to be successful, both alone or as adjunct therapy together with oral medication, and with a formulation having even reached the market in 2019, Spravato® [74–79]. This further proves the potential of the intranasal route for the treatment of these pathologies and leaves space for the future study of new drugs and formulations to be delivered intranasally.

Despite all the proven potential of the reported nanoparticles for antidepressant and anxiolytic drug delivery, some limitations can hinder the translation of these formulations into the pharmaceutical market. In general, nanoparticles can have scalability issues, meaning that what works at a small laboratory scale might not work on a larger industrial scale, with problems arising in what concerns controlling the formulations desired characteristics (particle size, PDI, zeta potential, EE, etc.) and stability. Furthermore, the complexity of these systems' composition and production methods could be quite costly and, hence, non-profitable for these companies [67,80]. Moreover, very few nanoparticles for the treatment of depression and/or anxiety have gone as far as clinical trials (and hence none have reached the market), and none using intranasal administration [81]. Yet, nanoformulations for the treatment of several other diseases, such as cancer, multiple sclerosis, or hepatitis, have been successfully developed and approved for commercialization [67,82]. Therefore, further investigation should be done in order to obtain nanosystems with simpler production methods, less expensive components, and scale-up studies could be done to better understand what could happen at an industrial scale so that someday nanoparticles containing antidepressant and/or anxiolytic drugs can reach the market and improve the therapeutic outcomes of these diseases.

Hence, despite the number of studies still being small, in general, the intranasal administration of nanoparticles presents high potential as an alternative to the currently available therapies for the treatment of depression and anxiety. However, the analyzed studies presented only in vitro and in vivo data. Therefore, it is relevant that future research is done in order to compare these animal studies with studies carried out in humans in order to verify the true potential of these formulations when administered intranasally. The focus on research and development of this type of formulation can make treatments increasingly more effective for pathologies that directly interfere with the daily lives of patients, affecting their quality of life.

4. Conclusions

In conclusion, the intranasal delivery of nanoparticles for the treatment of depression and anxiety disorders has been proven to be a quite promising approach, allowing to overcome the unavoidable disadvantages of oral administration, reducing the number of administrations necessary for effective treatment, which may increase patient compliance, and also allowing a faster onset of action, with increased and prolonged brain drug concentrations and, consequently, therapeutic effect.

Author Contributions: Conceptualization, P.C.P., A.C.P.-S. and F.V.; Formal analysis, investigation and data curation, M.A., P.C.P. and A.C.P.-S.; writing—original draft preparation, M.A., P.C.P. and

A.C.P.-S.; writing—review and editing, P.C.P., A.C.P.-S. and F.V. All authors have read and agreed to the published version of the manuscript.

Funding: This research received no external funding.

Institutional Review Board Statement: Not applicable.

Informed Consent Statement: Not applicable.

Data Availability Statement: Not applicable.

Conflicts of Interest: The authors declare no conflict of interest.

Abbreviations

AUC	Area under the curve
CUMS	Chronic Unpredictable Mild Stress
DTE%	Drug targeting efficiency
DTP%	Direct transport percentage
EDTA	Ethylenediaminetetraacetic acid
EE%	Encapsulation efficiency
GABA	γ-aminobutyric acid
HPMC	Hydroxypropyl methylcellulose
MAOi	Monoamine oxidase inhibitors
NLC	Nanostructured lipid carriers
PDI	Polydispersity index
PLGA	Poly lactic-co-glycolic acid
PVA	Poly(vinyl alcohol)
SLN	Solid lipid nanoparticles
CNS	Central nervous system
$t_{1/2}$	Half life time
Tf	transferrinT
fRp	specific peptide against Tf receptor
TPP	Sodium tripolyphosphate

References

1. World Health Organization Mental Health. Available online: https://www.who.int/health-topics/mental-health#tab=tab_1 (accessed on 31 October 2022).
2. Zhao, Y.F.; Verkhratsky, A.; Tang, Y.; Illes, P. Astrocytes and Major Depression: The Purinergic Avenue. *Neuropharmacology* **2022**, *220*, 109252. [CrossRef]
3. Gabriel, F.C.; de Melo, D.O.; Fráguas, R.; Leite-Santos, N.C.; Mantovani da Silva, R.A.; Ribeiro, E. Pharmacological Treatment of Depression: A Systematic Review Comparing Clinical Practice Guideline Recommendations. *PLoS ONE* **2020**, *15*, e0231700. [CrossRef]
4. Nemeroff, C.B. The State of Our Understanding of the Pathophysiology and Optimal Treatment of Depression: Glass Half Full or Half Empty? *Am. J. Psychiatry* **2020**, *177*, 671–685. [CrossRef] [PubMed]
5. Qian, H.; Shu, C.; Xiao, L.; Wang, G. Histamine and Histamine Receptors: Roles in Major Depressive Disorder. *Front. Psychiatry* **2022**, *13*, 825591. [CrossRef] [PubMed]
6. Jiang, Y.; Zou, D.; Li, Y.; Gu, S.; Dong, J.; Ma, X.; Xu, S.; Wang, F.; Huang, J.H. Monoamine Neurotransmitters Control Basic Emotions and Affect Major Depressive Disorders. *Pharmaceuticals* **2022**, *15*, 1203. [CrossRef] [PubMed]
7. Lenox, R.H.; Frazer, A. Mechanism of Action of Antidepressants and Mood Stabilizers. In *Neuropsychopharmacology: The Fifth Generation of Progress*; American College of Neuropsychopharmacology: Phoenix, AZ, USA, 2002; pp. 1139–1163, ISBN 9780781728379.
8. Kircanski, K.; Joormann, J.; Gotlib, I.H. Cognitive Aspects of Depression. *Wiley Interdiscip. Rev. Cogn. Sci.* **2012**, *3*, 301–313. [CrossRef]
9. Katzman, M.A.; Bleau, P.; Blier, P.; Chokka, P.; Kjernisted, K.; van Ameringen, M.; Antony, M.M.; Bouchard, S.; Brunet, A.; Flament, M.; et al. Canadian Clinical Practice Guidelines for the Management of Anxiety, Posttraumatic Stress and Obsessive-Compulsive Disorders. *BMC Psychiatry* **2014**, *14*, S1. [CrossRef]
10. Won, E.; Kim, Y.K. Neuroinflammation—Associated Alterations of the Brain as Potential Neural Biomarkers in Anxiety Disorders. *Int. J. Mol. Sci.* **2020**, *21*, 6546. [CrossRef] [PubMed]
11. Penninx, B.W.; Pine, D.S.; Holmes, E.A.; Reif, A. Anxiety Disorders. *Lancet* **2021**, *397*, 914–927. [CrossRef]

12. Chesnut, M.; Harati, S.; Paredes, P.; Khan, Y.; Foudeh, A.; Kim, J.; Bao, Z.; Williams, L.M. Stress Markers for Mental States and Biotypes of Depression and Anxiety: A Scoping Review and Preliminary Illustrative Analysis. *Chronic Stress* **2021**, *5*, 24705470211000338. [CrossRef]
13. Hu, P.; Lu, Y.; Pan, B.-X.; Zhang, W.-H. New Insights into the Pivotal Role of the Amygdala in Inflammation-Related Depression and Anxiety Disorder. *Int. J. Mol. Sci.* **2022**, *23*, 11076. [CrossRef]
14. Kilts, C.D. Potential New Drug Delivery Systems for Antidepressants: An Overview. *J. Clin. Psychiatry* **2003**, *64*, 31–33.
15. Nutt, D.J. Relationship of Neurotransmitters to the Symptoms of Major Depressive Disorder. *J. Clin. Psychiatry* **2008**, *69*, 4–7. [PubMed]
16. Jogani, V.; Jinturkar, K.; Vyas, T.; Misra, A. Recent Patents Review on Intranasal Administration for CNS Drug Delivery. *Recent Pat. Drug Deliv.* **2008**, *2*, 25–40. [CrossRef]
17. Bahadur, S.; Pathak, K. Physicochemical and Physiological Considerations for Efficient Nose-to-Brain Targeting. *Expert Opin. Drug Deliv.* **2012**, *9*, 19–31. [CrossRef]
18. Pires, P.C.; Santos, A.O. Nanosystems in Nose-to-Brain Drug Delivery: A Review of Non-Clinical Brain Targeting Studies. *J. Control. Release* **2018**, *270*, 89–100. [CrossRef] [PubMed]
19. Selvaraj, K.; Gowthamarajan, K.; Karri, V.V.S.R. Nose to Brain Transport Pathways an Overview: Potential of Nanostructured Lipid Carriers in Nose to Brain Targeting. *Artif. Cells Nanomed. Biotechnol.* **2018**, *46*, 2088–2095. [CrossRef] [PubMed]
20. Pardeshi, C.V.; Belgamwar, V.S. Direct Nose to Brain Drug Delivery via Integrated Nerve Pathways Bypassing the Blood-Brain Barrier: An Excellent Platform for Brain Targeting. *Expert Opin. Drug Deliv.* **2013**, *10*, 957–972. [CrossRef]
21. Mainardes, R.M.; Cocenza Urban, M.C.; Oliveira Cinto, P.; Vinícius Chaud, M.; Evangelista, R.C.; Palmira, M.; Gremião, D. Liposomes and Micro/Nanoparticles as Colloidal Carriers for Nasal Drug Delivery. *Curr. Drug Deliv.* **2006**, *3*, 275–285. [CrossRef]
22. Cunha, S.; Amaral, M.H.; Sousa Lobo, J.M.; Silva, A.C. Lipid Nanoparticles for Nasal/Intranasal Drug Delivery. *Crit. Rev. Drug Carr. Syst.* **2017**, *34*, 257–282. [CrossRef] [PubMed]
23. Battaglia, L.; Panciani, P.P.; Muntoni, E.; Capucchio, M.T.; Biasibetti, E.; de Bonis, P.; Mioletti, S.; Fontanella, M.; Swaminathan, S. Lipid Nanoparticles for Intranasal Administration: Application to Nose-to-Brain Delivery. *Expert Opin. Drug Deliv.* **2018**, *15*, 369–378. [CrossRef] [PubMed]
24. Scherließ, R. Nasal Formulations for Drug Administration and Characterization of Nasal Preparations in Drug Delivery. *Ther. Deliv.* **2020**, *11*, 183–191. [CrossRef]
25. Gadhave, D.; Rasal, N.; Sonawane, R.; Sekar, M.; Kokare, C. Nose-to-Brain Delivery of Teriflunomide-Loaded Lipid-Based Carbopol-Gellan Gum Nanogel for Glioma: Pharmacological and in Vitro Cytotoxicity Studies. *Int. J. Biol. Macromol* **2021**, *167*, 906–920. [CrossRef] [PubMed]
26. Taweel, M.M.E.; Aboul-Einien, M.H.; Kassem, M.A.; Elkasabgy, N.A. Intranasal Zolmitriptan-Loaded Bilosomes with Extended Nasal Mucociliary Transit Time for Direct Nose to Brain Delivery. *Pharmaceutics* **2021**, *13*, 1828. [CrossRef]
27. El-Shenawy, A.A.; Mahmoud, R.A.; Mahmoud, E.A.; Mohamed, M.S. Intranasal In Situ Gel of Apixaban-Loaded Nanoethosomes: Preparation, Optimization, and In Vivo Evaluation. *AAPS PharmSciTech* **2021**, *22*, 147. [CrossRef] [PubMed]
28. Pires, P.C.; Peixoto, D.; Teixeira, I.; Rodrigues, M.; Alves, G.; Santos, A.O. Nanoemulsions and Thermosensitive Nanoemulgels of Phenytoin and Fosphenytoin for Intranasal Administration: Formulation Development and in Vitro Characterization. *Eur. J. Pharm. Sci.* **2020**, *141*, 105099. [CrossRef] [PubMed]
29. Pires, P.C.; Santos, L.T.; Rodrigues, M.; Alves, G.; Santos, A.O. Intranasal Fosphenytoin: The Promise of Phosphate Esters in Nose-to-Brain Delivery of Poorly Soluble Drugs. *Int. J. Pharm.* **2021**, *592*, 120040. [CrossRef]
30. Sood, S.; Jain, K.; Gowthamarajan, K. Intranasal Therapeutic Strategies for Management of Alzheimer's Disease. *J. Drug Target.* **2014**, *22*, 279–294. [CrossRef]
31. Pires, P.C.; Fazendeiro, A.C.; Rodrigues, M.; Alves, G.; Santos, A.O. Nose-to-Brain Delivery of Phenytoin and Its Hydrophilic Prodrug Fosphenytoin Combined in a Microemulsion—Formulation Development and in Vivo Pharmacokinetics. *Eur. J. Pharm. Sci.* **2021**, *164*, 105918. [CrossRef]
32. Rautiola, D.; Maglalang, P.D.; Cheryala, N.; Nelson, K.M.; Georg, G.I.; Fine, J.M.; Svitak, A.L.; Faltesek, K.A.; Hanson, L.R.; Mishra, U.; et al. Intranasal Coadministration of a Diazepam Prodrug with a Converting Enzyme Results in Rapid Absorption of Diazepam in Rats. *J. Pharmacol. Exp. Ther.* **2019**, *370*, 796–805. [CrossRef]
33. Pires, A.; Fortuna, A.; Alves, G.; Falcão, A. Intranasal Drug Delivery: How, Why and What For? *J. Pharm. Pharm. Sci.* **2009**, *12*, 288–311. [CrossRef]
34. Mohaghegh, M.; Tafaghodi, M. Dextran Microspheres Could Enhance Immune Responses against PLGA Nanospheres Encapsulated with Tetanus Toxoid and Quillaja Saponins after Nasal Immunization in Rabbit. *Pharm. Dev. Technol.* **2011**, *16*, 36–43. [CrossRef] [PubMed]
35. Xia, Y.; Li, L.; Huang, X.; Wang, Z.; Zhang, H.; Gao, J.; Du, Y.; Chen, W.; Zheng, A. Performance and Toxicity of Different Absorption Enhancers Used in the Preparation of Poloxamer Thermosensitive in Situ Gels for Ketamine Nasal Administration. *Drug Dev. Ind. Pharm.* **2020**, *46*, 697–705. [CrossRef]
36. Li, Y.; Li, J.; Zhang, X.; Ding, J.; Mao, S. Non-Ionic Surfactants as Novel Intranasal Absorption Enhancers: In Vitro and in Vivo Characterization. *Drug Deliv.* **2016**, *23*, 2272–2279. [CrossRef]

37. Wang, J.; Lu, W.L.; Liang, G.W.; Wu, K.C.; Zhang, C.G.; Zhang, X.; Wang, J.C.; Zhang, H.; Wang, X.Q.; Zhang, Q. Pharmacokinetics, Toxicity of Nasal Cilia and Immunomodulating Effects in Sprague-Dawley Rats Following Intranasal Delivery of Thymopentin with or without Absorption Enhancers. *Peptides* **2006**, *27*, 826–835. [CrossRef]
38. Zhang, Y.; Zhang, Q.; Sun, Y.; Sun, J.; Wang, X.; Chen, M. Nasal Recombinant Hirudin-2 Delivery: Absorption and Its Mechanism in Vivo and in Vitro Studies. *Biol. Pharm. Bull.* **2005**, *28*, 2263–2267. [CrossRef] [PubMed]
39. Hassan, R.H.; Gad, H.A.; El-Din, S.B.; Shaker, D.S.; Ishak, R.A.H. Chitosan Nanoparticles for Intranasal Delivery of Olmesartan Medoxomil: Pharmacokinetic and Pharmacodynamic Perspectives. *Int. J. Pharm.* **2022**, *628*, 122278. [CrossRef] [PubMed]
40. Darwish, W.M.; Bayoumi, N.A.; Ebeid, N.H. Biocompatible Mucoadhesive Nanoparticles for Brain Targeting of Ropinirole Hydrochloride: Formulations. *Radiolabel. Biodistrib. Biopolym.* **2022**, *113*, e23489. [CrossRef]
41. Kiss, T.; Ambrus, R.; Abdelghafour, M.M.; Zeiringer, S.; Selmani, A.; Roblegg, E.; Budai-Szűcs, M.; Janovák, L.; Lőrinczi, B.; Deák, Á.; et al. Preparation and Detailed Characterization of the Thiomer Chitosan–Cysteine as a Suitable Mucoadhesive Excipient for Nasal Powders. *Int. J. Pharm.* **2022**, *626*, 122188. [CrossRef]
42. Teixeira, M.I.; Lopes, C.M.; Amaral, M.H.; Costa, P.C. Surface-Modified Lipid Nanocarriers for Crossing the Blood-Brain Barrier (BBB): A Current Overview of Active Targeting in Brain Diseases. *Colloids Surf. B Biointerfaces* **2023**, *221*, 112999. [CrossRef]
43. Cui, Y.; Zhang, M.; Zeng, F.; Jin, H.; Xu, Q.; Huang, Y. Dual-Targeting Magnetic PLGA Nanoparticles for Codelivery of Paclitaxel and Curcumin for Brain Tumor Therapy. *ACS Appl. Mater. Interfaces* **2016**, *8*, 32159–32169. [CrossRef] [PubMed]
44. Liu, H.-J.; Xu, P. Strategies to Overcome/Penetrate the BBB for Systemic Nanoparticle Delivery to the Brain/Brain Tumor. *Adv Drug Deliv. Rev.* **2022**, *114619*, 114619. [CrossRef]
45. Cui, Y.; Xu, Q.; Chow, P.K.H.; Wang, D.; Wang, C.H. Transferrin-Conjugated Magnetic Silica PLGA Nanoparticles Loaded with Doxorubicin and Paclitaxel for Brain Glioma Treatment. *Biomaterials* **2013**, *34*, 8511–8520. [CrossRef]
46. Terstappen, G.C.; Meyer, A.H.; Bell, R.D.; Zhang, W. Strategies for Delivering Therapeutics across the Blood–Brain Barrier. *Nat. Rev. Drug Discov.* **2021**, *20*, 362–383. [CrossRef] [PubMed]
47. Ulbrich, K.; Knobloch, T.; Kreuter, J. Targeting the Insulin Receptor: Nanoparticles for Drug Delivery across the Blood-Brain Barrier (BBB). *J. Drug Target.* **2011**, *19*, 125–132. [CrossRef] [PubMed]
48. Lombardo, R.; Musumeci, T.; Carbone, C.; Pignatello, R. Nanotechnologies for Intranasal Drug Delivery: An Update of Literature. *Pharm. Dev. Technol.* **2021**, *26*, 824–845. [CrossRef] [PubMed]
49. Gómez-Hens, A.; Fernández-Romero, J.M. Analytical Methods for the Control of Liposomal Delivery Systems. *Trends Anal. Chem.* **2006**, *25*, 167–178. [CrossRef]
50. Tenchov, R.; Bird, R.; Curtze, A.E.; Zhou, Q. Lipid Nanoparticles from Liposomes to MRNA Vaccine Delivery, a Landscape of Research Diversity and Advancement. *ACS Nano* **2021**, *15*, 16982–17015. [CrossRef]
51. Xu, J.; Tao, J.; Wang, J. Design and Application in Delivery System of Intranasal Antidepressants. *Front. Bioeng. Biotechnol.* **2020**, *8*, 626882. [CrossRef]
52. Singh, Y.; Meher, J.G.; Raval, K.; Khan, F.A.; Chaurasia, M.; Jain, N.K.; Chourasia, M.K. Nanoemulsion: Concepts, Development and Applications in Drug Delivery. *J. Control. Release* **2017**, *252*, 28–49. [CrossRef]
53. Costa, C.; Moreira, J.N.; Amaral, M.H.; Lobo, J.M.S.; Silva, A.C. Nose-to-Brain Delivery of Lipid-Based Nanosystems for Epileptic Seizures and Anxiety Crisis. *J. Control. Release* **2019**, *295*, 187–200. [CrossRef]
54. Xu, D.; Lu, Y.R.; Kou, N.; Hu, M.J.; Wang, Q.S.; Cui, Y.L. Intranasal Delivery of Icariin via a Nanogel-Thermoresponsive Hydrogel Compound System to Improve Its Antidepressant-like Activity. *Int. J. Pharm.* **2020**, *586*, 119550. [CrossRef] [PubMed]
55. Xu, D.; Qiao, T.; Wang, Y.; Wang, Q.S.; Cui, Y.L. Alginate Nanogels-Based Thermosensitive Hydrogel to Improve Antidepressant-like Effects of Albiflorin via Intranasal Delivery. *Drug Deliv.* **2021**, *28*, 2137–2149. [CrossRef] [PubMed]
56. Vitorino, C.; Silva, S.; Gouveia, F.; Bicker, J.; Falcão, A.; Fortuna, A. QbD-Driven Development of Intranasal Lipid Nanoparticles for Depression Treatment. *Eur. J. Pharm. Biopharm.* **2020**, *153*, 106–120. [CrossRef] [PubMed]
57. Jani, P.; Vanza, J.; Pandya, N.; Tandel, H. Formulation of Polymeric Nanoparticles of Antidepressant Drug for Intranasal Delivery. *Ther. Deliv* **2019**, *10*, 683–696. [CrossRef]
58. Haque, S.; Md, S.; Fazil, M.; Kumar, M.; Sahni, J.K.; Ali, J.; Baboota, S. Venlafaxine Loaded Chitosan NPs for Brain Targeting: Pharmacokinetic and Pharmacodynamic Evaluation. *Carbohydr. Polym.* **2012**, *89*, 72–79. [CrossRef]
59. Haque, S.; Md, S.; Sahni, J.K.; Ali, J.; Baboota, S. Development and Evaluation of Brain Targeted Intranasal Alginate Nanoparticles for Treatment of Depression. *J. Psychiatr. Res.* **2014**, *48*, 1–12. [CrossRef]
60. Cayero-Otero, M.D.; Gomes, M.J.; Martins, C.; Álvarez-Fuentes, J.; Fernández-Arévalo, M.; Sarmento, B.; Martín-Banderas, L. In Vivo Biodistribution of Venlafaxine-PLGA Nanoparticles for Brain Delivery: Plain vs. Functionalized Nanoparticles. *Expert Opin. Drug Deliv.* **2019**, *16*, 1413–1427. [CrossRef]
61. Tong, G.F.; Qin, N.; Sun, L.W. Development and Evaluation of Desvenlafaxine Loaded PLGA-Chitosan Nanoparticles for Brain Delivery. *Saudi Pharm. J.* **2017**, *25*, 844–851. [CrossRef]
62. Singh, D.; Rashid, M.; Hallan, S.S.; Mehra, N.K.; Prakash, A.; Mishra, N. Pharmacological Evaluation of Nasal Delivery of Selegiline Hydrochloride-Loaded Thiolated Chitosan Nanoparticles for the Treatment of Depression. *Artif. Cells Nanomed. Biotechnol.* **2016**, *44*, 865–877. [CrossRef]
63. Kaur, P.; Garg, T.; Vaidya, B.; Prakash, A.; Rath, G.; Goyal, A.K. Brain Delivery of Intranasal in Situ Gel of Nanoparticulated Polymeric Carriers Containing Antidepressant Drug: Behavioral and Biochemical Assessment. *J. Drug Target.* **2015**, *23*, 275–286. [CrossRef] [PubMed]

64. Bari, N.K.; Fazil, M.; Hassan, M.Q.; Haider, M.R.; Gaba, B.; Narang, J.K.; Baboota, S.; Ali, J. Brain Delivery of Buspirone Hydrochloride Chitosan Nanoparticles for the Treatment of General Anxiety Disorder. *Int. J. Biol. Macromol.* **2015**, *81*, 49–59. [CrossRef] [PubMed]
65. Nabi, B.; Rehman, S.; Fazil, M.; Khan, S.; Baboota, S.; Ali, J. Riluzole-Loaded Nanoparticles to Alleviate the Symptoms of Neurological Disorders by Attenuating Oxidative Stress. *Drug Dev. Ind. Pharm.* **2020**, *46*, 471–483. [CrossRef] [PubMed]
66. Samaridou, E.; Alonso, M.J. Nose-to-Brain Peptide Delivery—The Potential of Nanotechnology. *Bioorg. Med. Chem.* **2018**, *26*, 2888–2905. [CrossRef]
67. Ahmad, A.; Imran, M.; Sharma, N. Precision Nanotoxicology in Drug Development: Current Trends and Challenges in Safety and Toxicity Implications of Customized Multifunctional Nanocarriers for Drug-Delivery Applications. *Pharmaceutics* **2022**, *14*, 2463. [CrossRef] [PubMed]
68. Bose, M.; Farias Quipildor, G.; Ehrlich, M.E.; Salton, S.R. Intranasal Peptide Therapeutics: A Promising Avenue for Overcoming the Challenges of Traditional CNS Drug Development. *Cells* **2022**, *11*, 3629. [CrossRef] [PubMed]
69. Nojoki, F.; Ebrahimi-Hosseinzadeh, B.; Hatamian-Zarmi, A.; Khodagholi, F.; Khezri, K. Design and Development of Chitosan-Insulin-Transfersomes (Transfersulin) as Effective Intranasal Nanovesicles for the Treatment of Alzheimer's Disease: In Vitro, In Vivo, and Ex Vivo Evaluations. *Biomed. Pharmacother.* **2022**, *153*, 113450. [CrossRef]
70. Sahin, H.; Yucel, O.; Emik, S.; Senturk, G.E. Protective Effects of Intranasally Administrated Oxytocin-Loaded Nanoparticles on Pentylenetetrazole-Kindling Epilepsy in Terms of Seizure Severity, Memory, Neurogenesis, and Neuronal Damage. *ACS Chem. Neurosci.* **2022**, *13*, 1923–1937. [CrossRef]
71. Vitaliano, G.D.; Kim, J.K.; Kaufman, M.J.; Adam, C.W.; Zeballos, G.; Shanmugavadivu, A.; Subburaju, S.; McLaughlin, J.P.; Lukas, S.E.; Vitaliano, F. Clathrin-Nanoparticles Deliver BDNF to Hippocampus and Enhance Neurogenesis, Synaptogenesis and Cognition in HIV/NeuroAIDS Mouse Model. *Commun. Biol.* **2022**, *5*, 236. [CrossRef]
72. Oppong-Damoah, A.; Zaman, R.U.; D'Souza, M.J.; Murnane, K.S. Nanoparticle Encapsulation Increases the Brain Penetrance and Duration of Action of Intranasal Oxytocin. *Horm. Behav.* **2019**, *108*, 20–29. [CrossRef]
73. Tashima, T. Shortcut Approaches to Substance Delivery into the Brain Based on Intranasal Administration Using Nanodelivery Strategies for Insulin. *Molecules* **2020**, *25*, 5188. [CrossRef]
74. Lofts, A.; Abu-Hijleh, F.; Rigg, N.; Mishra, R.K.; Hoare, T. Using the Intranasal Route to Administer Drugs to Treat Neurological and Psychiatric Illnesses: Rationale, Successes, and Future Needs. *CNS Drugs* **2022**, *36*, 739–770. [CrossRef]
75. Takahashi, N.; Yamada, A.; Shiraishi, A.; Shimizu, H.; Goto, R.; Tominaga, Y. Efficacy and Safety of Fixed Doses of Intranasal Esketamine as an Add-on Therapy to Oral Antidepressants in Japanese Patients with Treatment-Resistant Depression: A Phase 2b Randomized Clinical Study. *BMC Psychiatry* **2021**, *21*, 526. [CrossRef] [PubMed]
76. Jha, M.K.; Williamson, D.J.; Magharehabed, G.; Turkoz, I.; Daly, E.J.; Trivedi, M.H. Intranasal Esketamine Effectively Treats Treatment-Resistant Depression in Adults Regardless of Baseline Irritability. *J. Affect. Disord.* **2023**, *321*, 153–160. [CrossRef] [PubMed]
77. Turkoz, I.; Daly, E.; Singh, J.; Lin, X.; Tymofyeyev, Y.; Williamson, D.; Salvadore, G.; Nash, A.I.; Macaluso, M.; Wilkinson, S.T.; et al. Treatment Response with Esketamine Nasal Spray Plus an Oral Antidepressant in Patients with Treatment-Resistant Depression without Evidence of Early Response: A Pooled Post Hoc Analysis of the TRANSFORM Studies. *J. Clin. Psychiatry* **2021**, *82*, 20m13800. [CrossRef] [PubMed]
78. Jones, R.R.; Freeman, M.P.; Kornstein, S.G.; Cooper, K.; Daly, E.J.; Canuso, C.M.; Nicholson, S. Efficacy and Safety of Esketamine Nasal Spray by Sex in Patients with Treatment-Resistant Depression: Findings from Short-Term Randomized, Controlled Trials. *Arch. Womens Ment. Health* **2022**, *25*, 313–326. [CrossRef]
79. Canuso, C.M.; Ionescu, D.F.; Li, X.; Qiu, X.; Lane, R.; Turkoz, I.; Nash, A.I.; Lopena, T.J.; Fu, D.J. Esketamine Nasal Spray for the Rapid Reduction of Depressive Symptoms in Major Depressive Disorder with Acute Suicidal Ideation or Behavior. *J. Clin. Psychopharmacol.* **2021**, *41*, 516–524. [CrossRef]
80. Paliwal, R.; Babu, R.J.; Palakurthi, S. Nanomedicine Scale-up Technologies: Feasibilities and Challenges. *AAPS PharmSciTech* **2014**, *15*, 1527–1534. [CrossRef]
81. Asadi, S.; Gholami, M.S.; Siassi, F.; Qorbani, M.; Sotoudeh, G. Beneficial Effects of Nano-Curcumin Supplement on Depression and Anxiety in Diabetic Patients with Peripheral Neuropathy: A Randomized, Double-Blind, Placebo-Controlled Clinical Trial. *Phytother. Res.* **2020**, *34*, 896–903. [CrossRef]
82. Bobo, D.; Robinson, K.J.; Islam, J.; Thurecht, K.J.; Corrie, S.R. Nanoparticle-Based Medicines: A Review of FDA-Approved Materials and Clinical Trials to Date. *Pharm. Res.* **2016**, *33*, 2373–2387. [CrossRef]

pharmaceutics

MDPI

Article

Safety in Rats of a Novel Nasal Spray Formulation for the Prevention of Airborne Viral Infections

Mirella Tanori [1], Michele Pitaro [2,*], Emiliano Fratini [1], Eleonora Colantoni [1], Angela Amoresano [2,3], Simona Celentano [3], Barbara Chiaramonte [4] and Mariateresa Mancuso [1]

1 Laboratory of Biomedical Technologies, Italian National Agency for New Technologies, Energy and Sustainable Economic Development (ENEA), Via Anguillarese 301, 00123 Rome, Italy
2 INBB–Biostructures and Biosystems National Institute, Viale delle Medaglie d'Oro 305, 00136 Rome, Italy
3 Department of Chemical Sciences, University of Naples Federico II, Via Cinthia 26, 80126 Naples, Italy
4 Istituto Nazionale per l'Assicurazione Contro Gli Infortuni sul Lavoro (INAIL), P.le Pastore 6, 00144 Rome, Italy
* Correspondence: michele.pitaro@inbb.it

Abstract: Hexedra+® is a nasal spray containing hydroxypropyl methylcellulose, beta-cyclodextrin, and usnic acid. It has been developed with the aim of reducing the risk of transmission of airborne viral infections, with particular reference to influenza and COVID-19. As part of the preclinical development of the product, we carried out a study on thirty male Wistar rats divided into three study groups and treated with Hexedra+, an alternative formulation containing a double concentration of usnic acid (0.015% instead of 0.0075%) or saline solution. Products were administered at the dose of 30 μL into each nostril, three times a day for seven consecutive days by means of a micropipette. By the end of the treatment period, no significant changes were observed in body weight. Histological examination of nasal mucosa and soft organs did not show any significant difference in the three study groups. Serum transaminase level remained in the normal limit in all the animals treated. The serum level of usnic acid was measured in order to assess the absorption of the molecule through the nasal mucosa. By the end of the study period, the usnic acid serum level was negligible in all the animals treated. In conclusion, the safety profile of Hexedra+ appears favorable in the animal model studied.

Keywords: respiratory viral infections; nasal spray; medical device; usnic acid

1. Introduction

A recent European Parliament resolution states that respiratory infectious diseases still represent a considerable threat to society, with a huge burden in terms of human life and economy [1]. For example, the cost of influenza in US prior to the COVID-19 pandemic was estimated in 11.2 USD billion annually, with 3.7 million outpatient visits, 247,000 hospital admissions, 36,300 deaths and more than twenty million working days lost [2].

Between 2002 and 2003, a new disease called SARS (Severe Acute Respiratory Syndrome) affected 8098 people in 26 different countries, most of them in the Guangdong province of China. The epidemic caused 774 deaths in 17 different countries, corresponding to a fatality rate of 10% [3]. The etiologic agent was a new beta coronavirus called SARS-CoV, transmitted from bats to humans through intermediate hosts identified in some wild animals sold in Chinese markets, like civets and raccoons. The overall economic burden of SARS was estimated between 30 and 100 billion USD [4]. Someone said, prophetically, that this epidemic would have been the dry run for a larger calamity in the future.

Swine flu affected the American continent in 2009 [5]. The etiologic agent was a H1N1 strain of orthomyxovirus which infected 59 million people and caused 265,000 hospitalizations in US alone.

Between April 2012 and January 2020, MERS (Middle East Respiratory Syndrome), an interstitial pneumonia caused by another new coronavirus called MERS-CoV, affected 2519 people and caused 866 deaths, corresponding to a fatality rate of 34.3% [6]. These figures are not conclusive, since the epidemic is still ongoing. A study carried out in South Korea estimated that the economic burden of MERS in 2005 was $ 2.6 billion [7]. To the best of our knowledge, no data have been published on the economic burden of MERS in other countries.

On the 31st of December 2019, the Chinese Health Authorities announced a suspected increase of interstitial pneumonia in the Hubei province, and mainly in its capital Wuhan [8]. It was the beginning of the COVID-19 pandemic caused by a third new coronavirus called SARS-CoV-2. According to the World Health Organization (WHO), by the 29th of January 2023, 752,517,552 people have been affected by the disease with 6,804,491 deaths (fatality rate: 0.9%) [9]. So far, the economic burden of COVID-19 has been dramatic. In 2020, the gross domestic product (GDP) in the European Union dropped by 7.4% [10].

Experts believe that respiratory viral infections will be more frequent in the future due to the expansion of large urban centers, the increase of air traffic and the climate changes linked to global warming [11]. Large urban centers facilitate virus transmission due to the close interindividual contiguity [12]. Air traffic moves every day large masses from one continent to another [13]. Finally, climate changes may have a direct impact on virus viability and host responses [14]. In fact, low temperatures increase the stability of many viruses [15]. A dry climate decreases the host's mucociliary clearance, whereas high relative humidity increases the permanence of viral particles in the air [16].

Interindividual transmission of pathogens depends on four basic mechanisms: direct contact between people; indirect contact through fomites (i.e., contaminated objects); droplets falling on mucous membranes; and aerosol inhalation [17]. Until recently, it was believed that respiratory viruses were transmitted by droplets [18]. These particles, characterized by a diameter > 100 µm, fall within 50 cm if the infected subject coughs or sneezes (20 cm if the infected subject speaks). Infection transmission depends on droplet deposition on the oral or nasal mucosa, as well as the ocular conjunctiva.

Extensive researches carried out on SARS-CoV-2 have highlighted the role of aerosol in interindividual transmission of the infection [19]. Significant viral loads have also been measured in the aerosol of patients with measles [20], influenza [21], SARS [22], and MERS [23]. Aerosol particles are characterized by a diameter < 100 µm (usually < 5 µm). They are produced not only by coughing and sneezing, but also by breathing, talking, singing, or playing wind instruments. Aerosol remains suspended in the air for more than 5 s (sometimes for hours) and can be inhaled through the respiratory tract (airborne transmission) [24]. Nasal sprays, which create a physical barrier on epithelial cells, can be a useful complement to personal protective equipment for the prevention of airborne viral infections. They could trap viral particles and eliminate them through the mucociliary clearance. A carrageenan-based nasal spray showed to be safe and effective in preventing the common cold [25]. A surfactant (lecithin phospholipid) was able to bind the SARS-CoV-2 receptor-binding domain (RBD) in an *in-silico* study, prompting the development of lecithin-based nasal sprays to decrease the risk of COVID-19 transmission [26]. A polysaccharide-based nasal spray prevented in vitro the infection of Vero cells by SARS-CoV-2 [27]. A nasal spray based on magnesium aluminum silicate significantly decreased the titers of SARS-CoV-2 Delta variant in a 3D model of human nasal mucosa without toxic effects [28]. Finally, a nasal spray was able to decrease by 62% the transmission rate of SARS-CoV-2 in a high-risk population of healthcare workers [29].

Hexedra+ is an innovative nasal spray based on hydroxypropyl methylcellulose (HPMC), beta cyclodextrin (b-CD), and usnic acid (UA). HPMC produces a hydrogel on the nasal mucosa which blocks the access to epithelial cells of viral particles [30], as well allergens [31]. B-CD has been added to the formulation in order to increase UA solubility [32,33]. However, this molecule has intrinsic antiviral properties that could potentially contribute to the overall efficacy of the product [34].

UA is a natural compound characterized by antibacterial and antiviral activities. It inhibits the growth of several Gram-positive bacteria, including Staphylococcus aureus [35] and Staphylococcus epidermidis [36]. Noteworthy, it is also effective against methicillin-resistant Staphylococcus aureus [37,38], several multidrug-resistant Gram-positive bacteria [39], and some Gran-negative bacteria, including vancomycin-resistant enterococci [37].

UA possess also a significant inhibitory activity against several strains of influenza virus [40,41]. Surprisingly, two recent in silico studies have shown a strong binding affinity of UA for residues of the SARS-CoV-2 Spike protein RBD (i.e., the region of the protein which binds to ACE2 on the epithelial cell surface) [42,43]. By binding SARS-CoV-2 Spike protein, UA could contribute to the retention of viral particles into the hydrogel produced by HPMC. UA and remdesivir (a product recently approved for the treatment of COVID-19) showed a similar activity in a SARS-CoV-2 binding assay [44]. Finally, an in vitro study performed on Vero E6 cells showed a significant activity of UA against three different strains of SARS-CoV-2, namely Wuhan, Delta, and Omicron [45].

UA inhibits oxidative phosphorylation in mitochondria without affecting the respiratory chain and ATP synthase [46]. These properties probably explain its broad-spectrum antibacterial activity and represent the rationale for the inclusion of UA in several slimming formulations sold in the past as over-the-counter products. However, high oral doses of UA for slimming purposes have been related to the development of hepatotoxicity in a limited number of subjects. For this reason, the US Food and Drug Administration (FDA) sent a warning letter, followed by the withdrawal of the products from the market in November 2001 [47]. On the other hand, the topical use of UA appears to be safe and well tolerated [48], making the product an appealing ingredient to be included in nasal spray formulations aimed at decreasing the risk of transmission of airborne infections.

It is well known that nasal formulations have been used for a long time to deliver active ingredients into the circulation through the nasal mucosa. Therefore, part of the UA included in the formulation of Hexedra+ could potentially reach the liver, raising concern about the possible risk of hepatotoxicity. For this reason, the main purpose of the present study was the evaluation of the safety profile of Hexedra+ administered intranasally for one week to Wistar male rats. In order to rule out the risk of hepatotoxicity, the plasma level of UA was assessed at the end of the treatment period by liquid chromatography-mass spectrometry (LC-MS).

2. Materials and Methods

2.1. Animals

Wistar male rats (body weight 200–300 g) were purchased from Charles River Laboratories (Lecco, Italy). Animals were housed under conventional conditions with ad libitum feeding and artificial 12 h light/dark cycle. Their general health status was monitored and, during the experiment, body weight was registered daily. The study was carried out according to the European Community Council Directive 2010/63/EU. It was approved by the local Ethical Committee for Animal Experiments of the ENEA, and authorized by the Italian Ministry of Health (883/2021-PR).

2.2. Study Procedures

Rats were randomized in 3 groups (10 for each group) treated with Hexedra+, an alternative formulation called H150 or physiological solution (PS). Hexedra+ is a nasal spray containing HPMC, b-CD, tocotrienols, and UA (0.0075%). H150 has the same composition of Hexedra+, the only difference being a double concentration of UA (0.015% instead of 0.0075%).

Products were administered at the dose of 30 μL into each nostril, three times a day for seven consecutive days by means of a micropipette. The dose of 30 μL was chosen according to the data provided in Table 1.

Table 1. Nasal cavity characteristics in different species [49]. The volume to be administered has been adjusted according to the maximum recommended dose of Hexedra+ (300 μL per nostril).

Species	Surface of Nasal Mucosa	Volume of Nasal Cavity	Volume to Be Administered
Man	160 cm^2	20 mL	300 μL
Rat	14 cm^2	0.4 mL	26 μL
Mouse	2.8 cm^2	0.03 mL	6 μL

In summary, the average area of nasal mucosa is 160 cm^2 and 14 cm^2 in man and rat, respectively (i.e., 11 times wider in men compared to rat). Since the recommended dose of Hexedra+ is 2–3 sprays per nostril (i.e., 200–300 μL per nostril), the corresponding dose in rat should be 18–27 μL per nostril. Therefore, a dose of 30 μL is 10% higher compared to the upper limit of the above-mentioned range in rat.

2.3. Histology, Morphometric Analysis and Immunohistochemistry

The day after the last treatment, the organs designed for morphological analysis (liver, brain, heart, spleen, kidneys and lungs) were quickly removed and fixed in formalin 10%. The diagonal section of the liver, lung, and spleen as well as the longitudinal section of the kidney, brain, and heart was obtained and processed for light microscopy, i.e., embedded in paraffin, sectioned at 4 μm, and stained with hematoxylin and eosin (H&E).

Skulls were also removed, and after fixation in 10% formalin for 24 h, they were incubated in a decalcifying solution (5% formic acid/4% hydrochloric acid) for 4 days. Transverse sections of nasal cavity were trimmed as follows: level 1, immediately posterior to the upper incisor teeth; level 2, at the incisive papilla; level 3, at the second palatine ridge; and level 4, at the level of the first upper molar teeth [50]. The sections of nasal cavity were then processed for light microscopy.

Nasal cavity sections stained with H&E were analyzed for the presence of edematous changes. Both the thickness of the olfactory epithelium and the proportion of glandular layer (relative to the thickness of the entire wall of mucosa) were measured. These measurements were all focused on the olfactory epithelium from the nasal septum in the region of the dorsal meatus. The thickness was quantified as the average of ten measurements, five from the right side and five from the left side of the septum, in nasal cavity sections of PS (n = 7), Hexedra+ (n = 6) and H150 (n = 6) rats.

Sections (4 μm) of paraffin-embedded nasal mucosa were also prepared to evaluate eventual presence of an inflammation status. Briefly, sections were dewaxed with Heat Mediated Antigen Retrieval Solution ("HMARS", Abcam, Germania, Germany), washed in water for 5 min, and peroxidase inhibited by incubation in 3% H_2O_2 for 10 min. After incubation with 5% bovine serum albumin (Santa Cruz Biotechnology, Santa Cruz, CA, USA) diluted in phosphate-buffered saline (PBS) for 30 min, they were incubated at 4 °C overnight with an antibody against ionized calcium-binding adaptor molecule 1 (Iba-1; Wako Pure Chemical Industries sections, Osaka, Japan, 1:500), a well-known marker of macrophage activation. After incubation with the secondary anti-rabbit antibody (Abcam, Cambridge, UK; 1:200), the antigen-antibody reaction was revealed by DAB detection kit (Dako, North America, Inc., Carpinteria, CA, USA). Finally, sections were counterstained with hematoxylin. Iba-1 quantification was performed counting manually by the NIS-Elements BR 4.00.05 software (Nikon Instruments S.p.A., Florence, Italy) and the positive cell density was expressed as activated macrophages per area (mm^2).

2.4. Enzyme-Linked Immunosorbent Assay (ELISA)

From each rat, a blood sample was collected into serum separator tube. After clot formation, serum was obtained by centrifugation (3000× g 15 min at 4 °C) and stored at −20 °C for the subsequent assay of alanine aminotransferase (ALT). Quantitative measurement of ALT protein was performed in duplicate by ELISA assay (Rat ALT SimpleStep ELISA® Kit; Abcam) according to the manufacturer's instructions.

2.5. Liquid Chromatography-Mass Spectrometry

Serum UA concentration was measured by precipitating 200 µL of serum with 600 µL of methanol. Samples were centrifugated for 10 min at 10000 rpm. Then, the supernatant was dried and resuspended in 100 µL of methanol. Using an Agilent 6420 Triple Quadrupole LC-MS/MS system with a HPLC 1100 series binary pump (Agilent Technologies, Waldbronn, Germany), 1 µL was analyzed by LC-MS/MS. The analytical column was a Phenomenex Kinetex 5 µm 100 A C18. The mobile phase was generated by mixing eluent A (0.1% Formic Acid in water) and eluent B (0.1% Formic Acid in methanol) for negative polarity. The flow rate was 0.2 mL/min. Elution gradient was from 20% to 80% solvent B in 5 min. Standard mixtures of 100 mg/L was diluted in MeOH/H_2O 50:50. The calibration standards of 0.25–0.5–1–5–25–50–100 µg/L were prepared by serial dilution. Tandem mass spectrometry was performed using a turbo ion spray source operated in mode, and the multiple reaction monitoring (MRM) mode was used for the selected analytes. Extracted mass chromatogram peaks of metabolites were integrated using MassHunter Quantitative Analysis software rev. B.05.00 (Agilent Technologies, Santa Clara, CA, USA).

2.6. Statistical Analysis

Statistical tests were performed with GraphPad Prism software v.7 (GraphPad, San Diego, CA, USA). p values were determined using a two-tailed t test; * $p < 0.05$; ** $p < 0.01$; *** $p < 0.001$; **** $p < 0.0001$. Data were expressed as mean ± standard deviation (SD).

3. Results

3.1. Body Weight

The general health status of animals was monitored during the experiment and the body weight was measured every day. Figure 1 shows the mean values of body weight at day 8 of treatment compared to baseline for each rat. No significant difference was observed in rats treated with Hexedra+ compared to H150 and PS.

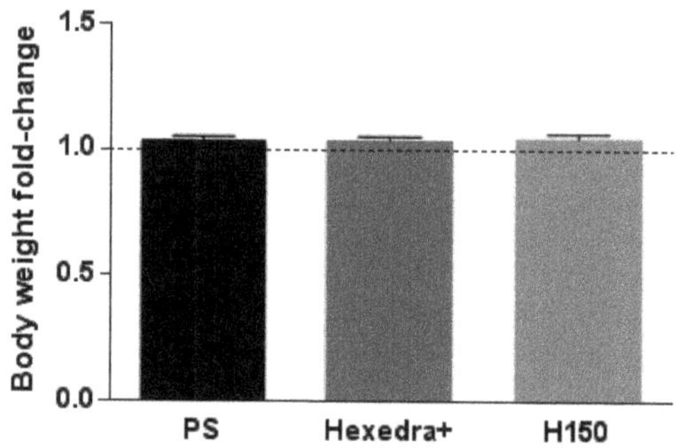

Figure 1. Rat body weight. Body weight change at the end of treatment with respect to baseline in rats treated with Hexedra+ compared to the alternative formulation with double quantity of UA (H150) and physiological solution (PS).

3.2. Histological Analysis

At the macroscopic level, no variation in terms of size and color were observed in all soft organs (liver, brain, heart, spleen, kidneys and lungs) collected from rats treated with Hexedra+ compared to H150 and PS. At the microscopic level, all organs showed a normal architecture, with an absence of inflammatory infiltrate as well as of any type of positive and/or negative adaptation (hypertrophy, hyperplasia, metaplasia and dysplasia) typically associated to tissue injury. Furthermore, no signs of reversible (swelling or enlarged size) or irreversible (apoptosis and necrosis) cell injury were detected. Representative images of liver and lung sections are shown in Figure 2.

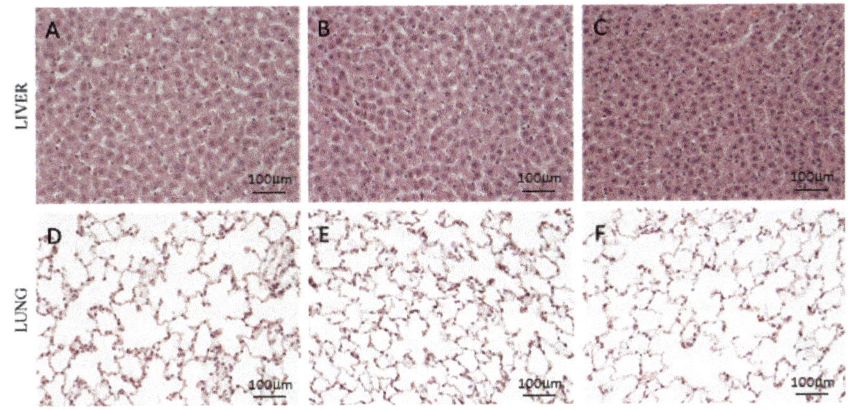

Figure 2. Histological analysis of rat liver and lung. Representative images of liver (**A–C**) and lung (**D–F**) of rats treated with PS (**A**,**D**), Hexedra+ (**B**,**E**) and H150 (**C**,**F**). PS: physiological solution; H150: alternative formulation with double quantity of UA.

In the nasal mucosa, three types of epithelia were analyzed in depth, in order to exclude any possible tissue reaction after in situ Hexedra+ application: squamous, respiratory, and olfactory epithelia.

The squamous epithelium (boxed in Figure 3) has an essentially defensive function, protecting the underlying tissues from the potential action of exogenous agents.

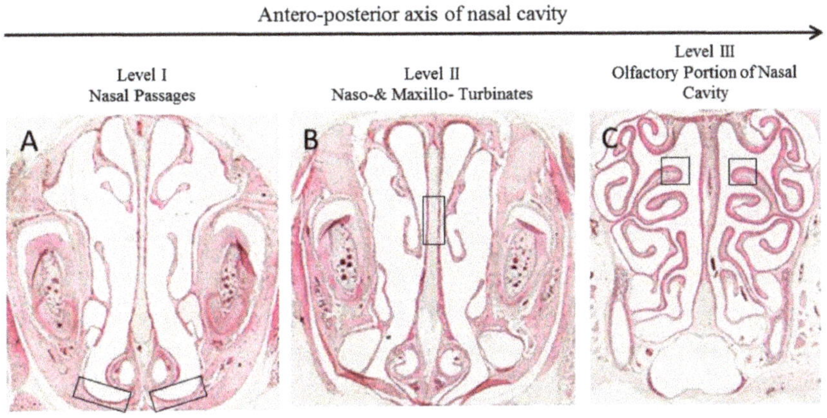

Figure 3. Distribution of the different types of epithelium within the nasal cavity of rats. At level I (**A**) of nasal passages is present the squamous epithelium; at level II (**B**) in naso- & maxillo turbinates there is the respiratory epithelium; finally, level III (**C**) is lined with the olfactory portion of nasal cavity. Boxes highlight the tract of epithelia analyzed.

Similarly to rats treated with PS and H150, the squamous epithelium of rats treated with Hexedra+ appeared lightly keratinized and stratified, consisting of a layer of basal cells and a few layers of squamous cells that become flatter toward the surface (Figure 4A–C).

The respiratory epithelium includes four main cell types: ciliated, nonciliated, basal, and goblet cells. Since the density of these cells changes depending on the location of the respiratory epithelium in the nasal cavity, to avoid mistakes in the evaluation of their distribution level, the same tract of epithelium was analyzed for each sample (boxed in Figure 3B). The mucociliary compartment of the animals treated with Hexedra+ was well-organized, with the ratio of goblet cells to ciliated cells similar among groups. No inflammatory phenomena were observed in the submucosa (Figure 4D–F).

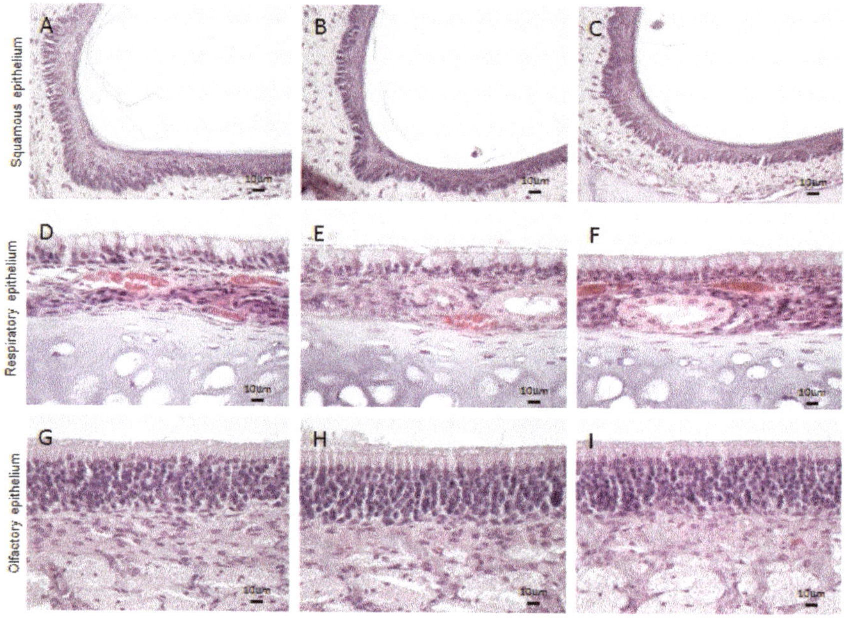

Figure 4. Histological analysis of nasal mucosa. Representative images of squamous (**A–C**), respiratory (**D–F**) and olfactory epithelium (**G–I**) of rats treated with PS (**A,D,G**), Hexedra+ (**B,E,H**), H150 (**C,F,I**). PS: physiological solution; H150: alternative formulation with double quantity of UA.

Finally, the olfactory epithelium of the nasal cavity was analyzed (boxed in Figure 3C). Three types of cells compose the olfactory epithelium: olfactory sensory neurons, supporting cells and basal cells. In rats treated with Hexedra+, the nuclei of all cells were aligned from the basal lamina to the apical surface similarly to the counterpart treated with PS or H150. In addition, Bowman's glands and their respective ducts, extending from the lamina propria to the epithelial surface, did not show alterations (Figure 4G–I). Moreover, no inflammatory cells were observed in the submucosa.

3.3. Morphometric Changes and Inflammation Assessment in the Olfactory Mucosa

To further investigate the presence of inflammation and edematous changes in the olfactory mucosa of the nasal cavity, both the thickness of epithelium and glandular layer and the expression of the activated macrophage marker Iba-1 were analyzed. To evaluate morphometric changes of the olfactory mucosa, the nasal septum in the region of dorsal meatus of the nasal passage was considered, as highlighted in Figure 5A.

Both treated groups showed no significant differences in the thickness of epithelium (PS: 55.54 μm ± 4.14; Hexedra+: 58.71 μm ± 1.51; H150: 57.98 μm ± 5.73) (Figure 5B,C) and in the glandular proportion of the mucosa (PS: 66.29% ± 1.6; Hexedra+: 65.83% ± 1.47; H150: 66.67% ± 1.03) (Figure 5B,D) compared to the control group. Furthermore, immunohistochemical analysis of Iba-1 revealed no difference in the activation of macrophages in the olfactory mucosa of treated groups with respect to control group (Figure 5E–H).

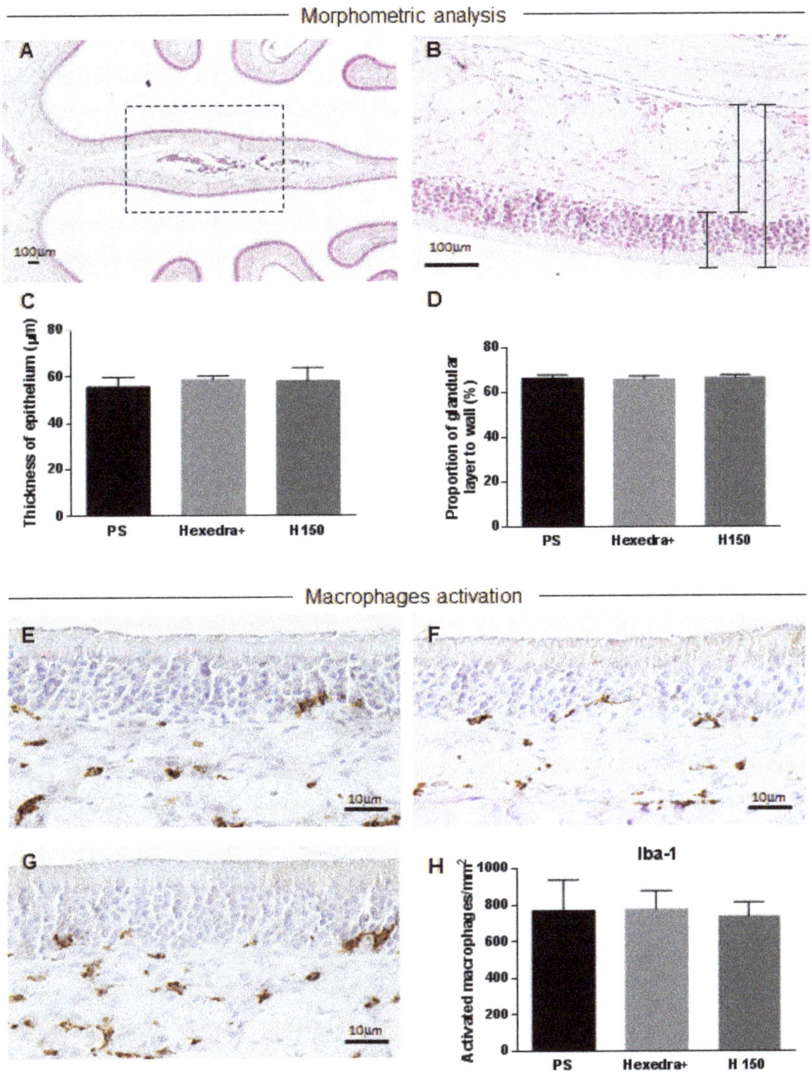

Figure 5. Morphometric analysis and macrophages activation in the olfactory mucosa. Representative image of nasal septum in the region of the dorsal meatus (dashed box) considered for measurements (**A**) and, at higher magnification, image of the thickness of olfactory epithelium and glandular layer (black lines in (**B**). Graphs with comparisons between treated and control groups for thickness of epithelium (**C**) and proportion of glandular layer to entire mucosa (**D**). Representative images of activated macrophage marker Iba-1 in the olfactory mucosa of rats treated with PS (**E**), Hexedra+ (**F**) and H150 (**G**) and relative quantitative representation (**H**). PS: physiological solution; H150: alternative formulation with double quantity of UA.

3.4. Serum ALT

ALT level is considered a sensitive and specific preclinical and clinical biomarker of hepatotoxicity [51]. However, an increase in serum ALT has also been associated with other organ toxicities, thus indicating that the enzyme has specificity beyond the liver in the absence of correlative histomorphological alteration in the liver. Results obtained from the

ELISA assay (Figure 6) show that ALT activity was not statistically different in the three study groups.

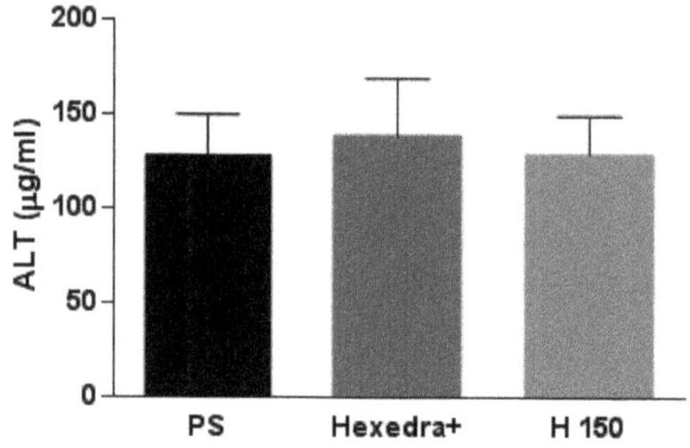

Figure 6. Rat serum ALT. Evaluation of ALT concentration level in rats treated with Hexedra+ compared to H150 and PS. PS: physiological solution; H150: alternative formulation with double quantity of UA.

3.5. Serum UA

Table 2 shows the serum concentration of UA in rats by the end of the study treatment. As expected, UA concentration was higher in rats treated with H150 (0.116 µM ± 0.006) compared to Hexedra+ (0.035 µM ± 0.004), while no UA was found in serum of rats treated with PS.

Table 2. Serum UA concentration. Analysis of UA levels in serum from each rat by the end of the study treatment (data are expressed in µM). PS: physiological solution; Hexedra+; H150: alternative formulation with double quantity of usnic acid.

PS				Hexedra+				H150			
No.	**S1**	**S2**	**Av.**	**No.**	**S1**	**S2**	**Av.**	**No.**	**S1**	**S2**	**Av.**
1	<1	<1	<1	1	0.032	0.034	0.033	1	0.115	0.111	0.113
2	<1	<1	<1	2	0.044	0.036	0.040	2	0.121	0.116	0.119
3	<1	<1	<1	3	0.039	0.040	0.039	3	0.112	0.107	0.109
4	<1	<1	<1	4	0.031	0.036	0.034	4	0.126	0.117	0.121
5	<1	<1	<1	5	0.030	0.028	0.029	5	0.116	0.119	0.117
6	<1	<1	<1	6	0.030	0.040	0.035	6	0.126	0.119	0.123
7	<1	<1	<1	7	0.033	0.036	0.034	7	0.114	0.107	0.111
8	<1	<1	<1	8	0.033	0.034	0.034	8	0.135	0.109	0.122
9	<1	<1	<1	9	0.033	0.028	0.031	9	0.112	0.102	0.107
10	<1	<1	<1	10	0.032	0.042	0.037	10	0.120	0.111	0.116
Av.			<1	Av.			0.035	Av.			0.116
SD			n.a.	SD			0.004	SD			0.006

4. Discussion

Hexedra+ is an innovative nasal spray based on HPMC, b-CD, and UA aimed at blocking the access of viral particles, as well as allergens, to epithelial cells of nasal mucosa HPMC and b-CD are known to be safe and well tolerated. The former is currently used as an excipient in spray formulations for the administration of active ingredients through the nasal route [52]. The latter is also widely used as an excipient in several pharmaceutical formulations [53].

Lichen extracts with a high content of UA have been used for a long time in traditional medicine [54]. The first documented use of UA dates back to the first century BC. when dried lichen extracts were officially included in traditional Chinese medicine texts. The product was used for the treatment of malaria, wounds, and snake bites at the recommended dose of 6–9 g of dried lichen taken as a tea or decoction, corresponding to a daily dose of 60–120 mg of UA. Currently, UA is widely used in cosmetics, deodorants, toothpaste and medicinal creams, and studies published so far on the topical use of UA (mainly for the treatment of skin ulcers) have demonstrated a good safety and tolerability profile.

On the other hand, UA deserves a particular attention, due to the development in the past of hepatotoxicity in a limited number of subjects treated orally for slimming purposes. The content of UA in these formulations was particularly high, ranging from 600 to 1300 mg daily (around ten times the daily dose described in traditional medicine) [46]. Biopsy performed in the subjects who developed liver failure showed acute hepatocellular necrosis and inflammation, with a marked elevation of alanine aminotransferase (ALT) and minimal increase in alkaline phosphatase levels.

Due to the small dimension of the molecule, UA administered intranasally could potentially enter the blood circulation and reach the liver. For this reason, we performed an in vivo study in order to identify any possible damage to the nasal mucosa and other systemic districts (mainly liver, brain, and lungs). Our study demonstrated that Hexedra+ administered in rats by the nasal route three times a day for seven consecutive days is safe and well tolerated, without significant changes in body weight and damage or inflammation in nasal mucosa. The morphological analysis of all organs did not highlight visible alterations. In particular, no signs of hepatotoxicity were observed in any of the animals treated. Serum ALT levels at the end of the treatment period were in the normal range, with no statistical differences in the three study groups.

UA serum concentrations at the end of the treatment period were negligible and well below the concentrations found to be toxic for hepatocytes in toxicology studies. H150 (the alternative formulation containing twice the amount of UA) produced a UA serum level below the toxic concentrations as well. Noteworthy, in vitro toxicology studies have shown that UA concentrations < 1 μM are safe and well tolerated, while concentrations > 5 μM are toxic for hepatocytes [46]. To the best of our knowledge, this is the first assessment of UA absorption through the nasal mucosa into the circulation.

5. Conclusions

Hexedra+ is safe and well tolerated in rats after one week of treatment by the nasal route of administration. The treatment did not induce any change in body weight, nor damage or inflammation to the nasal mucosa. UA serum concentrations following the absorption of the molecule through the nasal mucosa were negligible and well below the concentrations found to be toxic for hepatocytes. Product safety was confirmed by the maintenance of a normal ALT level and the absence of any sign of liver damage, not only in rats treated with Hexedra+, but also in animals treated with an alternative formulation containing double the concentration of UA.

Author Contributions: Conceptualization, M.P. and M.M.; methodology, M.P. and B.C.; software, M.T.; formal analysis, B.C.; investigation, M.T., E.F., E.C., A.A. and S.C.; resources, M.P.; data curation, M.T.; writing—original draft preparation, M.P. and M.T.; writing—review and editing, M.T., M.M. and A.A.; project administration, M.M. All authors have read and agreed to the published version of the manuscript.

Funding: This research is part of the registration dossier of Hexedra+ and it has been founded by Vivatis Pharma Italia S.r.l.

Institutional Review Board Statement: The animal study protocol was approved by the Institutional Review Board of ENEA and the Italian Ministry of Health (Prot. No. EE25E.20; authorization No. 883/2021-PR; date of authorization 18 November 2021).

Informed Consent Statement: Not applicable.

Data Availability Statement: Not applicable.

Conflicts of Interest: The authors declare no conflict of interest. The funder (Vivatis Pharma Italia S.r.l.) had no role in the design of the study; in the collection, analyses, or interpretation of data; in the writing of the manuscript; or in the decision to publish the results.

References

1. Delivorias, A.; Scholz, N.; EPRS (European Parliamentary Research Service). Economic Impact of Epidemics and Pandemics. Available online: https://www.europarl.europa.eu/thinktank/en/document/EPRS_BRI(2020)646195 (accessed on 27 February 2020).
2. Putri, W.C.W.S.; Muscatello, D.J.; Stockwell, M.S.; Newall, A.T. Economic burden of seasonal influenza in the United States. *Vaccine* **2018**, *27*, 3960–3966. [CrossRef] [PubMed]
3. Wang, J.T.; Chang, S.C. Severe acute respiratory syndrome. *Curr. Opin. Infect. Dis.* **2004**, *2*, 143–148. [CrossRef] [PubMed]
4. Keogh-Brown, M.R.; Smith, R.D. The economic impact of SARS: How does the reality match the predictions? Health Policy. *Health Policy* **2008**, *88*, 110–120. [CrossRef] [PubMed]
5. Neumann, G.; Kawaoka, Y. The first influenza pandemic of the new millennium. *Influenza Other Respir. Viruses* **2011**, *3*, 157–166. [CrossRef]
6. World Health Organization; Regional Office for the Eastern Mediterranean. MERS Situation Update, January 2020. Available online: http://www.emro.who.int/pandemic-epidemic-diseases/mers-cov/mers-situation-update-january-2020.html (accessed on 15 January 2023).
7. Joo, H.; Maskery, B.A.; Berro, A.D.; Rotz, L.D.; Lee, Y.K.; Brown, C.M. Economic Impact of the 2015 MERS Outbreak on the Republic of Korea's Tourism-Related Industries. *Health Secur.* **2019**, *2*, 100–108. [CrossRef]
8. Patel, A.; Jernigan, D.B. 2019-nCoV CDC Response Team. Initial Public Health Response and Interim Clinical Guidance for the 2019 Novel Coronavirus Outbreak—United States, 31 December 2019–4 February 2020. *MMWR Morb. Mortal. Wkly. Rep.* **2020**, *5*, 140–146. [CrossRef]
9. World Health Organization. WHO Coronavirus (COVID-19) Dashboard. Available online: https://covid19.who.int/ (accessed on 15 January 2023).
10. Clark, D. GDP Growth Rate Forecasts in Europe 2020–2021. Available online: https://www.statista.com/statistics/686147/gdp-growth-europe/ (accessed on 16 May 2022).
11. Neiderud, C.J. How urbanization affects the epidemiology of emerging infectious diseases. *Infect. Ecol. Epidemiol.* **2015**, *5*, 27060. [CrossRef]
12. Aguilar, J.; Bassolas, A.; Ghoshal, G.; Hazarie, S.; Kirkley, A.; Mazzoli, M.; Meloni, S.; Mimar, S.; Nicosia, V.; Ramasco, J.J.; et al. Impact of urban structure on infectious disease spreading. *Sci. Rep.* **2022**, *1*, 3816. [CrossRef]
13. Grobusch, M.P.; Weld, L.; Goorhuis, A.; Hamer, D.H.; Schunk, M.; Jordan, S.; Mockenhaupt, F.P.; Chappuis, F.; Asgeirsson, H.; Caumes, E.; et al. Travel-related infections presenting in Europe: A 20-year analysis of EuroTravNet surveillance data. *Lancet Reg. Health Eur.* **2020**, *1*, 100001. [CrossRef]
14. Mahmud, A.S.; Martinez, P.P.; He, J.; Baker, R.E. The Impact of Climate Change on Vaccine-Preventable Diseases: Insights from Current Research and New Directions. *Curr. Environ. Health Rep.* **2020**, *4*, 384–391. [CrossRef]
15. Moriyama, M.; Hugentobler, W.J.; Iwasaki, A. Seasonality of respiratory viral infections. *Annu. Rev. Virol.* **2020**, *7*, 83–101. [CrossRef]
16. Marr, L.C.; Tang, J.W.; Van Mullekom, J.; Lakdawala, S.S. Mechanistic insights into the effect of humidity on airborne influenza virus survival, transmission and incidence. *J. R. Soc. Interface* **2019**, *16*, 20180298. [CrossRef]
17. Randall, K.; Ewing, E.T.; Marr, L.C.; Jimenez, J.L.; Bourouiba, L. How did we get here: What are droplets and aerosols and how far do they go? A historical perspective on the transmission of respiratory infectious diseases. *Interface Focus* **2021**, *11*, 20210049. [CrossRef]
18. Wang, C.C.; Prather, K.A.; Sznitman, J.; Jimenez, J.L.; Lakdawala, S.S.; Tufekci, Z.; Marr, L.C. Airborne transmission of respiratory viruses. *Science* **2021**, *373*, 981. [CrossRef]
19. Santarpia, J.L.; Herrera, V.L.; Rivera, D.N.; Ratnesar-Shumate, S.; Reid, S.P.; Ackerman, D.N.; Denton, P.W.; Martens, J.W.S.; Fang, Y.; Conoan, N.; et al. The size and culturability of patient-generated SARS-CoV-2 aerosol. *J. Expo. Sci. Environ. Epidemiol.* **2021**, *32*, 706–711. [CrossRef]
20. Bloch, A.B.; Orenstein, W.A.; Ewing, W.M.; Spain, W.H.; Mallison, G.F.; Herrmann, K.L.; Hinman, A.R. Measles outbreak in a pediatric practice: Airborne transmission in an office setting. *Pediatrics* **1985**, *75*, 676–683. [CrossRef]
21. Yan, J.; Grantham, M.; Pantelic, J.; Bueno de Mesquita, P.J.; Albert, B.; Liu, F.; Ehrman, S.; Milton, D.K.; EMIT Consortium. Infectious virus in exhaled breath of symptomatic seasonal influenza cases from a college community. *Proc. Natl. Acad. Sci. USA* **2018**, *5*, 1081–1086. [CrossRef]
22. Yu, I.T.S.; Li, Y.; Wong, T.W.; Tam, W.; Chan, A.T.; Lee, J.H.W.; Leung, D.Y.C.; Ho, T. Evidence of airborne transmission of the severe acute respiratory syndrome virus. *N. Engl. J. Med.* **2004**, *17*, 1731–1739. [CrossRef]

23. Kim, S.H.; Chang, S.Y.; Sung, M.; Park, J.H.; Kim, H.B.; Lee, H.; Choi, J.P.; Choi, W.S.; Min, J.Y. Extensive Viable Middle East Respiratory Syndrome (MERS) Coronavirus Contamination in Air and Surrounding Environment in MERS Isolation Wards. *Clin. Infect. Dis.* **2016**, *3*, 363–369. [CrossRef]
24. Chen, W.; Zhang, N.; Wei, J.; Yen, H.L.; Li, Y. Short-range airborne route dominates exposure of respiratory infection during close contact. *Build. Environ.* **2020**, *176*, 106859. [CrossRef]
25. Bichiri, D.; Rente, A.R.; Jesus, Â. Safety and efficacy of iota-carrageenan nasal spray in treatment and prevention of the common cold. *Med. Pharm. Rep.* **2021**, *1*, 28–34. [CrossRef] [PubMed]
26. Qaisrani, M.N.; Belousov, R.; Rehman, J.U.; Goliaei, E.M.; Girotto, I.; Franklin-Mergarejo, R.; Güell, O.; Hassanali, A.; Roldán, E. Phospholipids dock SARS-CoV-2 spike protein via hydrophobic interactions: A minimal in-silico study of lecithin nasal spray therapy. *Eur. Phys. J. E Soft Matter* **2021**, *11*, 132. [CrossRef] [PubMed]
27. Moakes, R.J.A.; Davies, S.P.; Stamataki, Z.; Grover, L.M. Formulation of a Composite Nasal Spray Enabling Enhanced Surface Coverage and Prophylaxis of SARS-CoV-2. *Adv. Mater.* **2021**, *26*, e2008304. [CrossRef] [PubMed]
28. Fais, F.; Juskeviciene, R.; Francardo, V.; Mateos, S.; Guyard, M.; Viollet, C.; Constant, S.; Borelli, M.; Hohenfeld, I.P. Drug-Free Nasal Spray as a Barrier against SARS-CoV-2 and Its Delta Variant: In Vitro Study of Safety and Efficacy in Human Nasal Airway Epithelia. *Int. J. Mol. Sci.* **2022**, *7*, 4062. [CrossRef] [PubMed]
29. Balmforth, D.; Swales, J.A.; Silpa, L.; Dunton, A.; Davies, K.E.; Davies, S.G.; Kamath, A.; Gupta, J.; Gupta, S.; Masood, M.A.; et al. Evaluating the efficacy and safety of a novel prophylactic nasal spray in the prevention of SARS-CoV-2 infection: A multi-centre, double blind, placebo-controlled, randomised trial. *J. Clin. Virol.* **2022**, *155*, 105248. [CrossRef]
30. Bentley, K.; Stanton, R.J. Hydroxypropyl Methylcellulose-Based Nasal Sprays Effectively Inhibit In Vitro SARS-CoV-2 Infection and Spread. *Viruses* **2021**, *12*, 2345. [CrossRef]
31. Popov, T.A.; Åberg, N.; Emberlin, J.; Josling, P.; Ilyina, N.I.; Nikitin, N.P.; Church, M. Methyl-cellulose powder for prevention and management of nasal symptoms. *Expert Rev. Respir. Med.* **2017**, *11*, 885–892. [CrossRef]
32. Jin, J.Q.; Rao, Y.; Bian, X.l. Solubility of (+)-Usnic Acid in Water, Ethanol, Acetone, Ethyl Acetate and n-Hexane. *J. Solution Chem.* **2013**, *42*, 1018–1027. [CrossRef]
33. Dos Santos, P.H.; Mesquita, T.; Miguel-Dos-Santos, R.; Melo de Almeida, G.K.; Andrade de Sá, L.; Dos Passos Menezes, P.; Antunes de Souza Araujo, A.; Lauton-Santos, S. Inclusion complex with β-cyclodextrin is a key determining factor for the cardioprotection induced by usnic acid. *Chem. Biol. Interact.* **2020**, *332*, 109297. [CrossRef]
34. Garrido, P.F.; Calvelo, M.; Blanco-González, A.; Veleiro, U.; Suárez, F.; Conde, D.; Cabezón, A.; Piñeiro, A.; Garcia-Fandino, R. The Lord of the NanoRings: Cyclodextrins and the battle against SARS-CoV-2. *Int. J. Pharm.* **2020**, *588*, 119689. [CrossRef]
35. Gupta, V.K.; Verma, S.; Gupta, S.; Singh, A.; Pal, A.; Srivastava, S.K.; Singh, S.C.; Darokar, M.P. Membrane-damaging potential of natural L-(-)-usnic acid in Staphylococcus aureus. *Eur. J. Clin. Microbiol. Infect. Dis.* **2012**, *31*, 3375–3383. [CrossRef]
36. Francolini, L.; Taresco, V.; Crisante, F.; Martinelli, A.; D'Ilario, L.; Piozzi, A. Water soluble usnic acid-polyacrylamide complexes with enhanced antimicrobial activity against Staphylococcus epidermidis. *Int. J. Mol. Sci.* **2013**, *14*, 7356–7369. [CrossRef]
37. Elo, H.; Matikainen, J.; Pelttari, E. Potent activity of the lichen antibiotic (+)-usnic acid against clinical isolates of vancomycin-resistant enterococci and methicillin-resistant Staphylococcus aureus. *Naturwissenschaften* **2007**, *94*, 465–468. [CrossRef]
38. Pompilio, A.; Riviello, A.; Crocetta, V.; Di Giuseppe, F.; Pomponio, S.; Sulpizio, M.; Di Ilio, C.; Angelucci, S.; Barone, L.; Di Giulio, A.; et al. Evaluation of antibacterial and antibiofilm mechanisms by usnic acid against methicillin-resistant Staphylococcus aureus. *Future Microbiol.* **2016**, *11*, 1315–1338. [CrossRef]
39. Tozatti, M.G.; Ferreira, D.S.; Flauzino, L.G.B.; Moraes, T.D.S.; Martins, C.H.G.; Groppo, M.; Silva, M.L.A.E.; Januário, A.H.; Pauletti, P.M.; Cunhaa, W.R. Activity of the lichen Usnea steineri and its major metabolites against Gram-positive, multidrug-resistant bacteria. *Nat. Prod. Commun.* **2016**, *11*, 493–496. [CrossRef]
40. Shtro, A.A.; Zarubaev, V.V.; Luzina, O.A.; Sokolov, D.N.; Salakhutdinov, N.F. Derivatives of usnic acid inhibit broad range of influenza viruses and protect mice from lethal influenza infection. *Antivir. Chem. Chemother.* **2015**, *24*, 92–98. [CrossRef]
41. Sokolov, D.N.; Zarubaev, V.V.; Shtro, A.A.; Polovinka, M.P.; Luzina, O.A.; Komarova, N.I.; Salakhutdinov, N.F.; Kiselev, O.I. Anti-viral activity of (-)- and (+)-usnic acids and their derivatives against influenza virus A(H1N1). *Bioorg. Med. Chem. Lett.* **2012**, *22*, 7060–7064. [CrossRef]
42. Guthappa, R. Docking Studies of Usnic Acid and Sodium Usnate on SARS-CoV-2 Main Protease and Spike Protein RBD. *Chemrxiv* **2020**, 12638906. [CrossRef]
43. Prateeksha, G.; Rana, T.S.; Ashthana, A.K.; Barik, S.K.; Singh, B.N. Screening of cryptogamic secondary metabolites as putative inhibitors of SARS-CoV-2 main protease and ribosomal binding domain of spike glycoprotein by molecular docking and molecular dynamics approaches. *J. Mol. Struct.* **2021**, *1240*, 130506. [CrossRef]
44. Oh, E.; Wang, W.; Park, K.H.; Park, C.; Cho, Y.; Lee, J.; Kang, E.; Kang, H. (+)-Usnic acid and its salts, inhibitors of SARS-CoV-2, identified by using in silico methods and in vitro assay. *Sci. Rep.* **2022**, *12*, 13118. [CrossRef]
45. Filimonov, A.S.; Yarovaya, O.I.; Zaykovskaya, A.V.; Rudometova, N.B.; Shcherbakov, D.N.; Chirkova, V.Y.; Baev, D.S.; Borisevich, S.S.; Luzina, O.A.; Pyankov, O.V.; et al. (+)-Usnic Acid and Its Derivatives as Inhibitors of a Wide Spectrum of SARS-CoV-2 Viruses. *Viruses* **2022**, *14*, 2154. [CrossRef] [PubMed]
46. Croce, N.; Pitaro, M.; Gallo, V.; Antonini, A. Toxicity of Usnic Acid: A Narrative Review. *J. Toxicol.* **2022**, *2022*, 8244340. [CrossRef] [PubMed]

47. FDA Warns Against Use of the Dietary Supplement LipoKinetix. Available online: https://www.medscape.com/viewarticle/411150 (accessed on 21 November 2001).
48. Macedo, D.C.S.; Almeida, F.J.F.; Wanderley, M.S.O.; Ferraz, M.S.; Santos, N.P.S.; López, A.M.Q.; Santos-Magalhães, N.S.; Lira-Nogueira, M.C.B. Usnic acid: From an ancient lichen derivative to promising biological and nanotechnology applications. *Phytochem. Rev.* **2021**, *20*, 609–630. [CrossRef]
49. Gizurarson, S. The relevance of nasal physiology to the design of drug absorption studies. *Adv. Drug Deliv. Rev.* **1993**, *11*, 329–347. [CrossRef]
50. Young, J.T. Histopathologic examination of the rat nasal cavity. *Fundam. Appl. Toxicol.* **1981**, *4*, 309–312. [CrossRef]
51. Ozer, J.; Ratner, M.; Shaw, M.; Bailey, W.; Schomaker, S. The current state of serum biomarkers of hepatotoxicity. *Toxicology* **2008**, *3*, 194–205. [CrossRef]
52. Burdock, G.A. Safety assessment of hydroxypropyl methylcellulose as a food ingredient. *Food Chem. Tox.* **2007**, *45*, 2341–2351. [CrossRef]
53. Crini, G. Review: A history of cyclodextrins. *Chem. Rev.* **2014**, *114*, 10940–10975. [CrossRef]
54. Guo, L.; Shi, Q.; Fang, J.L.; Mei, N.; Ali, A.A.; Lewis, S.M.; Leakey, J.E.A.; Frankos, V.H. Review of Usnic Acid and Usnea Barbata Toxicity. *J. Environ. Sci. Health C Environ. Carcinog. Ecotoxicol. Rev.* **2008**, *26*, 317–338. [CrossRef]

pharmaceutics MDPI

Article

Visualization and Estimation of Nasal Spray Delivery to Olfactory Mucosa in an Image-Based Transparent Nasal Model

Amr Seifelnasr [1], Xiuhua April Si [2] and Jinxiang Xi [1,*]

[1] Department of Biomedical Engineering, University of Massachusetts, Lowell, MA 01854, USA; amr_seifelnasr@student.uml.edu

[2] Department of Mechanical Engineering, California Baptist University, Riverside, CA 92504, USA; asi@calbaptist.edu

* Correspondence: jinxiang_xi@uml.edu; Tel.: +1-978-934-3259

Abstract: Background: Nose-to-brain (N2B) drug delivery offers unique advantages over intravenous methods; however, the delivery efficiency to the olfactory region using conventional nasal devices and protocols is low. This study proposes a new strategy to effectively deliver high doses to the olfactory region while minimizing dose variability and drug losses in other regions of the nasal cavity. **Materials and Methods:** The effects of delivery variables on the dosimetry of nasal sprays were systematically evaluated in a 3D-printed anatomical model that was generated from a magnetic resonance image of the nasal airway. The nasal model comprised four parts for regional dose quantification. A transparent nasal cast and fluorescent imaging were used for visualization, enabling detailed examination of the transient liquid film translocation, real-time feedback on input effect, and prompt adjustment to delivery variables, which included the head position, nozzle angle, applied dose, inhalation flow, and solution viscosity. **Results:** The results showed that the conventional vertex-to-floor head position was not optimal for olfactory delivery. Instead, a head position tilting 45–60° backward from the supine position gave a higher olfactory deposition and lower variability. A two-dose application (250 mg) was necessary to mobilize the liquid film that often accumulated in the front nose following the first dose administration. The presence of an inhalation flow reduced the olfactory deposition and redistributed the sprays to the middle meatus. The recommended olfactory delivery variables include a head position ranging 45–60°, a nozzle angle ranging 5–10°, two doses, and no inhalation flow. With these variables, an olfactory deposition fraction of 22.7 ± 3.7% was achieved in this study, with insignificant discrepancies in olfactory delivery between the right and left nasal passages. **Conclusions:** It is feasible to deliver clinically significant doses of nasal sprays to the olfactory region by leveraging an optimized combination of delivery variables.

Keywords: nasal spray; soft-mist inhaler; nose-to-brain (N2B); intranasal drug delivery; head position; vertex-to-floor; liquid film translocation

1. Introduction

Nasal drug delivery has gained significant attention as a non-invasive method of delivering therapeutic agents to the brain. Drug administrations from the nose directly to the brain (known as N2B) have become an attractive substitute for conventional treatments of neurological disorders [1–4]. The olfactory mucosa, which is located in the upmost region of the nasal cavity, has been identified as a promising target for the administration of medications to the central nervous system (CNS). Neurological medications that are administered to the olfactory region have the ability to reach the CNS through the olfactory pathways and circumvent the Blood–Brain Barrier [5,6]. Nevertheless, the efficacy of N2B has been restricted due to the difficulties in administering clinically effective quantities of medication to the olfactory cleft using conventional nasal devices [7–10]. Thus, drug delivery to the brain through the nasal route is not commonly used in clinical settings due to the low amount of medication that can reach the olfactory region with conventional nasal delivery devices.

The complex anatomy of the nasal cavity creates various obstacles that hinder the effective delivery of drugs through the olfactory route. As illustrated in Figure 1a, the inadequate delivery of drugs to the olfactory region results from the restricted airflow through this area, as well as the intricate structure of the nose, which screens out most intranasally delivered drugs well before they even get to the olfactory mucosa [11]. The nasal valve, the narrowest part of the nasal passage, acts as a filter that prevents most inhaled spray droplets from passing through. Those droplets that do make it past the valve tend to deposit within the labyrinthine turbinate area. As the airway transitions between the nasal valve and the turbinate region, the cross-sectional area increases, which reduces the respiratory flow velocity and facilitates the settling of large particles in the inferior and middle nasal cavity passages. The tortuous and restricted pathway of the turbinate area further promotes the deposition of administered droplets through direct interception and inertia-driven impaction. The superior meatus, situated at the uppermost part of the nasal cavity, has a narrower passage, making it difficult for respiratory air and particles to reach the olfactory mucosa [12]. Prior research has shown that the olfactory region receives less than 1% of aerosol medications that are administered intranasally [13]. González-Botas et al. found that when utilizing a typical radial-hole inhaler that dispenses 140 mL per application, most of the medication was deposited within the nasal valve and inferior meatus, with very little deposited in the olfactory cleft [14]. Accordingly, the significantly low amount of medication that can reach the brain through the nose has hindered the clinical use of N2B drug delivery and has become a significant obstacle in the advancement of neurological therapies via the nasal route [15].

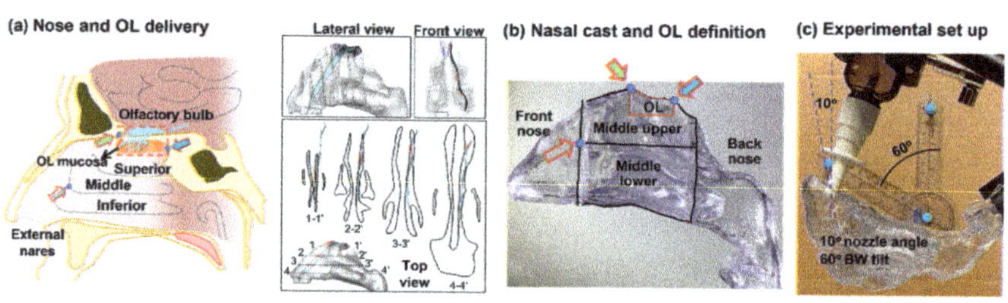

Figure 1. Nasal model and delivery experimental setup: (**a**) diagram of the human nose and olfactory (OL) region with anatomical features preventing effective olfactory delivery viewed from lateral, front, and top directions; (**b**) transparent nasal cast with four sections (front nose, middle upper (UpM), middle lower (LowM), back nose) and the delineated olfactory (OL) region using two landmarks (solid green and blue arrows); and (**c**) delivery experimental setup with adjustable nozzle angle (left panel) and head orientation (right panel).

The deposition of particles within the human nasal cavity has been extensively researched in human participants, as well as using in vitro nasal cavity models and computational simulations [16–18]. Although significant inter-subject variability exists in nasal morphology, research in this area has consistently demonstrated that several aspects—including the type of intranasal device used, medication formulation, delivery methods, as well as a patient's inhalation pattern—can all have an impact on nasal deposition. Reliable techniques are available to determine the overall deposition fractions in hollow nasal replica casts, although substantiated techniques for visualizing and quantifying deposition fractions in specific regions or local areas are rare. However, when predicting clinical effects or assessing negative health outcomes, localized deposition is of greater clinical significance than total deposition. Computational models can predict deposition patterns, but the limited validation of these models and their inability to directly correlate with medical outcomes have hindered their use in clinical settings. Additionally, since multiple factors can impact spray deposition, and no single factor has been predominantly correlated with intranasal dosimetry, experimental testing is essential for validating targeted drug deliveries [6].

The bioequivalence of drugs administered within a specific region has been evaluated using techniques that make use of dyes such as methylene blue to inspect the intensity of staining [19]. However, these techniques have certain drawbacks, including the inability to quantify dosage accurately, as well as the diffusion and dripping of the solution. Some investigations employed gamma scintigraphy to visualize the distributions of deposition within human nasal cavities by using particles labeled with technetium-99m (99mTc) [20–22]. Gamma scintigraphy has also been utilized with in vitro nasal airway models [23–25]. In this method, a gamma camera is used to capture images of the deposition of radioactive aerosols, which are later analyzed and converted into dosage measurements based on color intensity. One major limitation of gamma scintigraphy is that its effectiveness is sensitive to the weakening of gamma rays as they pass through the body, resulting in up to 50% of photons either being dispersed or blocked by the surrounding tissue [26]. The scattering of photons can cause distortions in scintigraphy images and lead to inaccurate dose quantification, with around 30% of photons being scattered and causing measurement errors. Other factors that can affect accuracy include the dosage administered before the study, aerosol radiolabeling quality control, and radioactivity recovery [27]. Furthermore, scintigraphy images are only 2D and cannot distinguish between multiple layers of deposition. A cost-effective and efficient method was developed by Dalby and partners that utilized a water-detecting paste (Sar-Gel) to observe and measure the distribution of deposited water droplets. Kundoor and Dalby [28,29] have shown that Sar-Gel, which undergoes a color transformation from white to purple after coming into contact with water, is capable of detecting a volume of water as small as 0.5 μL, which corresponds to the minimum water droplet size found in nasal sprays. Sar-Gel was employed by Xi et al. to visualize and measure deposition in the nasal cavity and olfactory region in a sectional model of an adult nasal airway [6].

Different nasal devices and delivery methods have been studied to improve the delivery of therapeutic medication to the olfactory mucosa. Several important factors, such as exiting velocity, spray plume angle, droplet size, and angle of administration, affect the deposition location of nasal sprays [29–32]. Cheng et al. [30] examined the resulting deposition pattern from nasal spray pumps in a human nasal airway model and found that frontal nasal deposition was higher when larger spray particles and a wider spray angle were used, whereas smaller droplet sizes and a narrow spray cone angle resulted in a larger number of administered droplets passing through the nasal valve. Kundoor and Dalby [29] conducted a study to determine how nozzle orientation, ranging from 0 to 90°, affects olfactory delivery. They found that the most optimal deposition in the olfactory mucosa occurred when the nasal spray nozzle was oriented between 60° and 75°. Wang et al. [32] devised a method that involved intubation of the nozzle into the middle or superior meatus and administration of the spray directly below the olfactory mucosa. Although this approach had the potential to improve olfactory dosing, it involved invasive procedures that posed risks of tissue injury. As a result, this and similar techniques have not become popular. Gizurarson [31] proposed a less invasive technique that involved using an intranasal spray pump with a narrow cone angle to deliver medications to the olfactory region through the superior meatus. This method involved applying a relatively high-pressure spray to facilitate droplet penetration into the olfactory cleft. Nevertheless, the improvements in delivery to the olfactory region achieved through this approach were limited.

While there have been numerous test-based and computational studies into the deposition pattern of spray droplets, only a limited number of investigations explored the ensuing mobilization of these droplets once they have adhered to the walls of the nasal airway [12]. The migration of a liquid film due to gravity and/or flow shear following the application of a spray can result in a notable enhancement of delivering drugs to the olfactory mucosa. The effectiveness of topical treatments, such as intranasal drops, in reaching the olfactory cleft depends heavily on the position of the head during administration [33]. Merkus et al. [34] utilized methylene blue dye and nasal endoscopy to examine and compare four distinct head positions: upright, lying with the head tilted backward (Mygind), lying in a lateral position (Kaiteki), and head facing downward (vertex-to-floor, also known as Mecca). The researchers concluded that the vertex-to-floor orientation was the most effective in delivering spray doses to the upper nasal cavity and suggested it as the preferred one for intranasal spray administration targeting the olfactory cleft, particularly for individuals with nasal polyposis [34]. Likewise, when Cannady et al. [35] administered three dexamethasone drops intranasally to the vestibules of patients who had undergone endoscopic sinus surgery, they found that maintaining a vertex-to-floor head orientation resulted in effective delivery to the maxillary, ethmoid, and sphenoid sinuses, as well as the olfactory mucosa in a consistent manner. Furthermore, it was found that holding the vertex-to-floor head orientation for a 5 min duration resulted in higher levels of olfactory deposition compared to retaining the position for only 1 min, which suggests that the translocation of the liquid film can occur within the first 5 min following the application of the nasal drop [35]. In a study conducted by Milk et al. [33], they compared the delivery of intranasal drops to the olfactory region using two separate head positions: lying with the head tilted backward and vertex-to-floor. The study found that these two head positions resulted in similar levels of drug delivery to the olfactory mucosa [33]. Mori et al. [36] performed a study in which they evaluated the effectiveness of the Kaiteki orientation (which involves lying in a lateral position tilting the head and lifting the chin) for delivering intranasal sprays to the olfactory mucosa in healthy individuals. The results showed that the nasal spray was able to get to the olfactory cleft among 96% of decongested subjects and in 75% of those who did not receive treatment [36].

The above-mentioned studies utilized a variety of techniques to visualize the distribution and deposition patterns of sprays administered into the nasal cavity, which makes it challenging to compare them to one another [23]. Moreover, the evaluation of subregional doses in some of those studies was based on subjective evaluations by the researchers, which can make it difficult to compare results across different groups. This qualitative approach to assessing doses can create further confusion in interpreting the data [37]. Additionally, in order to establish a correlation between dose and therapeutic response for the treatment of olfactory impairment or neurological disorders, it is crucial to have accurate quantitative information about the dose delivered to the olfactory region. An alternative method to overcome these challenges involves utilizing transparent multipiece nasal cavity casts in studies pertaining to in vitro intranasal drug delivery, similar to the one used in this study. Such models provide clear and detailed views of the deposition patterns of administered nasal sprays. They allow for visualization of the distribution of nasal sprays throughout the different parts of the nasal cavity, as well as more accurate quantification of the deposition pattern of nasal sprays. Making use of such nasal cavity casts can allow researchers to assess the nasal spray distribution pattern throughout the nasal cavity with greater precision, better optimize nasal spray delivery, and evaluate the effectiveness of different drug formulations.

A good delivery protocol for olfactory (OL) delivery should (1) deliver clinically significant doses to the OL region, (2) have low variability in OL dosimetry, (3) minimize wastes in other regions, and (4) be easy to use. In our previous studies, it has been demonstrated that the dosimetry of nasal spray delivery was determined not only by the initial deposition of spray droplets but also by the subsequent liquid film translocation, which further depends on many factors such as gravity, fluid viscosity, wall angle, etc. [38]. With a transparent nasal cast and fluorescence, it now becomes feasible to visualize the dynamic process of the liquid formation and translocation under different delivery scenarios and thus identify the optimal delivery protocol to the target. Specific to the challenges that have precluded effective OL drug delivery, this visualization method allows a detailed examination of the spray liquid film migration toward the OL region in a fine spatiotemporal manner. It is thus promising to (1) evaluate the relative effects of individual delivery variables on the dynamic spray liquid film behavior and final OL dosimetry, and then (2) put together the acquired knowledge and recommend a new delivery method for improved OL delivery.

The objective of this study was to establish a technique using a soft-mist inhaler that can effectively administer medications to the olfactory mucosa for the treatment of neurological disorders and brain tumors. An anatomically accurate, transparent nasal cavity model was used to test the influence of a variety of delivery parameters, including the head position, nozzle angle, dose number, flow rate, and solution viscosity, on the spray deposition pattern and identify the optimum spray delivery method targeting the olfactory region. Specific aims include:

(1) Visualize the deposition distribution of intranasally administered sprays and subsequent liquid film translocation in the nasal cavity using different angles of administration, head positions, number of spray applications, and inhalation flow rates.
(2) Visualize the effect of formulation viscosity on the dosimetry of intranasal sprays.
(3) Quantify the deposition of intranasal sprays in the olfactory cleft, the turbinate region, the front nose, as well as the nasopharynx.
(4) Examine the results and compare the performance between the different test cases to determine the optimal combination of factors that lead to maximum bioavailability in the olfactory region (i.e., delivery of clinically significant doses).

2. Materials and Methods

2.1. Nasal Cast Model

The nasal airway model that had been reconstructed from MRI scans of a 53-year-old male was used for the in vitro deposition tests [39]. This nose model has been extensively used in previous studies for deposition experiments [39–45] and computational simulations [46–49]. Transparent hollow casts were fabricated with a Polyjet 3D printer (Stratasys, Inc., Rehovot, Israel) with a printing resolution of 30 μm and a Somos WaterShed XC 11122 stereolithography (SLA) material (Figure 1). To measure regional deposition, each cast was separated into four parts, i.e., the front nose (vestibule and valve), upper middle (superior meatus), middle lower (middle and inferior meatus), and back nose (caudal turbinate and nasopharynx). To secure a good seal, a stepped groove was created at all connecting ends in each part. The olfactory region was defined as the area that houses the olfactory nerves and enables nose-to-brain drug transport (Figure 1a). Two landmarks were used, with the nose apex defining the front and the second peak defining the back of the olfactory region (red line, Figure 1b). The area of the olfactory region was around 20% of the middle upper nose and 8.7% of the middle nose.

2.2. Study Design

To study the effects of the head position on OL delivery, the vertex-to-floor was first tested with four nozzle angles (0°, 5°, 10°, 15°) counterclockwise from the nostril normal. This position has been commonly assumed to be optimal for OL delivery based on the intuition that nasal sprays would settle down to the OL region, which is presumably the lowest point in the nasal cavity, by gravity. The spray solution was a water solution with 0.4% *w*/*v* methyl cellulose (MC). Two doses would be applied in the nose with no inhalation flow. A video camera operating at 30 frames per second was used to document the motion and deposition of the spray liquid film in each test. Both the deposition fraction (DF) and variability in the OL region were quantified.

Three other head positions were then tested: 60°, 45°, and 30° backward (BW) tilt from the supine position. Note that the vertex-to-floor position was equivalent to tilting 90° BW from supine, even though it was more often practiced by taking a praying position. Four nozzle angles (0°, 5°, 10°, 15°) were tested with a 60° BW tilt head position in order to narrow down the optimal delivery variables for the head position and nozzle angle through the comparison of liquid film transient behavior, OL dose/variability, and drug losses in other regions. Two nozzle angles (5°, 10°) were tested for the head positions of 45° and 30° BW tilt. Considering that the slope of the nasal roof became increasingly steeper from the vertex-to-floor to 30° BW tilt, it was hypothesized that a steeper slope would increase the liquid film flowability and OL delivery, but it would also increase the risk of liquid overflow from the OL region and thus the drug loss in the nasopharynx.

To study the inhalation flow effects on the spray liquid film behavior and fate, two flow rates, 10 and 20 L/min, were tested separately with the head tilted BW 45° and 60°. Considering that the increased flow shear could facilitate the liquid film motion, the OL DFs were quantified following a single-dose administration as well as a two-dose administration. This would help answer whether a combination of head position, nozzle angle, and flow shear is sufficient to effectively deliver nasal sprays to the OL region.

Considering that the solution viscosity could affect the liquid film translocation and thus OL delivery, four more spray solutions with different methyl cellulose (MC) concentrations (0.1%, 0.2%, 0.3%, and 0.5% *w*/*v*) were considered in addition to the baseline case (0.4% *w*/*v* MC). The solution viscosity of varying MC concentrations was measured using a digital rotational viscometer (Cgoldenwall, NDJ-5S, Hangzhou, China).

Considering that the liquid film translocation was sensitive to the nasal anatomy, differences in OL delivery between the right and left nasal passage were tested in the left nose with a head 60° position and two nozzle angles (5° and 10°). The nasal cast used in this study was created from MRI images of a 53-year-old male, and the two nasal passages had different morphologies [50]. The right–left discrepancy in transient liquid film behavior and eventual OL deposition would shed light on the OL DF variability due to geometry variations.

Considering the liquid evaporation effects, the following procedures were taken to estimate and minimize the evaporation effect on the olfactory dosimetry. Prior to the in vitro tests, the spray mass per application from the inhaler was quantified by weighing (1) the mass difference of the inhaler before and after the application, and (2) the mass of sprays collected in the in vitro cast model with no inhalation flow immediately after the application. In the second case, all administered sprays would be deposited in the cast model. We observed an insignificant difference (<1%) between these two cases. Considering that a longer time was needed for in-deposition tests with sectional cast models (i.e., model dissembling and part weighing), evaporation was more likely to happen. Immediately after each test, the model parts were promptly disassembled and weighed to minimize evaporation. In addition, evaporation occurred for all parts. Thus, its impact on the relative deposition (i.e., deposition fraction) presented hereof was expected to be insignificant.

2.3. *Inhaler and Spray Solutions*

A refillable soft-mist spray inhaler (Hengni) was used to atomize a spray solution with 0.4% *w*/*v* methyl cellulose (MC) concentration. The spray discharge from the inhaler and subsequent spray plume development in the open space were captured at a rate of 2000 frames per second with a Phantom VEO 1310 camera (Vision Research Inc., Wayne, NJ, USA).

2.4. *Protocol for Nasal Spray Delivery*

The experimental setup is shown in Figure 1c. Soldering clamps were used to fix the assembled nasal cast and soft mist inhaler to prescribed head positions and nozzle angles. The inhaler nozzle was inserted 1 cm into the right nostril. The nozzle angle was defined as counterclockwise from the nostril normal and was controlled using a protractor prior to spray administration, as illustrated in Figure 1c. Similarly, the head position was defined as a backward (BW) tilt from the supine position and was controlled using a protractor. When multiple doses were applied, a waiting period of 5 s was observed between the two spray applications. A vacuum (Robinair 3 CFM, Warren, MI, USA) was employed to generate the inhalation flow, and a flow meter (Omega, FL-510, Stamford, CT, USA) was utilized to regulate the flow rate.

In order to examine the transient liquid film translocation within the nasal cavity, a solution containing 0.5% fluorescent dye (GLO Effex, Murrieta, CA, USA) was used for visualization, which exhibited a bright green color when exposed to a 385–395 nm LED light. The entire process, from nasal administration to one minute after spray administration, was captured with a video camera at 30 frames per second.

To quantify the deposited doses in different regions of the nose (i.e., front, middle upper, middle lower, and back), the masses before and after each run were measured with an electronic scale with a range/resolution of 120 g/0.0001 g (Bonvoisin, San Jose, CA, USA). The deposition fraction (DF) was calculated as the percentage of the regional dose over the applied dose. To calculate the mean and variability, each test was conducted a minimum of three times.

2.5. Image-Based Estimation of Olfactory Dosimetry

There were challenges in quantifying the olfactory (OL) dose using the current mass-measuring method. When a continuous liquid film covered the olfactory region and its neighboring region, potential liquid film relocation during disassembly would make the dose measurement unreliable. As a result, an image-based method was applied in this study to estimate the OL dose. First, the projected area of the liquid-covered region (A1) in the middle upper nose was quantified on an image using a user-defined MATLAB code. The dose per unit liquid-covered area was calculated as the deposited dose in this region over A1. Similarly, the liquid-covered region (A2) in the OL region was also quantified. The OL dosimetry was then estimated as the product of A2 and dose per unit area in the liquid-covered region, i.e., A2 × (middle-upper-dose/A1). This method was based on an assumption of equal (or similar) dose per unit area in the liquid-covered region between the middle upper nose and olfactory region; this assumption appeared reasonable based on the deposition images, which are presented in later sections.

2.6. Statistical Analysis

Minitab (State College, PA, USA) was employed to perform statistical analyses of the deposition results (outputs) and determine the importance of different delivery variables (inputs). The deposition fraction variability was assessed using one-way analysis of variance (ANOVA). A mean and standard deviation were calculated for the deposition fractions.

3. Results

3.1. Characterization of Spray Viscosity and Aerosol Generation

Figure 2 presents the measured viscosity of nasal spray solutions with varying methyl cellulose (MC) concentrations (% *w*/*v*). The solution viscosity increased nonlinearly with increasing MC concentration. The viscosity was measured to be 1.9 mPa·s at an MC concentration of 0.1% *w*/*v*, 16.1 mPa·s at 0.4% *w*/*v*, and 31.8 mPa's at 0.5% *w*/*v*.

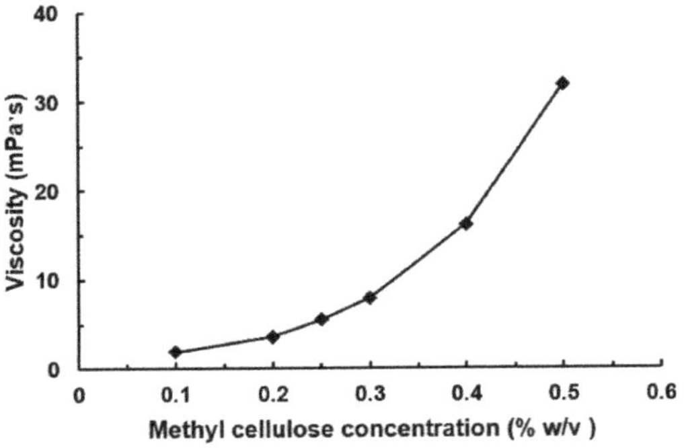

Figure 2. Measured viscosity of nasal spray solutions with varying methyl cellulose concentrations (% *w*/*v*).

Figure 3 shows the high-speed images (recorded at 2000 fps) of the spray aerosols from the soft mist inhaler during the first 300 ms after actuation. Two stages were observed: the forceful discharge of spray droplets during 0–30 ms, and the spray plume decay during the remaining 30–300 ms. At the very beginning of the actuation (2.2–4 ms), polydisperse spray droplets were generated, with liquid filaments immediately outside of the nozzle orifice (red arrow) and occasional large droplets further downstream (yellow arrow). Due to the resistance of the ambient air, a vortex ring was observed to form at the front of the soft mist at 2.8 ms (blue arrow), which moved forward at a slower pace (blue arrows, 2.8–10 ms) in comparison to the large droplets or even the soft mist as a whole (Figure 3a).

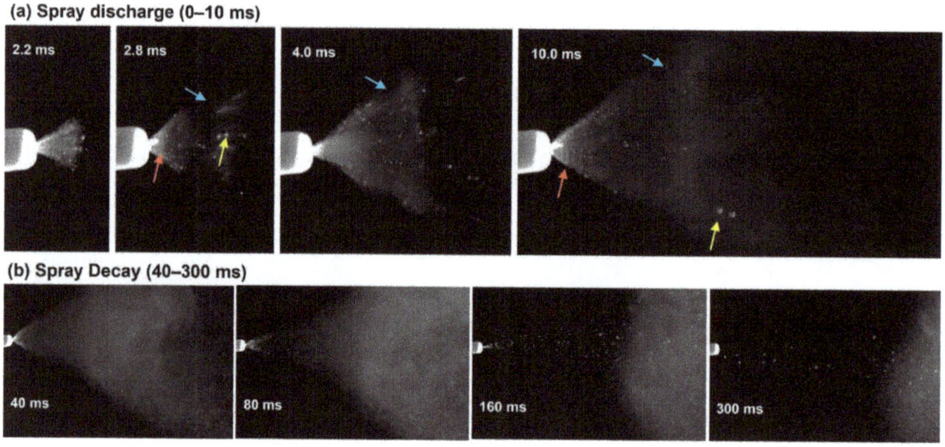

Figure 3. High-speed images of the spray droplets from the soft mist inhaler during the first 300 ms after actuation in two stages: (**a**) spray discharge (0–30 ms) and (**b**) spray plume decay (30–300 ms).

At the spray decay stage (40–300 ms), the spray plume angle decreased gradually, and the fraction of large spray droplets increased (Figure 3b), indicating decreasing actuation energy. From 160 ms, the actuation energy was no longer sufficient to generate a soft mist, leaving only large droplets being released. At 300 ms, even the generation of large droplets stopped.

3.2. *Vertex-To-Floor Head Position for Olfactory Delivery*

Figure 4 shows the spray dosimetry in a nasal cast with a vertex-to-floor head position with four nozzle angles (i.e., 0°, 5°, 10°, 15° relative to the nostril's normal direction). It was observed that one dose only was not enough to dispense drugs to the OL region, with nearly all sprays stuck in the top front nose (first row, Figure 4a). This might result from the narrow passages of this region, as well as the high liquid viscosity (cohesive inter-molecular force), wall adhesion (liquid–wall), and surface tension (liquid–air). The nasal vestibule and valve were very confined spaces. Due to the high inertia of discharged spray droplets, they were deposited on the lateral walls (white arrow) and roof of the top front nose (yellow arrow), particularly those of the nasal valve. The deposited droplets coalesced into a focused continuous liquid film, which, with collective gravity and interfacial forces, could behave differently from those of individual droplets. Once stability was reached, the gravity and inertia of the liquid film were insufficient to break this stability and mobilize the liquid film.

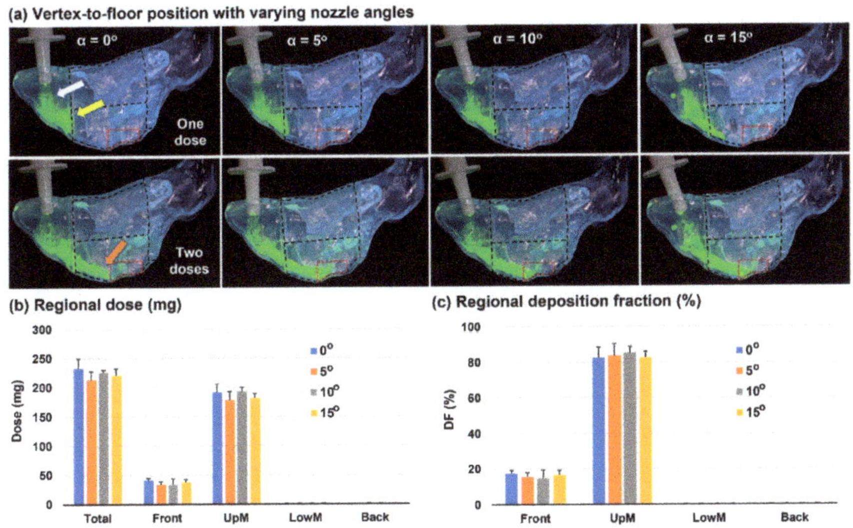

Figure 4. Nozzle angle effects on the nasal spray dosimetry in a nasal cast with a vertex-to-floor head position: (**a**) fluorescent visualization of the spray distributions after one and two actuations using different nozzle angles (α: 0–15°); (**b**) quantification of total and regional deposition after two doses; and (**c**) deposition fractions (DF) in four nasal regions using different nozzle angles (α: 0–15°). UpM: middle upper; LowM: middle lower.

The second row of Figure 4a shows the spray distribution one minute after applying the second dose. The added mass destabilized and mobilized the liquid film. Once the film translocation started, its own inertia would keep it moving forward till the stabilizing forces slowed it down, and a new force equilibrium was reached. It was noted that a dynamic shear was often smaller than its static counterpart. As the liquid film expanded further, its thickness decreased, and the added mass effect dwindled until the liquid stopped moving (brown arrow). It was further noted that the gravity effect depended on the local incline angle. As illustrated in Figure 4a, at a vertex-to-floor position, the superior meatus acted as an inclined furrow, which became progressively flatter from the nasal valve to the nasal crest. After the crest, the furrow reverted to an upward angle so that gravity would slow down the film motion and stabilize it to the furrow valley (nasal crest herein).

A quantitative comparison of total and regional deposition among different nozzle angles is shown in Figure 4b. Overall, similar doses were delivered to the front nose and the middle upper nose (UpM). Nearly no dose was deposited in the middle lower nose (LowM) and back nose. Figure 4c shows the normalized deposition by the total dose (i.e., deposition fraction, DF). In this case, about 82.6–85.2% of the applied dose reached the middle upper nose. Only a small fraction reached the olfactory region, which was quantified, as will be shown later, using an image-based method.

3.3. *Head Position: 60° Backward Tilt from the Supine Position*

3.3.1. Deposition Distribution

To improve OL delivery, the head position was adjusted to be 60° backward tilt from the supine position (referred to as 60° BW tilt hereafter). At this position, the roof of the front nose had a larger incline angle and, thus, a larger gravitational effect. As expected, the liquid film after the first dose moved slightly further downward than the corresponding vertex-to-floor position (Figure 5a vs. Figure 4a, first row). Furthermore, the liquid film after the second dose reached the posterior OL region (brown arrow) and, therefore, improved the delivery to the OL region more than the vertex-to-floor head position, given all other factors the same (Figure 5a vs. Figure 4a, second row).

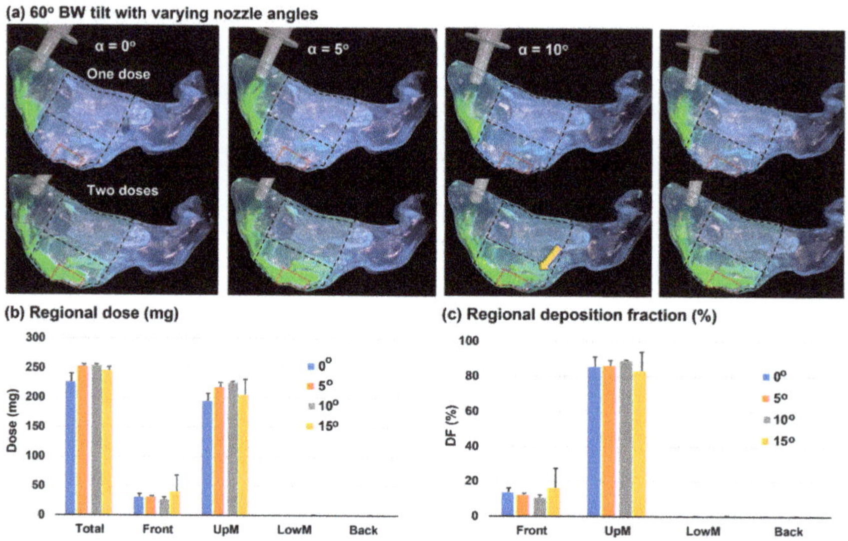

Figure 5. Nozzle angle effects on the nasal spray dosimetry in a nasal cast with a head position tilted backward 60° from the supine position (i.e., 60° BW tilt): (**a**) spray distribution after one and two actuations for nozzle angles α of 0–15°; (**b**) quantified depositions after applying two doses; and (**c**) deposition fractions (DF) in four nasal regions for nozzle angles α: 0–15°. UpM: middle upper; LowM: middle lower.

Similar to the vertex-to-floor position, nearly no deposition was observed in the middle lower nose or the back nose (Figure 5b,c). A slightly higher percentage of applied dose reached the middle upper nose (i.e., UpM DF: 83.3–88.8%) than the vertex-to-floor position (Figure 5c vs. Figure 4c). For the nozzle angle of 5–10°, the 60° BW tilt head position led to much lower variability in the UpM DF than the vertex-to-floor position, as evident by the lower standard deviation of 0.7–3.0% in Figure 5c vs. 3.5–6.7% in Figure 4c.

The liquid film coverage appeared to be sensitive to the nozzle angle when adopting a 60° BW tilt head position. From Figure 5a, there was more coverage of the olfactory region at the nozzle angle of 5–15° than at 0°. The nozzle angle affected the initial deposition position and perhaps the initial liquid film inertia as well. The spray plume traveled longer in the nose before deposition when discharged from a more inclined nozzle, which might increase the liquid film flowability and allow it to move further (Figure 5a).

3.3.2. Dynamic Formation and Translocation of Liquid Film

To better understand the dynamic process of the formation and translocation of liquid film, a time series of spray deposition snapshots are plotted in Figure 6a,b at varying instants after applying the first and second dose, respectively. The head position was 60° BW tilt, the nozzle angle was 10°, and the images were acquired at 30 fps. During the first 0–67 ms, the high-speed spray impinged on the two lateral walls and roof of the front nose (yellow arrows, Figure 6a). A liquid film formed on the inclined wall of the front nose roof upon contact (0 ms, Figure 6a). With continuous sprays from 33 ms to 67 ms, the liquid film grew in size and started to move downward along the inclined wall due to the self-weight and the impaction inertia. A large, rounded liquid front formed because of the liquid–wall adhesion and liquid–air surface tension. From 133 ms, when the spray discharge was completed, the liquid front continued to move along the inclined wall, but at a much slower speed. After the completion of the spray discharge at 100 ms, the liquid front continued to advance along the inclined wall, albeit at a significantly reduced pace (Figure 6a, 0.133–3.5 s). Only a short distance (less than 1 cm) was traveled within the next

4 to 5 s, reflecting an equilibrium state between the destabilizing gravitational force and the resistant forces such as wall adhesion, viscosity, and surface tension.

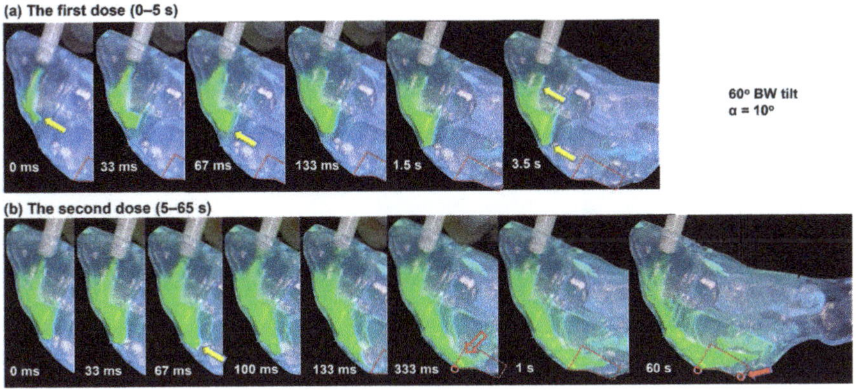

Figure 6. Snapshots of the dynamic liquid translocation in the nasal cast with a 60° BW tilt head position from supine and a nozzle angle of 10° from the nostril normal (**a**) after the first dose (0–4 s), and (**b**) after the second dose (0–60 s, or 4–64 s if counted from the first dose).

The dynamic progression of the liquid film after the second dose is displayed in Figure 6b within one minute. Around 125 mg of the spray formulation was added to the existing liquid film between 0 and 100 ms (yellow arrow). The added mass and kinetic energy mobilized the otherwise static liquid film, which was observed to move at an increasing speed from 100 to 333 ms, followed by a deceleration. At 333 ms after the second dose (hollow red arrow, Figure 6b), the liquid film reached the nasal crest, which was also one of the two landmarks defining the olfactory region. After 60 s, the liquid film crawled beyond the second landmark (solid red arrow, Figure 6b) and covered the entire OL region.

3.4. Head Positions of 45° and 30° Backward Tilt from the Supine Position

Further tests were conducted with the head position being adjusted to 45° and 30° BW tilt from the supine position, as shown in Figure 7a. Both had a nozzle angle of 10° and an inhalation flow rate of 0 L/min. For all 45° BW tilt cases, the liquid film went beyond the second landmark of the OL region. This improved liquid flowability was presumably because of a steeper inclined wall than the 60° BW tilt cases. The flowability difference was particularly apparent in the liquid film morphology and translation distance after the first dose, with a tapered shape about 2 cm beyond the nasal valve for 45° BW tilt versus a rounded shape that barely went beyond the nasal valve (Figure 7a vs. Figure 6a).

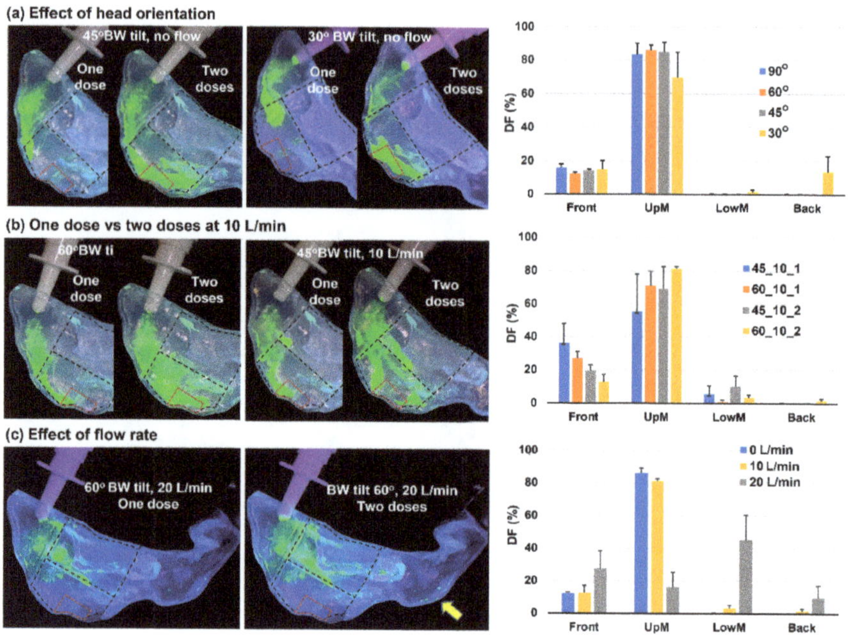

Figure 7. Effects of delivery variables (head orientation, dose number, and inhalation flow rate) on the regional spray dosimetry: (**a**) head orientation of 45° and 30° BW tilt from the supine position (no flow); (**b**) effect of 10 L/min inhalation flow rate and dose number; (**c**) spray dosimetry at 20 L/min. Here, 45_10_1: head orientation of 45°, inhalation rate of 10 L/min, and 1 dose; 45_10_2: head orientation of 45°, inhalation rate of 10 L/min, and 2 doses; similarly for 60_10_1 and 60_10_2.

Significant differences were observed in the spray distribution between 30° and 45° BW tilt head positions (second panel vs. first panel in Figure 7a). Because of a steeper slope at a 30° tilt head position, the gravitational component after the first dose became stronger than the wall adhesion force, causing the liquid to move straight down along the side walls instead of adhering to the nasal roof like in all other cases considered earlier (second panel, Figure 7a). After applying the second dose, the steeper slope also led to lower retention in the front nose and a perceivable deposition in the back nose (second and third panels, Figure 7a).

3.5. *Effect of Inhalation Flow Rate*

The effect of inhalation flow rate on spray deposition was tested by considering 10 and 20 L/min. At 10 L/min (Figure 7b), the liquid film after the first dose traveled a greater distance because of the increased flow shear, which disrupted and mobilized the otherwise stagnant liquid film when there was no flow. A notable difference in deposition pattern was observed following the second dose administered at 10 L/min, with the sprays effectively covering most of the middle upper nose, as opposed to the coverage of the nasal roof solely with no flow. A quantitative comparison of the regional DF following one dose and two doses administrated at 10 L/min is shown in the rightmost panel of Figure 7b. As expected, the front nose retention rate following one dose was much higher than that following two doses for both head positions (45° and 60° BW tilt) considered. As a result, lower DFs in the middle upper nose were obtained following one dose than two doses. Spray deposition in the middle lower nose was observed following both one dose and two doses administrated at 10 L/min with a head position of 45° BW tilt (Figure 7b, middle and right panels). Its steeper slope of the nasal roof wall and the flow shear diverted a fraction of sprays to the middle lower passage. This was in contrast to the 60 BW tilt head position at 10 L/min, where no or negligible sprays were deposited in the middle lower passage following one dose and two doses. Therefore, spray deposition was more sensitive to the head position with a non-zero flow rate. Likewise, the DF variability at 10 L/min was much higher than without a flow (Figure 7b vs. Figure 5c).

Figure 7c shows the spray dosimetry at 20 L/min. The high flow through the middle meatus transported the majority of the sprays to the middle lower nose, and only a small fraction to the middle upper nose. There was even a small amount of spray droplets deposited in the nasopharynx (yellow arrow, Figure 7c). Furthermore, a much higher degree of variability in dosimetry was observed at 20 L/min compared to 0 and 10 L/min, as evident by the quantitative dosimetry comparison in Figure 7c (right panel).

3.6. Effects of Solution Viscosity

Figure 8 shows the effects of solution viscosity on spray dosimetry by varying the methyl cellulose (MC) concentration (0.1–0.5% w/v) in the solution. The correlation between the solution viscosity and the methyl cellulose concentration is shown in Figure 2. Following a single-dose application, the liquid film of a lower MC concentration traveled a greater distance along the nasal roof (solid yellow arrows, upper panel of Figure 8a). The remnant liquid films on the vestibular side walls appeared much thinner for 0.1% and 0.2% solutions than for the 0.5% solution (hollow red arrows, upper panel of Figure 8a).

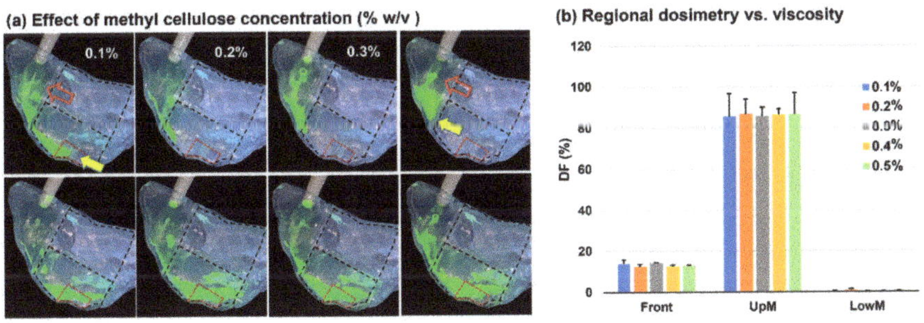

Figure 8. Effects of solution viscosity on the regional spray dosimetry with varying methyl cellulose concentrations (% w/v): (**a**) spray deposition distributions; (**b**) regional dosimetry vs. viscosity.

The spray dosimetries following the second dose of 0.1–0.5% w/v MC concentrations are visualized in the lower panel of Figure 8a and quantified in Figure 8b. Surprisingly, the two-dose DFs appeared to be insensitive to the solution MC concentration, with insignificant differences in both the front nose and middle-upper nose among the five solutions (Figure 8b). All liquid films reached or went beyond the posterior OL region, indicating a good coverage of the OL mucosa. Considering the 0.5% solution, its viscosity nearly doubled that of the 0.4% solution (16.1 vs. 31.8 mPa·s, Figure 2). However, the added mass from the second dose successfully mobilized the liquid dam accumulated in the front nose, which subsequently entered the superior meatus and ultimately reached the olfactory region.

3.7. Left-Right Discrepancy in Dosimetry

A comparison of the spray dosimetry between the left and right nasal passages with a 60° BW tilt head position is shown in Figure 9 for a nozzle angle of 10° at two flow rates (0 and 20 L/min). The solution utilized had an MC concentration of 0.4% w/v. Overall, given all other variables being the same, the two passageways yielded comparable deposition distributions (Figure 9a,b) and regional DFs (Figure 9c,d). Note that the nasal cast model was developed from patient-specific MRI scans, and the two passages had different morphologies. At 0 L/min, the liquid film in the left passage, much like that in the right passage, extended over the olfactory region after two doses (Figure 9a). Distinct deposition patterns were observed at 20 L/min. The right passage had predominant coverage in the middle lower nose, while the left passage exhibited more coverage in the middle upper nose (Figure 9b).

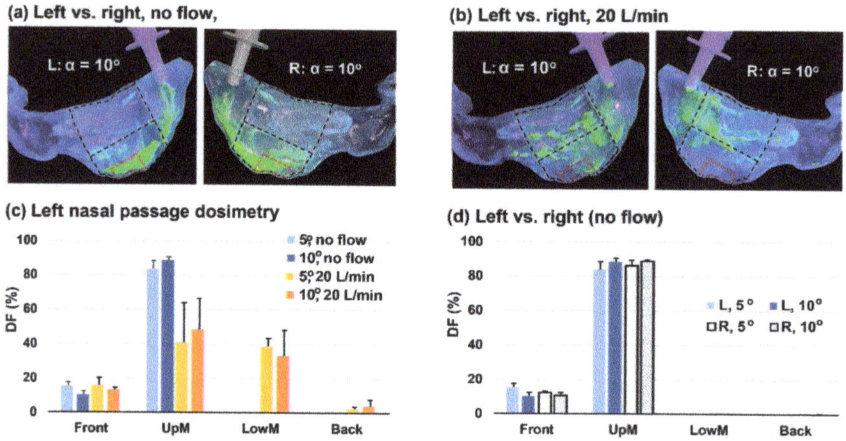

Figure 9. Comparison of nasal spray deposition between the left and right nasal passages: (**a**) surface deposition at the nozzle angle of 10° with no flow; (**b**) surface deposition at the nozzle angle of 10° at an inhalation flow rate of 20 L/min; (**c**) quantified regional dosimetry in the left passage at 0 and 20 L/min with nozzle angles of 5° and 10°; (**d**) comparison of dosimetry between the left and right nasal passages at 0 L/min.

3.8. Image-Based Olfactory Dosimetry Estimation

The deposition fraction (DF) in the olfactory region was calculated as (A2/A1) times the DF in the middle upper nose, where A2 and A1 were the liquid-covered area in the OL region and middle-upper nose, respectively (Figure 10a). Figure 10b compares the OL DFs and standard deviations vs. the head position, nozzle angle, dose number, flow rate, MC concentration, and passage geometry.

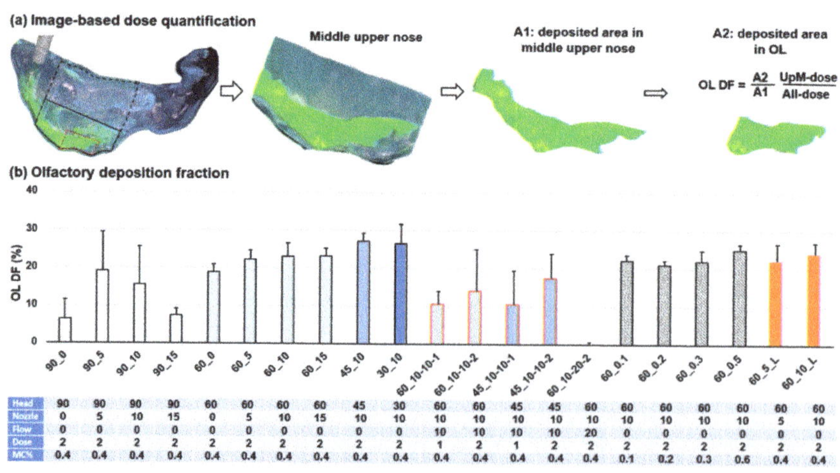

Figure 10. Image-based dosimetry: (**a**) estimation diagram and (**b**) olfactory deposition fraction.

It was observed that the vertex-to-floor (90°) head position failed to yield the optimal OL DF and, at the same time, had a large variability in OL DF (the first four bars, Figure 10b). By contrast, the head position of 60° and 45° gave satisfactory OL DFs except for the nozzle angle of 0° (60°: four light blue bars and 45°: one blue bar in Figure 10b). Their standard deviations were also lower. Thus, a head position ranging 45–60° and a nozzle angle ranging 5–10° (with two-dose application and no inhalation flow) were proposed for effective delivery of nasal spray to the OL region. The head position of 30° also had the potential to dispense high doses to the OL region (deep blue bar, Figure 10b); however, it was not recommended because of its relatively high variability in OL DF and high DF in other regions, as previously explained in Figure 7a.

A lower magnitude and higher variability in the OL DF were observed for the inhalation flow rate of 10 L/min and 20 L/min, and for single-dose applications (red boundary bars). With two-dose applications, the OL DF and variability did not exhibit high sensitivity to the solution viscosity ranging 1.9–32 mPa·s, nor to the left or right nasal passage in this study (rightmost six bars, Figure 10b). After putting everything together, it was suggested that for optimal delivery of nasal spray to the OL region, a head position between 45° and 60° BW tilt from supine and a nozzle angle between 5° and 10° normal to the nostril angle should be used, along with a two-dose application and no inhalation flow.

3.9. Deposition Sensitivity Analysis to Delivery Variables

Figure 11a shows the box plots of the nasal spray dosimetry variability among five regions based on the recommended delivery variables. Based on the nasal model used in this study, a DF of 22.7 ± 3.7% was achieved in the strictly defined OL region that was bounded by two landmarks, as illustrated in Figure 1a. It is worth noting that in previous studies, the OL region had been defined to cover varying extents of the top nose, and the defined OL area/location could significantly affect the OL dose estimation. Further examination of Figure 11a revealed that the two worst outliers (black arrows) came from one single test case, which had a 60° tilt head position and a nozzle angle of 15°. This was consistent with the abnormally large DF variability in Figure 5c for the front nose and middle-upper nose.

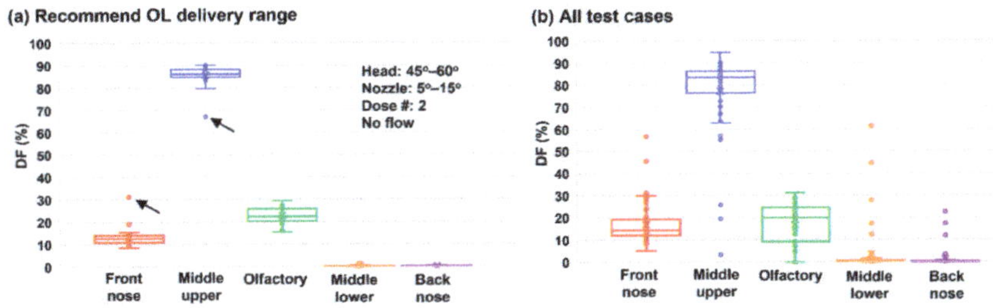

Figure 11. Box plots: (**a**) middle-upper nose coverage variability (overall, vs. head orientation, and vs. nozzle degree), and (**b**) comparison of deposition variability among five regions.

The DF variability based on all test cases is shown in Figure 11b. As expected, a much higher variability and more outliers were observed for the DF in all five regions. Individual checks of these outliers showed that they mainly came from test cases with 20 L/min or single-dose administration, suggesting that these two categories should be excluded.

Sensitivity analyses of the regional DF to individual delivery variables are presented in Figure 12a–e for the dose number, flow rate, head position, nozzle angle, and MC concentration, respectively. The front nose DF was noted to be highly sensitive to the number of doses applied and the inhalation flow rate, both of which exhibited large variations in the mean value and box size (first column, Figure 12). By comparison, the front nose DF was relatively insensitive to the nozzle angle (0–15°) and solution viscosity (1.9–32 mPa·s). Considering the middle-upper nose DF (second column, Figure 12), the highest variability occurred when the flow rate varied, while the lowest variability occurred with varying nozzle angle and solution viscosity.

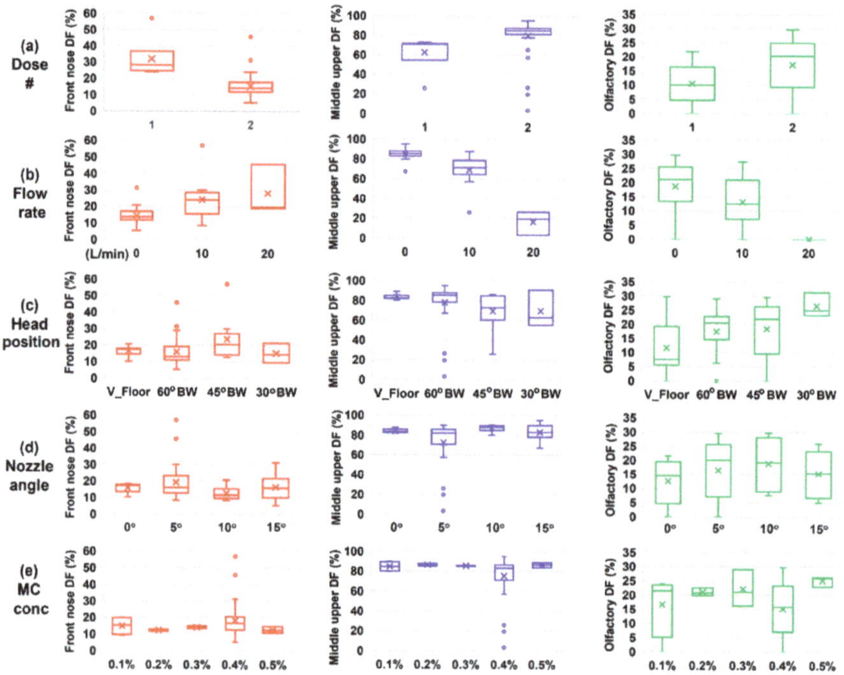

Figure 12. Box plots of the regional deposition fractions from sixty test cases in response to varying delivery variables: (**a**) the number of applied doses, (**b**) inhalation flow rate, (**c**) head orientation, (**d**) nozzle angle, and (**e**) spray solution viscosity by varying methyl cellulose concentrations. Regions of interest: front nose, middle-upper nose, and olfactory region.

The third column of Figure 12 shows the OL DF sensitivity analysis to input variables. Its y-coordinate range was 0–35% in contrast to 0–60% in the first column and 0–100% in the second column. It was clear that a two-dose application could significantly improve OL DF over a single-dose application (Figure 12a). Furthermore, the presence of an inhalation flow reduced the OL DF, and a flow rate of 20 L/min could completely preclude dispensing nasal sprays to the OL region (by diverting to the middle meatus), as shown in Figure 12b. No, or very slow, flow was expected to attain the optimal OL delivery, where the gravity-driven liquid film translocation along inclined walls was the major mechanism for delivering drugs to the OL region. In Figure 12c, the vertex-to-floor (V_Floor) head position was shown to deliver significantly lower doses to the OL region than the other three head positions and, thus, should not be used for future OL delivery. In Figure 12d, the nozzle angle of 5° and 10° overall performed better than 0° and 15° in OL delivery. Again, the OL DF in this study did not exhibit significant sensitivity to the viscosity of the solution (Figure 12e), given that two doses were applied, which triggered and facilitated the liquid film translocation.

4. Discussion

One major difference between nasal sprays and nebulizers is the large size and high speed of the spray droplets, which, upon deposition in the front nose, will form a liquid film and cause dripping [51]. Using a transparent nasal cast and fluorescent imaging allows a detailed examination of the film's dynamic behavior that had been previously veiled due to 3D printing materials. The real-time feedback on the input variables, in turn, enables prompt adjustments to individual delivery parameters. This interactive manner can notably expedite the design process for continuous improvement to reach an optimal delivery protocol. Similar delivery systems as in this study are promising as a test platform for other nasal spray applications such as para-sinus drug delivery and for studying the complex interactions among the patient-, device-, and administration-related variables.

Different levels of sensitivity to delivery variables were observed for the dynamic liquid film translocation and final olfactory deposition. Applying two doses from a soft-mist inhaler (~125 mg per dose) was needed to destabilize the accumulated liquid film in the front nose and mobilize the fluid along the inclined nasal roof toward the olfactory region. However, applying more than two doses would over-flood the olfactory and cause waste in the nasopharynx. The inhalation flow was observed to decrease the liquid film translocation to the OL region, which diverted a portion of the fluid to the middle meatus. At 20 L/min, almost no fluid reached the OL region. Considering the head position, our results showed that vertex-to-floor was not the best position for OL delivery, giving lower OL deposition and higher variability than the head position of 45–60° tilted backward from the supine position. Considering the nozzle angle, a range of 5–10° gave rise to higher OL deposition and lower variability than 0° and 15°. As a result, the following parameters were proposed to effectively deliver nasal sprays to the OL region: a head position tilting 45–60° backward from the supine position, a nozzle angle ranging 5–10° counterclockwise from the nostril normal, two doses, and no inhalation flow. In practice, the patient should breathe slowly during the spray application and hold their head position for at least 60 s to allow the liquid film to translocate to the OL region.

The results of this study demonstrated that delivering clinically significant doses to the olfactory (OL) region is feasible by leveraging the liquid film translocation after nasal spray administration. With recommended delivery parameters, a delivery efficiency of 22.7 ± 3.7% was achieved in the strictly defined OL region. Note that the OL area hereof was around 20% of the middle upper nose and 8.7% of the middle nose. Different definitions of the olfactory region have been used in previous studies. While the general consensus is that the olfactory mucosa is situated at the top of the nose, there is no agreement on the precise location and extent where drug molecules can enter the brain. The absence of agreement makes it challenging to compare findings among various studies. Various areas have been reported for the olfactory region, which ranged from 5.0–6.8 cm^2 [39,52], 10 cm^2 [53], and 35 cm^2 [47]. Similarly, the location and extent of the olfactory region have been defined differently. Si et al. [54] and Shi et al. [55] defined a crescent-shaped olfactory region at the apex of the nose. Schroeter et al. [47] defined an olfactory region with a similar area but different locations, which was slightly posterior to the nasal apex and was similar to the definition in this study. An OL delivery efficiency of 5% was reported using 10.3 μm particles. On the other hand, gamma scintigraphy studies commonly regarded the superior meatus as synonymous with the olfactory zone [56–59]. Using a nasal cast composed of three parts (lower, middle, and top) and a nasal pump, Wang et al. [32] measured a remarkable delivery efficiency of 73.5% to the top part, which had been described as the olfactory zone. This high percentage, however, was close to the spray deposition fraction of 80% in the middle upper nose in this study. More recently, Si et al. [12] numerically studied the liquid film translocation in the nose and predicted a 6.2% delivery efficiency to the olfactory region with the same definition as in this study. However, the liquid film translocation path in [12], which was linear from the vestibule to OL, was different from this study (along the nasal crest). A standard definition of the location and scope of the olfactory region is necessary for nose-to-brain drug delivery and especially for the performance evaluation of nasal devices targeting the olfactory region.

In this study, we observed that two doses were sufficient to mobilize the liquid films of all methyl cellulose (MC) concentrations (0.1–0.5% w/v) considered with appropriate head and device orientations. Theoretically, the added mass to mobilize the liquid film formed from the first dose would vary for formulations of different MC concentrations (or viscosities). In this study, the formulation viscosity ranged 1.9–31.8 mPa·s (Figure 2), which covered most nasal spray formulations. It was thus expected that two doses would be sufficient for olfactory delivery for most nasal sprays in practice. We have not quantified the exact mass needed to mobilize the first-dose film because the soft-mist inhaler could only release a specific mass (~125 mg) per dose. To this aim, a device that can release a small mass is needed by progressively adding incremental masses till the liquid film starts to move. This aim, however, was out of the scope of this study.

The limitations of this study include a single airway, 3D-printed rigid nasal casts, and a limited number of test cases. Both the initial deposition and subsequent liquid film translocation were sensitive to the geometrical details of the nasal cavity. Thus, inter-subject variability is expected. In this study, the geometrical effects were evaluated by comparing the liquid film translocation and OL delivery between the right and left nasal passages of the nasal cast. It was observed that despite the large differences in the transient behaviors of the liquid film motion, the final dosimetry (and even variability) in the OL region were similar between the two passages. Future studies are needed in a sufficiently large cohort of nasal models that are representative of the targeted patient group, such as age, gender, race, and health condition. Not all factors were explicitly investigated, such as fluid density and surface tension, despite these two factors varying with MC concentrations. Another interesting question that needs further investigation is the liquid film stability on an inclined wall of different materials. The liquid film behavior on the nasal epithelium will differ from that of the 3D printing SLA material because of their differences in surface energy, roughness, and interactions with the fluid [60]. This question was partially answered in this study by considering the spray solutions of varying methyl cellulose (MC) concentrations (0.1–0.5% w/v). It was demonstrated that with a sufficiently steep slope (45–60° head position) and two-dose application (i.e., large enough weight to trigger the film motion), the MC concentration had an insignificant effect on the final OL dosimetry (Figure 8b). However, we also observed different shapes and motion speeds of the liquid film among different solutions after applying both the first and second doses. Future studies of the fluid and cast material effects on transient fluid translocation and OL deposition in different nasal airway models were needed. The soft-mist inhaler used in this study generated polydisperse droplets with a wide size distribution (Figure 3). Thus, deposition images with monodisperse aerosols were not available. We refer interested readers to a study by Perkins et al. [61], who computationally studied nasal deposition with different monodisperse aerosol sizes.

5. Conclusions

In summary, an in vitro system for nasal spray delivery was developed using sectional, transparent nasal casts and fluorescent imaging. A systemic study of the delivery parameters was conducted for effective olfactory (OL) delivery, which included head position, nozzle angle, dose number, inhalation flow rate, and spray solution viscosity. The transient liquid film translocation, the final deposition in the olfactory region, the deposition variability, and the input sensitivity were examined. Specific findings are:

(1) The OL dosimetry depended not only on the initial deposition of spray droplets but also on the liquid film translocation.
(2) A two-dose application from the soft-mist inhaler was needed to mobilize the liquid film and enable it to move to the olfactory region.
(3) Recommended OL delivery parameters included: a head position tilting 45–60° backward from the supine position, a nozzle angle ranging 5–10° counterclockwise from the nostril normal, two doses, and no inhalation flow.
(4) With the recommended protocol, a delivery efficiency of 22.7 ± 3.7% was achieved in the strictly defined OL region.
(5) The presence of inhalation flow reduced the liquid film translocation to the OL region, with negligible OL doses at 20 L/min.
(6) The vertex-to-floor head position was not optimal for OL delivery, with lower OL delivery efficiency and higher variability.

Author Contributions: Conceptualization, A.S., X.A.S. and J.X.; methodology, A.S., X.A.S. and J.X.; validation, A.S., X.A.S. and J.X.; formal analysis, A.S., X.A.S. and J.X.; investigation, A.S. and J.X.; resources, X.A.S. and J.X.; data curation, J.X.; writing—original draft preparation, J.X.; writing—review and editing, A.S., X.A.S. and J.X. All authors have read and agreed to the published version of the manuscript.

Funding: This research received no external funding.

Institutional Review Board Statement: Not applicable.

Informed Consent Statement: Not applicable.

Data Availability Statement: The data presented in this study are available on request from the corresponding author.

Acknowledgments: Jacob Stover is gratefully acknowledged for reviewing this manuscript.

Conflicts of Interest: The authors declare no conflict of interest.

References

1. Badhan, R.K.; Kaur, M.; Lungare, S.; Obuobi, S. Improving brain drug targeting through exploitation of the nose-to-brain route: A physiological and pharmacokinetic perspective. *Curr. Drug Deliv.* **2014**, *11*, 458–471. [CrossRef] [PubMed]
2. Frey, W.H.; Liu, J.; Chen, X.; Thorne, R.G.; Fawcett, J.R.; Ala, T.A.; Rahman, Y.-E. Delivery of 125I-NGF to the Brain via the Olfactory Route. *Drug Deliv.* **1997**, *4*, 87–92. [CrossRef]
3. Jin, K.; Xie, L.; Childs, J.; Sun, Y.; Mao, X.O.; Logvinova, A.; Greenberg, D.A. Cerebral neurogenesis is induced by intranasal administration of growth factors. *Ann. Neurol.* **2003**, *53*, 405–409. [CrossRef] [PubMed]
4. Pardeshi, C.V.; Belgamwar, V.S. Direct nose to brain drug delivery via integrated nerve pathways bypassing the blood-brain barrier: An excellent platform for brain targeting. *Expert. Opin. Drug Deliv.* **2013**, *10*, 957–972. [CrossRef]
5. Born, J.; Lange, T.; Kern, W.; McGregor, G.P.; Bickel, U.; Fehm, H.L. Sniffing neuropeptides: A transnasal approach to the human brain. *Nat. Neurosci.* **2002**, *5*, 514–516. [CrossRef] [PubMed]
6. Xi, J.; Yuan, J.E.; Zhang, Y.; Nevorski, D.; Wang, Z.; Zhou, Y. Visualization and Quantification of Nasal and Olfactory Deposition in a Sectional Adult Nasal Airway Cast. *Pharm. Res.* **2016**, *33*, 1527–1541. [CrossRef] [PubMed]
7. Hanson, L.R.; Frey, W.H., 2nd. Strategies for intranasal delivery of therapeutics for the prevention and treatment of neuroAIDS. *J. Neuroimmune Pharmacol.* **2007**, *2*, 81–86. [CrossRef]
8. Illum, L. Is nose-to-brain transport of drugs in man a reality? *J. Pharm. Pharmacol.* **2004**, *56*, 3–17. [CrossRef]
9. Misra, A.; Kher, G. Drug delivery systems from nose to brain. *Curr. Pharm. Biotechnol.* **2012**, *13*, 2355–2379. [CrossRef]
10. Xi, J.; Lei, L.R.; Zouzas, W.; April Si, X. Nasally inhaled therapeutics and vaccination for COVID-19: Developments and challenges. *MedComm (2020)* **2021**, *2*, 569–586. [CrossRef]
11. Xi, J.; Longest, P.W. Characterization of submicrometer aerosol deposition in extrathoracic airways during nasal exhalation. *Aerosol Sci. Technol.* **2009**, *43*, 808–827. [CrossRef]
12. Si, X.A.; Sami, M.; Xi, J. Liquid Film Translocation Significantly Enhances Nasal Spray Delivery to Olfactory Region: A Numerical Simulation Study. *Pharmaceutics* **2021**, *13*, 903. [CrossRef]
13. Garcia, G.J.; Schroeter, J.D.; Kimbell, J.S. Olfactory deposition of inhaled nanoparticles in humans. *Inhal. Toxicol.* **2015**, *27*, 394–403. [CrossRef]
14. González-Botas, J.H.; Seara, A.P. Nasal gel and olfactory cleft. *Acta Otorrinolaringol. Esp.* **2012**, *63*, 370–375. [CrossRef] [PubMed]
15. Illum, L. Nasal drug delivery: New developments and strategies. *Drug Discov. Today* **2002**, *7*, 1184–1189. [CrossRef] [PubMed]
16. Basu, S. Computational characterization of inhaled droplet transport to the nasopharynx. *Sci. Rep.* **2021**, *11*, 6652. [CrossRef] [PubMed]
17. Basu, S.; Akash, M.M.H.; Lao, Y.; Balivada, P.A.; Ato, P.; Ka, N.K.; Mituniewicz, A.; Silfen, Z.; Suman, J.; Chakravarty, A.; et al. A model-based approach to improve intranasal sprays for respiratory viral infections. *medRxiv* **2022**. [CrossRef]
18. Basu, S.; Holbrook, L.T.; Kudlaty, K.; Fasanmade, O.; Wu, J.; Burke, A.; Langworthy, B.W.; Farzal, Z.; Mamdani, M.; Bennett, W.D.; et al. Numerical evaluation of spray position for improved nasal drug delivery. *Sci. Rep.* **2020**, *10*, 10568. [CrossRef]
19. Valentine, R.; Athanasiadis, T.; Thwin, M.; Singhal, D.; Weitzel, E.K.; Wormald, P.J. A prospective controlled trial of pulsed nasal nebulizer in maximally dissected cadavers. *Am. J. Rhinol.* **2008**, *22*, 390–394. [CrossRef]
20. Djupesland, P.G.; Skretting, A.; Winderen, M.; Holand, T. Breath actuated device improves delivery to target sites beyond the nasal valve. *Laryngoscope* **2006**, *116*, 466–472. [CrossRef]
21. Möller, W.; Schuschnig, U.; Celik, G.; Münzing, W.; Bartenstein, P.; Häussinger, K.; Kreyling, W.G.; Knoch, M.; Canis, M.; Becker, S. Topical drug delivery in chronic rhinosinusitis patients before and after sinus surgery using pulsating aerosols. *PLoS ONE* **2013**, *8*, e74991. [CrossRef] [PubMed]
22. Washington, N.; McGlashan, J.A.; Jackson, S.J.; Bush, D.; Pitt, K.G.; Rawlins, D.A.; Gill, D.A. The effect of nasal patency on the clearance of radiolabeled saline in healthy volunteers. *Pharm. Res.* **2000**, *17*, 733–736. [CrossRef] [PubMed]

23. Guo, Y.; Laube, B.; Dalby, R. The Effect of Formulation Variables and Breathing Patterns on the Site of Nasal Deposition in an Anatomically Correct Model. *Pharm. Res.* **2005**, *22*, 1871–1878. [CrossRef] [PubMed]
24. Laube, B.L.; Sharpless, G.; Shermer, C.; Nasir, O.; Sullivan, V.; Powell, K. Deposition of albuterol aerosol generated by pneumatic nebulizer in the Sophia Anatomical Infant Nose-Throat (SAINT) model. *Pharm. Res.* **2010**, *27*, 1722–1729. [CrossRef]
25. Suman, J.D.; Laube, B.L.; Dalby, R. Validity of in vitro tests on aqueous spray pumps as surrogates for nasal deposition, absorption, and biologic response. *J. Aerosol Med.* **2006**, *19*, 510–521. [CrossRef]
26. Fleming, J.S.; Conway, J.H.; Bolt, L.; Holgate, S.T. A comparison of planar scintigraphy and SPECT measurement of total lung deposition of inhaled aerosol. *J. Aerosol Med.* **2003**, *16*, 9–19. [CrossRef]
27. Bondesson, E.; Bengtsson, T.; Borgström, L.; Nilsson, L.E.; Norrgren, K.; Trofast, E.; Wollmer, P. Planar gamma scintigraphy--points to consider when quantifying pulmonary dry powder aerosol deposition. *Int. J. Pharm.* **2003**, *258*, 227–240. [CrossRef]
28. Kundoor, V.; Dalby, R.N. Assessment of nasal spray deposition pattern in a silicone human nose model using a color-based method. *Pharm. Res.* **2010**, *27*, 30–36. [CrossRef]
29. Kundoor, V.; Dalby, R.N. Effect of formulation- and administration-related variables on deposition pattern of nasal spray pumps evaluated using a nasal cast. *Pharm. Res.* **2011**, *28*, 1895–1904. [CrossRef]
30. Cheng, Y.S.; Holmes, T.D.; Gao, J.; Guilmette, R.A.; Li, S.; Surakitbanharn, Y.; Rowlings, C. Characterization of nasal spray pumps and deposition pattern in a replica of the human nasal airway. *J. Aerosol Med.* **2001**, *14*, 267–280. [CrossRef]
31. Gizurarson, S. Method for Administration of Active Substances to the Olfactory Region. Patents CA 2298596, 2 February 2000.
32. Wang, J.; Bentz, J.; Anderson, R. Nasal Device for Delivery to the Olfactory Region. U.S. Patent 20070119451A1, 31 May 2007.
33. Milk, D.G.; Khong, G.C.; Çam, O.H.; Alfaro-Iraheta, F.; Tierney, C.; Kassem, F.; Leong, S.C. A Comparison between Mygind and Kaiteki positions in administration of drops to the olfactory cleft. *Clin. Otolaryngol.* **2021**, *46*, 406–411. [CrossRef] [PubMed]
34. Merkus, P.; Ebbens, F.A.; Muller, B.; Fokkens, W.J. The 'best method' of topical nasal drug delivery: Comparison of seven techniques. *Rhinology* **2006**, *44*, 102–107.
35. Cannady, S.B.; Batra, P.S.; Citardi, M.J.; Lanza, D.C. Comparison of delivery of topical medications to the paranasal sinuses via "vertex-to-floor" position and atomizer spray after FESS. *Otolaryngol. Head Neck Surg.* **2005**, *133*, 735–740. [CrossRef] [PubMed]
36. Mori, E.; Merkonidis, C.; Cuevas, M.; Gudziol, V.; Matsuwaki, Y.; Hummel, T. The administration of nasal drops in the "Kaiteki" position allows for delivery of the drug to the olfactory cleft: A pilot study in healthy subjects. *Eur. Arch. Otorhinolaryngol.* **2016**, *273*, 939–943. [CrossRef] [PubMed]
37. Bäck, L.J.; Hytönen, M.L.; Malmberg, H.O.; Ylikoski, J.S. Submucosal bipolar radiofrequency thermal ablation of inferior turbinates: A long-term follow-up with subjective and objective assessment. *Laryngoscope* **2002**, *112*, 1806–1812. [PubMed]
38. Seifelnasr, A.; Talaat, M.; Ramaswamy, P.; Si, X.A.; Xi, J. A supine position and dual-dose applications enhance spray dosing to the posterior nose: Paving the way for mucosal immunization. *Pharmaceutics* **2023**, *15*, 359. [CrossRef]
39. Xi, J.; Kim, J.; Si, X.; Corley, R.A.; Zhou, Y. Modeling of inertial depositions in scaled models of rat and human nasal airways: Towards in vitro regional dosimetry in small animals. *J. Aerosol Sci.* **2016**, *99*, 78–93. [CrossRef]
40. Cheng, K.-H.; Cheng, Y.-S.; Yeh, H.-C.; Swift, D.L. Deposition of ultrafine aerosols in the head airways during natural breathing and during simulated breath holding using replicate human upper airway casts. *Aerosol Sci. Technol.* **1995**, *23*, 465–474. [CrossRef]
41. Kelly, J.T.; Asgharian, B.; Kimbell, J.S.; Wong, B. Particle depositon in human nasal airway replicas manufactured by different methds. Part II: Ultrafine particles. *Aerosol Sci. Technol.* **2004**, *38*, 1072–1079. [CrossRef]
42. Xi, J.; Wang, Z.; Si, X.A.; Zhou, Y. Nasal dilation effects on olfactory deposition in unilateral and bi-directional deliveries: In vitro tests and numerical modeling. *Eur. J. Pharm. Sci.* **2018**, *118*, 113–123. [CrossRef]
43. Xi, J.; Wang, Z.; Nevorski, D.; White, T.; Zhou, Y. Nasal and olfactory deposition with normal and bidirectional intranasal delivery techniques: In vitro tests and numerical simulations. *J. Aerosol Med. Pulm. Drug Deliv.* **2017**, *30*, 118–131. [CrossRef]
44. Zhou, Y.; Guo, M.; Xi, J.; Irshad, H.; Cheng, Y.-S. Nasal deposition in infants and children. *J. Aerosol Med.* **2014**, *26*, 110–116. [CrossRef]
45. Xi, J.; Yuan, J.E.; Alshaiba, M.; Cheng, D.; Firlit, Z.; Johnson, A.; Nolan, A.; Su, W.C. Design and testing of electric-guided delivery of charged particles to the olfactory region: Experimental and numerical Studies. *Curr. Drug Deliv.* **2016**, *13*, 265–274. [CrossRef] [PubMed]
46. Kimbell, J.S.; Overton, J.H.; Subramaniam, R.P.; Schlosser, P.M.; Morgan, K.T.; Conolly, R.B.; Miller, F.J. Dosimetry modeling of inhaled formaldehyde: Binning nasal flux predictions for quantitative risk assessment. *Toxicol. Sci.* **2001**, *64*, 111–121. [CrossRef] [PubMed]
47. Schroeter, J.D.; Tewksbury, E.W.; Wong, B.A.; Kimbell, J.S. Experimental measurements and computational predictions of regional particle deposition in a sectional nasal model. *J. Aerosol Med. Pulm. Drug Deliv.* **2015**, *28*, 20–29. [CrossRef] [PubMed]
48. Schroeter, J.D.; Kimbell, J.S.; Asgharian, B. Analysis of particle deposition in the turbinate and olfactory regions using a human nasal computational fluid dynamics model. *J. Aerosol Med.* **2006**, *19*, 301–313. [CrossRef] [PubMed]
49. Xi, J.; Si, X.A.; Peters, S.; Nevorski, D.; Wen, T.; Lehman, M. Understanding the mechanisms underlying pulsating aerosol delivery to the maxillary sinus: In vitro tests and computational simulations. *Int. J. Pharm.* **2017**, *520*, 254–266. [CrossRef]
50. Si, X.; Xi, J.; Kim, J. Effect of laryngopharyngeal anatomy on expiratory airflow and submicrometer particle deposition in human extrathoracic airways. *Open J. Fluid. Dyn.* **2013**, *3*, 286–301. [CrossRef]
51. Masiuk, T.; Kadakia, P.; Wang, Z. Development of a physiologically relevant dripping analytical method using simulated nasal mucus for nasal spray formulation analysis. *J. Pharm. Anal.* **2016**, *6*, 283–291. [CrossRef]

52. Gizurarson, S. Anatomical and histological factors affecting intranasal drug and vaccine delivery. *Curr. Drug Deliv.* **2012**, *9*, 566–582. [CrossRef]
53. Landis, M.S.; Boyden, T.; Pegg, S. Nasal-to-CNS drug delivery: Where are we now and where are we heading? An industrial perspective. *Ther. Deliv.* **2012**, *3*, 195–208. [CrossRef] [PubMed]
54. Si, X.A.; Xi, J.; Kim, J.; Zhou, Y.; Zhong, H. Modeling of release position and ventilation effects on olfactory aerosol drug delivery. *Respir. Physiol. Neurobiol.* **2013**, *186*, 22–32. [CrossRef] [PubMed]
55. Shi, H.; Kleinstreuer, C.; Zhang, Z. Laminar airflow and nanoparticle or vapor deposition in a human nasal cavity model. *J. Biomech. Eng.* **2006**, *128*, 697–706. [CrossRef] [PubMed]
56. Sengoku, R.; Matsushima, S.; Bono, K.; Sakuta, K.; Yamazaki, M.; Miyagawa, S.; Komatsu, T.; Mitsumura, H.; Kono, Y.; Kamiyama, T.; et al. Olfactory function combined with morphology distinguishes Parkinson's disease. *Park. Relat. Disord.* **2015**, *21*, 771–777. [CrossRef] [PubMed]
57. Shiga, H.; Taki, J.; Okuda, K.; Watanabe, N.; Tonami, H.; Nakagawa, H.; Kinuya, S.; Miwa, T. Prognostic value of olfactory nerve damage measured with thallium-based olfactory imaging in patients with idiopathic olfactory dysfunction. *Sci. Rep.* **2017**, *7*, 3581. [CrossRef] [PubMed]
58. Kikuchi, A.; Baba, T.; Hasegawa, T.; Sugeno, N.; Konno, M.; Takeda, A. Differentiating Parkinson's disease from multiple system atrophy by [123I] meta-iodobenzylguanidine myocardial scintigraphy and olfactory test. *Park. Relat. Disord.* **2011**, *17*, 698–700. [CrossRef]
59. Prado, G.L.; Itabashi, Y.; Noda, H.; Miura, H.; Mariya, Y.; Abe, Y. Olfactory neuroblastoma visualized by Technetium-99m-ECD SPECT. *Radiat. Med.* **2001**, *19*, 267–270.
60. Kolanjiyil, A.V.; Alfaifi, A.; Aladwani, G.; Golshahi, L.; Longest, W. Importance of spray-wall interaction and post-deposition liquid motion in the transport and delivery of pharmaceutical nasal sprays. *Pharmaceutics* **2022**, *14*, 956. [CrossRef]
61. Perkins, E.L.; Basu, S.; Garcia, G.J.M.; Buckmire, R.A.; Shah, R.N.; Kimbell, J.S. Ideal particle sizes for inhaled steroids targeting vocal granulomas: Preliminary study using computational fluid dynamics. *Otolaryngol. Head Neck Surg.* **2018**, *158*, 511–519. [CrossRef]

pharmaceutics

MDPI

Article

Chitosan-Based Thermogelling System for Nose-to-Brain Donepezil Delivery: Optimising Formulation Properties and Nasal Deposition Profile

Mirna Perkušić [1], Laura Nižić Nodilo [1], Ivo Ugrina [2], Drago Špoljarić [3], Cvijeta Jakobušić Brala [4], Ivan Pepić [1], Jasmina Lovrić [1], Maša Safundžić Kučuk [5], Marie Trenkel [6], Regina Scherließ [6,7], Dijana Zadravec [8], Livije Kalogjera [9] and Anita Hafner [1,*]

[1] Department of Pharmaceutical Technology, University of Zagreb Faculty of Pharmacy and Biochemistry, 10000 Zagreb, Croatia; mperkusic@pharma.hr (M.P.); lnizic@pharma.hr (L.N.N.); ipepic@pharma.hr (I.P.); jlovric@pharma.hr (J.L.)
[2] Intellomics Ltd., 21000 Split, Croatia; ivo.ugrina@intellomics.com
[3] Visage Technologies d.o.o., 10000 Zagreb, Croatia; dspoljaric@gmail.com
[4] Department of Physical Chemistry, University of Zagreb Faculty of Pharmacy and Biochemistry, 10000 Zagreb, Croatia; cjakobus@pharma.hr
[5] Jadran-Galenski Laboratorij d.d., 51000 Rijeka, Croatia; masa.safundzic@jglpharma.com
[6] Department of Pharmaceutics and Biopharmaceutics, Faculty of Mathematics and Natural Sciences, Kiel University, 24118 Kiel, Germany; mtrenkel@pharmazie.uni-kiel.de (M.T.); rscherliess@pharmazie.uni-kiel.de (R.S.)
[7] Priority Research Area Kiel Nano, Surface and Interface Sciences (KiNSIS), Kiel University, 24118 Kiel, Germany
[8] Department of Diagnostic and Interventional Radiology, University Hospital Center Sestre Milosrdnice, University of Zagreb School of Dental Medicine, 10000 Zagreb, Croatia; zadravec@sfzg.hr
[9] ORL/HNS Department, University Hospital Center Sestre Milosrdnice, Zagreb School of Medicine, 10000 Zagreb, Croatia; kalogjera@sfzg.hr
* Correspondence: anita.hafner@pharma.unizg.hr

Abstract: Donepezil nasal delivery strategies are being continuously investigated for advancing therapy in Alzheimer's disease. The aim of this study was to develop a chitosan-based, donepezil-loaded thermogelling formulation tailored to meet all the requirements for efficient nose-to-brain delivery. A statistical design of the experiments was implemented for the optimisation of the formulation and/or administration parameters, with regard to formulation viscosity, gelling and spray properties, as well as its targeted nasal deposition within the 3D-printed nasal cavity model. The optimised formulation was further characterised in terms of stability, in vitro release, in vitro biocompatibility and permeability (using Calu-3 cells), ex vivo mucoadhesion (using porcine nasal mucosa), and in vivo irritability (using slug mucosal irritation assay). The applied research design resulted in the development of a sprayable donepezil delivery platform characterised by instant gelation at 34 °C and olfactory deposition reaching a remarkably high 71.8% of the applied dose. The optimised formulation showed prolonged drug release ($t_{1/2}$ about 90 min), mucoadhesive behaviour, and reversible permeation enhancement, with a 20-fold increase in adhesion and a 1.5-fold increase in the apparent permeability coefficient in relation to the corresponding donepezil solution. The slug mucosal irritation assay demonstrated an acceptable irritability profile, indicating its potential for safe nasal delivery. It can be concluded that the developed thermogelling formulation showed great promise as an efficient donepezil brain-targeted delivery system. Furthermore, the formulation is worth investigating in vivo for final feasibility confirmation.

Keywords: donepezil; chitosan; nose-to-brain delivery; thermoresponsive in situ gelling system; 3D nasal cavity model; olfactory deposition

1. Introduction

Nasal drug delivery offers distinct advantages in brain-targeted therapy of neurologic disorders. Olfactory and trigeminal nerves innervating the olfactory and/or respiratory mucosa enable the direct transport of nasally administered drugs to the brain, bypassing the blood–brain barrier [1]. Nevertheless, the described potential is still scarcely utilised. The demands for a major step forward include the development of functional drug delivery systems and efficient drug deposition in specific nasal regions of interest [2]. Generally, research on the development of nasal delivery systems has addressed the issues of limited drug solubility, permeability, stability, and nasal residence time [3–5]. The potential of advanced delivery platforms of simple production and easy scale-up, such as in situ gelling liquid systems, is of particular interest [3,6]. These systems can incorporate mucoadhesive polymers, drug permeation enhancers, and/or nanocarriers, thus optimising nasal retention time, drug release, and absorption profile [7]. Formulation-related viscosity and/or reduced volume of administration may improve patient compliance, diminishing the potential for discomfort related to formulation run-off to the throat and unpleasant aftertaste [2,8].

Lately, drug delivery to the targeted region of the nasal cavity has become an inevitable milestone towards effective nasal therapy [4], and it emerged as one of the key elements in nasal product development [9]. Recently, our research team pioneered and extensively investigated the issue of coupling formulation and administration parameters employing the quality-by-design (QbD) approach to optimise the nasal deposition pattern in vitro in relation to the specific disease in adults [10]. Such an approach has been shown to hold great promise in promoting targeted nasal drug delivery [11,12].

Targeted nasal delivery can be considered a viable option for advancing drug therapy in Alzheimer's disease [13]. Alzheimer's disease is a progressive neurodegenerative disorder impairing memory, thinking, and behaviour, with rising prevalence corresponding to population ageing [14]. It is one of the leading indications of the demand for drug delivery strategies that overcome the blood–brain barrier [15]. Currently, donepezil is the first-line treatment in patients with mild to moderate Alzheimer's disease, which is available predominantly in oral solid dosage forms [16]. Donepezil oral delivery has several limitations including first-pass metabolism, gastrointestinal and peripheral adverse effects, and low brain bioavailability [17]. On the contrary, the nasal administration of donepezil offers the potential for its efficient and direct central nervous system delivery, reduced systemic bioavailability, and a lower risk of adverse effects [18]. The recognised advantages of nasal donepezil delivery have led to the development of several liquid pharmaceutical platforms including donepezil nanosuspension [19], donepezil-loaded liposomes [20,21], nanoemulsion [22], lipid nanoparticles [23], microemulsion [24], and in situ gel [17], improving donepezil solubility and/or its permeation profile and enhancing its brain bioavailability, as evidenced in animal models in vivo. However, no studies on their possible application mode in humans and deposition pattern within the nasal cavity have been performed.

The idea behind our study was to develop a donepezil-loaded advanced liquid formulation and harmonize its biopharmaceutical performance and nasal deposition profile while meeting all requirements for efficient brain-targeted delivery and keeping the formulating process simple.

In situ gelling thermoresponsive polymer/drug solutions bear the potential to fulfil the above-mentioned requirements. They present easy-to-produce and scale-up formulations that can be readily applied as sprays while ensuring prolonged residence time in the nasal cavity upon gelation triggered by nasal physiological temperature [6]. Ideally, gel-forming constituents could contribute to a sustained drug release and interact with biological barriers to increase drug absorption, altogether resulting in increased bioavailability of the nasally applied drug [25].

Chitosan is a cationic linear polysaccharide widely applied as a mucoadhesive agent and absorption enhancer in nasal formulations [26]. Moreover, chitosan can yield thermoresponsive physical gels in the presence of β-glycerophosphate [27]. An almost neutral aqueous solution of chitosan and β-glycerophosphate demonstrates a strong rise in the storage modulus upon heating [6].

The aim of this study was to develop the chitosan-based donepezil-loaded thermoresponsive in situ gelling system, considering all aspects of donepezil nasal delivery, including formulation stability, sprayability, gelation temperature and time, drug release profile, interaction with the biological barrier, and, in particular, nasal deposition pattern, which was included as a required complementary indicator of the brain-targeting potential in humans and studied using the model of the healthy adult nasal cavity.

To the best of our best knowledge, this is the first report on the development of a chitosan-based thermoresponsive system for nasal delivery of donepezil. Previously, only Gu et al. [17] reported the development of a thermogelling nasal donepezil system. In that study, two types of poloxamers were used as the thermogelling agent. The systems were characterised in terms of gelation properties, in vitro release, and in vivo pharmacokinetics in rats, and formulation potential to increase donepezil brain bioavailability was confirmed. Compared with the aforementioned study, the innovation in our approach refers to a comprehensive research design that allows an integrated formulation development, taking into account all features of the nasal delivery, including the challenges of brain targeting in humans.

The complex task of correlating the in situ gelling formulation properties and nasal deposition profile with formulation and/or nasal administration parameters was accomplished by employing a statistical design of experiments.

Thorough biopharmaceutical characterisation of the leading formulation, including studies on stability, in vitro release, in vitro biocompatibility and permeability (using Calu-3 cells), ex vivo mucoadhesion (using excised nasal mucosa), and in vivo irritability (using slug mucosal irritation assay), was performed to evaluate the overall potential of the developed formulation in donepezil nose-to-brain delivery.

Finally, the results on the nasal deposition of the leading in situ gelling formulation will be compared with the results obtained previously with optimised donepezil powder formulation [12] to account for the differences in accessibility of the olfactory region using two distinct formulation approaches.

2. Materials and Methods

2.1. Materials

Donepezil hydrochloride (further denoted as DH) was obtained from Carbosynth Ltd. (Compton, UK). β-glycerophosphoric acid disodium salt pentahydrate (denoted as β-glycerophosphate, BGP, further in the text) was purchased from Biosynth Ltd. (Bratislava, Slovakia). Low-molecular-weight chitosan (molecular weight 50–190 kDa, with 75–85% degree of deacetylation; further denoted as chitosan, C), medium-molecular-weight chitosan (molecular weight 190–310 kDa, with 75–85% degree of deacetylation), and high-molecular-weight chitosan (molecular weight 310–375 kDa, with >75% degree of deacetylation) were obtained from Sigma-Aldrich (Taufkirchen, Germany). Simulated nasal fluid (SNF) was prepared as an aqueous solution by dissolving the following solids: NaCl (150.0 mM; Kemig, Zagreb, Croatia), KCl (40.0 mM; Kemig, Zagreb, Croatia), and $CaCl_2 \times H_2O$ (5.3 mM; Sigma-Aldrich, Taufkirchen, Germany) [10]. Hank's balanced salt solution (HBSS; pH = 7.0) was prepared by dissolving the following in distilled water: KCl (5.4 mM), $NaHCO_3$ (4.2 mM), NaCl (136.9 mM), and D-glucose monohydrate (5.6 mM), all purchased from Kemig, Zagreb, Croatia; KH_2PO_4 (0.4 mM; Kemika, Zagreb, Croatia); $Na_2HPO_4 \times 2H_2O$ (0.3 mM; Fluka Chemie AG, Buchs, Switzerland); N-2-hydroxyethylpiperazine-N'-2-ethanesulfonic acid (HEPES; 30.0 mM; Sigma-Aldrich, Taufkirchen, Germany); and $CaCl_2 \times 2H_2O$ (1.3 mM; Sigma-Aldrich, Taufkirchen, Germany). The mixture was used for in vitro cell biocompatibility and permeability studies. Sar-gel® (Arkema, Colombes, France) was used for the determination of the fractional deposition pattern. All other chemicals or solvents used in the study were of analytical grade and purchased from Kemika (Zagreb, Croatia).

2.2. Preliminary Studies

Thorough preliminary studies were performed to select suitable excipients and appropriate settings of upper and lower limits of the in situ gelling formulation and administration parameters.

Preliminary samples were prepared according to the protocol described in Section 2.4. using chitosans of different molecular weight and different constituent concentrations as presented in the Supplementary Materials, Tables S2–S6.

Exclusion criteria included observed precipitation, inappropriate gelation time or temperature, and poor sprayability (determined as spray cone angle or droplet size distribution). Finally, administration parameters most common in the relevant literature were preliminarily tested within the design space of formulation parameters. The methods applied are described in Sections 2.6.2–2.8.

2.3. Design of Experiments (DoE)

Quality by design (QbD) principles were built into the donepezil–chitosan–β-glycerophosphate (DH-C-BGP) in situ gelling system development process. This approach was used for optimising formulation and administration parameters to achieve efficient DH nasal delivery. Two formulation (the concentration of DH and C) and two administration (the inspiratory flow rate and angle of administration from the horizontal plane) parameters were incorporated in the definite screening design developed with JMP 14.0 statistical software (JMP®, Version 14.0, SAS Institute Inc., Cary, NC, USA, 1989–2007). Settings of the parameters in the experimental design are listed in Table 1.

Table 1. Settings of the parameters considered in the experimental design.

Parameter	High (+1)	Medium (0)	Low (−1)
Donepezil hydrochloride (DH) concentration (mg mL^{-1})	0.50	0.40	0.30
Chitosan (C) concentration (mg mL^{-1})	9.23	7.69	6.15
Angle of administration from the horizontal plane, AAH (°)	75	60	45
Inspiratory flow rate, IFR (L min^{-1})	30	15	0

Gelation properties (i.e., gelation time and temperature), zero-shear viscosity, droplet size distribution, spray cone angle, and deposition in the turbinate and olfactory region of the nasal cavity were investigated as responses. The statistical software JMP 14.0 (JMP®, Version 14.0, SAS Institute Inc., Cary, NC, USA, 1989–2007) was used to perform data analysis.

2.4. Preparation of the DH-C-BGP In Situ Gelling Formulation

DH-C-BGP nasal formulations were prepared according to Gholizadeh et al. [28], with slight modifications. First, concentrated C solutions (1.0%, 1.5%, and 2.0%, *w*/*w*) were prepared by dissolving chitosan in 0.5% (*v*/*v*) acetic acid at room temperature, under stirring conditions for 24 h. Then, an appropriate amount of DH was dissolved in a C solution. A concentrated BGP solution (49%, *w*/*w*) was prepared by dissolving BGP in water at room temperature. At 4 °C (in an ice bath), the concentrated BGP solution was added dropwise to the DH-C solution, followed by 10 min of mixing. DH-C and BGP solutions were mixed in a 1.6:1 volume ratio. Final DH and C concentrations are listed in Table 2. The concentration of BGP in all DoE samples was 188 mg mL^{-1}. The pH value of all samples was also measured, using a S47 SevenMulti pH meter (Mettler Toledo, Greifensee, Switzerland).

2.5. Determination of DH Concentration in the DH-C-BGP Formulations

The DH concentrations in the prepared DoE samples were assessed via the high-performance liquid chromatography (HPLC) method, as detailed in Section 2.10. An aliquot of the DH-C-BGP sample was diluted with purified water. The diluted sample was filtered (0.2 µm pore size, Chromafil® Xtra PES-20/25, Macherey-Nagel GmbH & Co. KG, Düren, Germany), and then the drug concentration in the sample was determined. Measurements for each sample were performed in triplicate.

2.6. Rheological Characterisation

Rheological characteristics of the prepared DH-C-BGP formulations were assessed using a Modular Compact Rheometer MCR 102 (Anton Paar GmbH, Graz, Austria). The temperature on the rheometer was assured via a Peltier temperature control system. Oscillatory rheological tests were performed using a parallel plate (PP50; diameter 50 mm) and rotational rheological tests were performed using a cone plate (CP50; diameter 50 mm, cone slope 1°). Software RheoCompass™ Light Version 1.23.403 (Anton Paar GmbH, Graz, Austria) was used for the data analysis.

2.6.1. Zero-Shear Viscosity Determination

A rotational creep test, using a CP50 measuring system, was applied to determine zero-shear viscosity (η_0) of the prepared formulations, at 25 °C. The zero gap was set at 0.102 mm. Before the test, the sample was left on the lower plate to equilibrate at 25 °C for 3 min. During the test time of 5 min, a shear strain stress of 0.1 Pa was applied to the sample, and the shear strain was recorded as a function of time. Zero-shear viscosity was computed using RheoCompass software, fitting the shear stress vs. data on the shear rate and calculating the regression on the creep measuring data within the three retardation points [10]. Each sample was analysed in triplicate.

2.6.2. Measurement of Gelation Temperature

In order to determine the sol–gel transition point, an oscillatory temperature test was used. A PP50 measuring system was used and the test recorded the changes in storage (G') and loss modulus (G'') over a temperature range from 20 °C to 40 °C. The gap was set at 0.500 mm, the angular frequency was fixed at 6.28 rad s^{-1}, and the applied strain was 1%. The intersection of G' and G'' curves was recorded as the gelation temperature—T_{GEL} [29]. All measurements were performed in triplicate.

2.6.3. Measurement of Gelation Time

The time needed for the formulation to undergo sol–gel transition was determined using an oscillatory time test. A PP50 measuring system was used and the test was performed at 34 °C—the temperature of the nasal cavity [5]. Variations in G' and G'' were monitored as a function of time. The zero gap was fixed at 0.500 mm. The measurement was performed at an angular frequency of 6.28 rad s^{-1} and 1% strain. The cross point of G' and G'' curves was recorded as the time needed for the formulation to transit from the liquid to the gel state (t_{GEL}) [30]. Each formulation was analysed in triplicate.

2.7. Droplet Size Distribution (DSD)

Droplet size distribution (DSD) was determined via a Malvern Spraytec unit (Malvern Instruments, Malvern, Worcestershire, UK) via a laser diffraction technique. Samples were loaded into a VP7 spray pump equipped with a 232 NE actuator (dosing volume of 100 µL), kindly provided by AptarGroup Inc., Le Neubourg, France. Prior to the test, the spray pump was primed several times by discarding the actuations as waste. For the measurement, the tip of the device was placed 3 cm below the laser diffraction measurement zone. The focal distance from the lens was 300 mm. Each test was performed manually, in triplicate. The results were expressed as volume diameters D_v10, D_v50, and D_v90. Span, defined as $(D_v90 - D_v10)/D_v50$, was also calculated [31]. The analysis of the results was performed via Malvern Spraytec 3.20 software (Malvern Instruments, Malvern, Worcestershire, UK).

2.8. Spray Cone Angle Determination (SCA)

Spray cone angle (SCA) was determined by spraying the samples from the VP7 spray pump equipped with the 232 NE actuator (AptarGroup Inc., Le Neubourg, France) against the dark background. A Panasonic Lumix DMC-FZ1000 camera was used to record the spray plume under a set-up of 120 frames per second. The recorded spray plume was analysed using a virtual protractor. Each formulation was analysed in triplicate.

2.9. Assessment of the Deposition Pattern in the Nasal Cavity In Vitro

Nasal deposition pattern studies were performed using a multi-sectional 3D-printed nasal cast. The development of the nasal cavity model had been previously performed by our research group using anonymised Multislice Computer Tomography (CT) scan data of a 62-year-old patient [32], obtained from the Sestre milosrdnice University Hospital Center database. The protocol was carried out following the rules of the Declaration of Helsinki and was approved by the Ethics Committee of the Sestre milosrdnice University Hospital Center (Project identification code: EP-9941/19–3) and the Ethics Committee of the University of Zagreb Faculty of Pharmacy and Biochemistry (Class: 643–02/19–01/02; Registry number: 251–62-03–19-43). The model was made via stereolithography process using 3D Systems®ProX 800 (3D Systems, Inc., Rock Hill, SC, USA). Transparent rigid plastic Accura ClearVue was used to print the septum and the olfactory, respiratory, and posterior regions of the model. The anterior region was printed in a flexible material (Digital-Material FLX 9850, 60 ShoreA TangoBlackPlus and VeroWhitePlus) using a Stratasys Connex 350 printer (Stratasys Ltd., Rehovot, Israel) [32]. In order to observe a fractional deposition pattern, the model was divided into different regions of the nasal cavity: anterior region, turbinate region and septum—both with detachable olfactory fragments, and a posterior region (nasopharynx) with a connecting part for the respiratory pump. The model also contains the paranasal sinuses. The proper assembly and alignment of the model parts were ensured using bar pins, measuring 6.4 and 2.0 mm in diameter and 6.0 and 4.0 mm in height, and transverse coupling.

The fractional nasal deposition pattern was assessed by placing the 3D-printed nasal cast on a stand in order to properly connect the model to a respiratory pump (model 613; Hardvard Apparatus, Holliston, MA, USA). The respiratory pump was used to simulate breathing conditions in a range from 15 L min^{-1} (rest breathing) to 30 L min^{-1} (deep moderate breathing condition) [10]. The inspiration flow rate set by the respiratory pump was checked via the inspiratory flow meter (In-Check Nasal; Clement Clarke International Ltd., Harlow, UK). Prior to the administration of the sample, the model was uniformly coated with a thin layer of a Sar-gel® indicator paste (Arkema, Colombes, France) in order to visualise the deposition pattern and prevent the formulation from dripping. The Sar-gel® paste turns purple when in contact with the formulation. The formulation was administered into the model using a VP7 spray pump, equipped with the 232 NE actuator. The spray pump was inserted into the right nostril, at a depth of 5 mm, and the device was actuated at an angle 0° from the vertical plane, and 45°, 60°, and 75° from the horizontal plane, while the left nostril was blocked. The fractional spray deposition pattern was determined gravimetrically: each region of the right side of the model was weighed before and after formulation administration, using an electronic balance (precision 0.01 mg; Mettler Toledo, Greifensee, Switzerland) [11]. The assessment of the deposition pattern was performed in duplicate for each run of the experimental design.

2.10. HPLC Method for Quantitative Determination of DH

The quantitative determination of DH was performed via the HPLC method using a 1260 Infinity II LC System consisting of an auto-sampling system, controller unit, degasser, UV–VIS detector and column oven (Agilent Technologies, Santa Clara, CA, USA). OpenLab software (Agilent Technologies, Santa Clara, CA, USA) was used to process the data of all chromatographic analyses. The chromatographic separation was carried out using a Kinetex C18 (250 × 4.6 mm, 2.6 μm particle size) reverse-phase column with a suitable guard column, both obtained by Phenomenex (Torrance, CA, USA). The method was performed according to Pappa et al. [33], with a few minor adjustments. Briefly, the mobile phase was prepared by mixing 0.02 M buffer phosphate (pH 2.7), methanol, and triethylamine in a volume ratio of 50:50:0.5. The flow rate was set at 1.0 mL min^{-1} and the injection volume at 20 µL. The analysis was performed at 25 °C. The detection wavelength was 268 nm. The run time was 7 min and the DH retention time was 5 min. The above-described method was validated based on the International Conference on Harmonization (ICH) guideline Q2 (R1) [34]. The validation of the method was carried out for linearity, range of linearity, accuracy, repeatability, intermediate precision, the limit of detection (LOD), and the limit of quantification (LOQ) (Table S1). All measured concentration values were within the range of linearity of the method (Table S1).

2.11. *In-Depth Characterisation of the Leading DH-C-BGP Formulation*

The leading DH-C-BGP formulation (LF) was further characterised in terms of in vitro DH release profile, mucoadhesiveness, biocompatibility, and permeability. The stability profile was also assessed. The slug mucosal irritation assay was performed in order to predict the formulation's potential to cause nasal discomfort.

2.11.1. In Vitro Release Studies

The automated Franz diffusion cell testing system Phoenix™ RDS (Teledyne Hanson, Chatsworth, CA, USA) was used to determine the DH in vitro release profile from the LF. The Phoenix RDS platform consists of six vertical diffusion cells (volume of the receptor compartment: 15 mL) placed in the Peltier heating and stirring block. The cells were filled with SNF and the system was thermostated at 34 °C under a constant stirring of 500 rpm. A polyamide membrane with a pore size of 0.45 µm (Sartorius Stedim Biotech GmbH, Göttingen, Germany) was placed between the donor and acceptor compartment. Prior to the experiment, the membranes were conditioned in SNF for 15 min. The selected samples (500 µL) were pipetted into the donor compartment using a Multipette® E3 (Eppendorf, Hamburg, Germany) equipped with 1 mL ViscoTip® (Eppendorf, Hamburg, Germany). At predetermined time intervals, aliquots of 200 µL were drawn from the receptor compartment and replaced with fresh SNF, also heated to 34 °C. The total time of the experiment was 5 h and, during that time, the sink conditions were assured. The DH content in the collected samples was determined via the HPLC method, as detailed in Section 2.10. Donor compartments were also tested for DH content. All release experiments were performed in triplicate.

2.11.2. In Vitro Mucoadhesion Test

Mucoadhesive properties of the LF were tested using a porcine nasal mucosa, obtained from a local slaughterhouse. The nasal mucosa was isolated from porcine heads by splitting the heads in half by longitudinal incision, and then the mucosa was separated from the septum and conchae [35]. Prior to the experiments, the mucosa was kept at −20 °C. A texture analyser TA.XT Plus (Stable Micro Systems, Godalming, UK), equipped with a mucoadhesion rig, was used to test the mucoadhesiveness of the LF; this method was previously developed by our research group [11]. Prior to the experiment, the mucosa was soaked in SNF for approximately 30 s at 34 °C. Then, the mucosa was cut into a 10 mm diameter disk and adhered to the upper probe using cyanoacrylate glue. A selected sample (100 µL) was pipetted onto the lower platform (using Multipette® E3 (Eppendorf, Hamburg, Germany)) and thermostated at 34 °C for 30 s. The experimental parameters used were: pre-test, test, and post-test speeds of 0.5 mm s^{-1}, 0.1 mm s^{-1}, and 0.1 mm s^{-1}, respectively, with a contact time of 120 s and applied force of 0.1 N. Mucoadhesive properties were expressed as the maximum detachment force (F_{max}) and the work of adhesion (W_{adh}) [32]. The sample from the DoE with a chitosan concentration different from the leading concentration (control formulation—CF) and corresponding aqueous DH solution were used as controls. Filter paper soaked in SNF served as a negative control. Each sample was tested in triplicate.

2.11.3. Cell Culture Conditions

In order to examine in vitro biocompatibility and permeability of the formulations, Calu-3 cell line (ATCC® HTB-55TM, ATCC, Manassas, VA, USA) was used. The cells were cultured in Dulbecco's modified Eagle's medium (DMEM-F12) cell culture medium (Sigma Aldrich, Burlington, MA, USA) containing penicillin/streptomycin (1% *v*/*v*; Lonza, Basel, Switzerland) and fetal bovine serum (FBS; 1% *v*/*v*, Sigma Aldrich, Burlington, MA, USA). The cell cultures were maintained at 95% humidity and 37 °C in an atmosphere of 5% CO_2 (Sanyo CO_2 incubator, Osaka, Japan). The medium was changed every 2 days, and the cells were passaged when they reached 70–90% confluence, according to the ATCC recommended protocol. The detachment of the cells from the flasks was performed using a mixture of trypsin (0.25%) and EDTA (0.02%) solutions in phosphate-buffered saline (PBS; Lonza, Basel, Switzerland).

2.11.4. In Vitro Biocompatibility Study

The Calu-3 cells were seeded into 96-well plates (Corning Costar, Corning, NY, USA) at a density of 4×10^4 cells per well and allowed to reach confluence over 48 h. Biocompatibility was assessed using an MTT (3-[4,5-dimethylthiazol-2-yl]-2,5-diphenyl tetrazolium bromide, Sigma-Aldrich, Burlington, MA, USA) colorimetric test.

Before the experiment, the cell culture medium from the wells was withdrawn, and the cells were washed with HBSS/HEPES (pH = 7.0) and treated with the prepared samples. The leading formulation was mixed with HBSS/HEPES (pH = 7.0) in a volume ratio 1:1. The LF-HBSS/HEPES (pH = 7.0) mixture resulted in DH, C, and BGP concentrations of 0.15 mg mL^{-1}, 4.62 mg mL^{-1}, and 94.00 mg mL^{-1}, respectively. The cells incubated in HBSS/HEPES (pH = 7.0) were used as a negative control. The DH solution in HBSS/HEPES (pH = 7.0) (DH concentration ranging between 0.05 and 0.25 mg mL^{-1}) and the BGP solution in HBSS/HEPES (pH = 7.0) (94.00 mg mL^{-1}) served as controls. The cells were incubated with the prepared samples for 2 h at 37 °C. Afterwards, the samples were removed from the wells, and the wells were rinsed twice with HBSS/HEPES (pH = 7.0), followed by adding 100 µL of prepared MTT reagent in each well. The MTT reagent was prepared by dissolving MTT in PBS (MTT concentration of 2.5 mg mL^{-1}), and then the solution was further diluted with DMEM-F12 to a final MTT concentration of 0.5 mg mL^{-1}. The cells were incubated with MTT reagent for 2 h at 37 °C. After the incubation, the reagent was removed. Isopropanol (100 µL per well) was added to lyse the cells and to dissolve the formazan crystals. The amount of formazan product was determined using a spectrophotometer 1420 Multilabel counter VICTOR3, Perkin Elmer, Waltham, MA, USA, at 570 nm. Cell viability was calculated using the following equation:

$$\text{Viability (\%)} = \frac{A_{sample} - A_{ipr}}{A_c - A_{ipr}} \times 100 \quad (1)$$

where A_{sample} is the absorbance of the formazan crystal solution formed in cells treated with tested samples, A_{ipr} is the absorbance of pure isopropanol, and $A_{control}$ is the absorbance of a solution of formazan crystals formed in cells treated only with HBSS/HEPES (pH = 7.0).

2.11.5. In Vitro Permeability through the Epithelial Model Barrier

The Calu-3 epithelial cells were seeded into polycarbonate 12-well Transwell® inserts, with 0.4 µm mean pore size, and 1.12 cm^2 surface area (Corning Costar Inc., Corning, NY, USA) at a density of 5.5×10^5 cells per well in order to test in vitro permeability [32]. The volume of the cell culture medium in the apical and basolateral compartment was 0.5 mL and 1.5 mL, respectively. After an incubation period of 48 h, the medium from the apical compartment was aspirated and the cells were cultured at the air–liquid interface, with 800 µL of the culture medium in the basolateral compartment. The media in the basolateral compartment was replaced with a fresh medium every 48 h. The cells were grown for 14 days until a plateau in transepithelial electrical resistance (TEER) was reached (above 1000 Ω cm^2). An epithelial volt/ohm meter EVOM with STX-2 chopstick electrode (WPI Inc., Sarasota, FL, USA) was used to measure the TEER of the cell monolayers. Permeability studies included the following samples: (i) LF mixed with HBSS/HEPES (pH = 7.0) in a volume ratio of 1:1; (ii) solution of DH in HBSS/HEPES (pH = 7.0) (DH concentration = 0.25 mg mL^{-1}); (iii) DH solution in hyperosmotic HBSS/HEPES (pH = 7.0) (DH concentration = 0.15 mg mL^{-1}); and (iv) HBSS/HEPES (pH = 7.0) as the negative control. Osmolality of the hyperosmotic HBSS/HEPES (pH = 7.0) was equal to the leading formulation–HBSS/HEPES (pH = 7.0) mixture. The hyperosmotic HBSS/HEPES (pH = 7.0) was prepared according to Soni et al. [36]. An amount of 12 g of NaCl was added to 1 L of the prepared HBSS/HEPES (pH = 7.0), resulting in 2% NaCl (*w*/*v*) in the final hypertonic HBSS/HEPES (pH = 7.0) solution. Osmolality measurements were performed with an OsmoTECH® Single-Sample Micro-Osmometer (Advanced Instruments, Norwood, MA, USA).

Before the experiment, the cells were washed with HBSS/HEPES (pH = 7.0) and, afterwards, the HBSS/HEPES (pH = 7.0) was pipetted into apical and basolateral compartments and the plate was incubated at 37 °C, 5% CO_2, for 20 min. After the incubation, TEER was measured at the beginning of the permeability experiment. The HBSS/HEPES (pH = 7.0) was removed from the wells and 500 µL of each sample was added to the apical compartment. Each sample was tested in triplicate. Over the period of 120 min, 500 µL of the sample from the basolateral compartment was taken every 20 min and replaced with fresh HBSS/HEPES (pH = 7.0). All samples collected during the experiment, including the samples from the donor compartment at the 120 min final point of the experiment, were analysed for DH content using the HPLC method described in Section 2.10. In order to check cells' monolayer integrity, TEER values were recorded during and upon completion of the experiments. During the permeability test, cells were incubated at 37 °C and 50 rpm on a horizontal orbital shaker. The apparent permeability coefficient (P_{app}) was calculated according to the following equation:

$$P_{app} = \frac{dQ}{dt} \times \frac{1}{AC_0} \quad (2)$$

where dQ/dt is the permeability rate, A is the surface area of the permeation barrier, and C_0 is the initial concentration of DH in the apical compartment [27].

The attenuation factor was calculated as the ratio between the P_{app} value of the LF or the DH solution in the hyperosmolar HBSS/HEPES (pH = 7.0) and the P_{app} value of the DH solution in the HBSS/HEPES (pH = 7.0) [12].

2.11.6. Slug Mucosal Irritation Assay

The slug mucosal irritation (SMI) assay was used to evaluate the potential of the leading formulation to cause irritation on the nasal mucosa. The SMI was performed according to Trenkel et Scherließ [37]. Briefly, slugs of the species *Arion lusitanicus* were collected by wild harvesting. Prior to the experiment, the specimens were kept under laboratory conditions. The SMI assay was performed only with slugs with a body weight between 3 and 6 g. Slugs were weighed (BW) at the beginning of the experiment. An aliquot (100 µL) of the tested sample was transferred into a Petri dish and the mass of the dish and the sample was recorded. Slugs were placed on the liquid formulation for a contact period (CP) of 15 min. After the time of the first contact period expired, the slugs were placed on 1.5 mL of PBS in another dish, for a resting time of 60 min. During the resting time, the dish with the liquid formulation and the mucus produced after the first CP was weighed and recorded. This procedure was repeated two more times, so the total number of CPs was three. Total mucus production (TM) after three CPs was calculated according to the equation:

$$TM\ (\%) = \Sigma\ M \frac{(Mucus\ per\ CP,\ g)}{BW,\ g} \times 100\% \quad (3)$$

The same procedure was applied for negative control (100 µL of PBS) and positive control (100 µL of 1% (*w*/*v*) benzalkonium chloride (BAC) solution). Experiments were performed in triplicate. For each replicate, a separate slug was used.

2.11.7. Stability Studies

Stability studies of the LF were performed in time points of 30 and 90 days. The liquid was kept in an airtight container, at 5 ± 3 °C, which is the envisaged storage temperature for the product. The drug concentration, rheological properties, SCA, and in vitro drug release profile were measured and compared with the initial results, recorded right after the preparation of the leading sample. All experiments were performed in triplicate.

2.12. Statistical Analysis

JMP 14.0 software (JMP®, Version 14.0, SAS Institute Inc., Cary, NC, USA, 1989–2007) was used to perform statistical analysis related to DoE, with $p < 0.05$ set as the minimal level of significance. Mucoadhesive properties were analysed using GraphPad Prism (trial version, GraphPad Software, Inc., San Diego, CA, USA), using a one-way analysis of variance (ANOVA), followed by a Tukey's post hoc test. The similarity factor (f_2) was used to assert the similarity between in vitro release profiles [38]. The profiles were considered similar when the f_2 factor was greater than 50 [39].

3. Results and Discussion

The aim of this research was to develop a thermosensitive in situ gelling platform for efficient nose-to-brain delivery of DH. Thermosensitive hydrogels based on C-BGP have been studied for various purposes [29,40–42], but there are only a few studies aimed at the development of a C-BGP in situ gelling system for nasal delivery [28,43]. In this work, we focused on the development of a nasal C-BGP formulation that is safe, biocompatible, non-irritable, and efficient regarding delivery of DH to the brain.

A nasal in situ gelling DH formulation was developed with the aim to produce a platform that is easily administered as a spray but turns to gel at the temperature of the nasal mucosa, 33–35 °C [44]. The sol–gel transition results in prolonged residence time of the formulation at the mucosal surface, owing to reduced mucociliary clearance [45].

Chitosan (C) is a non-toxic, biocompatible, biodegradable, and bioadhesive polymer with penetration-enhancing properties [30]. On its own, chitosan does not exhibit thermosensitive properties. However, by mixing the chitosan with a polyol-phosphate, such as BGP, the C-BGP platform undergoes a sol–gel transition at the temperature of the nasal cavity. At room temperature, β-glycerophosphate interacts with the positively charged chitosan amine groups, keeping chitosan chains in the solution by forming a water-protective shield despite increasing the pH of the solution. The mechanism of thermoreversible sol–gel transition includes a loss of electrostatic repulsion, ionic crosslinking, hydrogen bonding, and hydrophobic interaction [6].

3.1. Selection of the Formulation and Administration Parameters for DH-Loaded In Situ Gelling Systems

In this study, the development of a DH-loaded in situ gelling formulation was performed employing a statistical design of experiments. Such an approach potentiates the development of a DH thermogelling delivery platform with built-in quality, maximizing the cost and time savings [46]. In order to set the appropriate design space, thorough preliminary studies were conducted to select the constituents and their concentrations, fulfilling the requirements for nasal delivery [5].

Donepezil concentration range in the preliminary studies (0.3–0.6 mg mL^{-1}; Table S2) was in line with the relevant references concerning donepezil nose-to-brain delivery [19]. Taking into account the dosing volume of 100 μL, the indicated concentration range provides delivering the dose per actuation equal to 0.6–1.2% (or 0.3–0.6%) of 5 (or 10) mg oral daily dose. The aforementioned fraction of the donepezil daily oral dose is considered appropriate to achieve its therapeutic potential via direct nose-to-brain delivery [47].

The starting BGP concentration was set at 188 mg mL^{-1} (Table S2), which is within the range usually reported for such systems [28,29,48]. In previous studies, the molecular weight of chitosan was shown to have a significant impact on thermogelling properties of the chitosan–BGP systems [41]. More particularly, it was observed that the increase in chitosan molecular weight resulted in faster system gelation [28,49,50]. In this study, DH-loaded systems prepared with the medium and high molecular weight chitosans at the gelation-promoting concentration (6.15 mg mL^{-1}) showed precipitation or poor sprayability (Tables S2 and S3), while at lower chitosan concentrations, the systems did not exhibit gelling properties. On the contrary, the chitosans of low molecular weight provided appropriate spray and gelation properties at the relevant range of DH concentrations (Table S3).

In the next step, a DH-loaded system (DH concentration 0.3 mg mL^{-1}) prepared with the low-molecular-weight chitosan (C concentration 6.15 mg mL^{-1}) was selected for the BGP concentration optimization. Based on the results obtained (Table S4), a fixed concentration of BGP was set. Namely, even a small shift in gelling agent concentration caused a great difference in the formulation's thermogelling properties [51]. Ranges in the BGP concentrations were previously reported in experimental designs for the development of similar systems [52,53]. However, susceptibility to the BGP concentration in this study may be related to the difference in the incorporated drug type and concentration.

The final step revealed concentration ranges for both the DH and the low molecular weight chitosan, defining the design space for formulation optimisation in relation to the studied responses (Tables S5 and S6).

It was previously shown that the angles of administration and inspiratory flow exhibit a pronounced impact on the nasal deposition pattern. According to the literature sources, administration parameters including the angle of administration from the horizontal plane ranging from 30 to 75° and inspiratory flow from 0 to 30 L min^{-1} were assessed in the preliminary deposition studies [10,54–57]. Only the angle of administration of 30° was discarded as inappropriate for targeted nasal delivery of tested formulations. Other parameters were included in the statistical design of experiments as presented in Table 1.

3.2. Design of Experiments: Optimisation of DH-C-BGP Formulation

The design of the experiments was successfully incorporated into the DH-C-BGP formulation development. The DoE generated 17 runs varying in formulation (DH and C concentration) and/or administration parameters (horizontal angle of administration and inspiratory flow rate). The design matrix is presented in Table 2.

The DH concentration in the prepared DoE samples ranged between 0.29 ± 0.00 and 0.52 ± 0.02 mg mL^{-1} (Table 2), providing complete DH dissolution in C-BGP systems and adequate DH dose with respect to nasal delivery [19]. The value of pH for all prepared samples ranged between 7.02 ± 0.00 and 7.35 ± 0.00 (Table 2). The observed pH values were expected due to the basic values of BGP systems [28] and are acceptable for nasal administration [58,59].

Within the DoE, the formulation of rheological and thermogelling properties (gelation time and temperature, and zero-shear viscosity), spray characteristics (droplet size distribution and spray cone angle), as well as olfactory and turbinate deposition assessed in the nasal cavity model were analysed as responses. The obtained results are presented in Table 2.

Regression modelling was applied to enlighten which formulation parameters (and their interactions) had the most influence on the responses and to select the parameter settings that resulted in the most convenient response values. Regression modelling equations are presented in standardised covariates that are normalised to unitless intervals $[-1, 1]$, an approach common in experimental design modelling [60]. Within the regression model equation, all statistically significant parameters ($p < 0.05$) are noted with an asterisk. The regression models and the analysis for the formulation of rheological, thermogelling, and spray properties as DoE responses are presented in Table 3. Nasal deposition modelling in relation to the formulation and administration parameters will be discussed in a separate section. Prediction profilers are presented in Figures S1–S7.

3.2.1. Formulation of Rheological, Thermogelling, and Spray Properties within the DoE Space

DH-C-BGP formulations prepared according to the design matrix were moderately viscous solutions with zero-shear viscosity ranging between 35.03 ± 0.82 and 232.21 ± 2.30 mPa s. The observed range of the viscosity values is appropriate for simple administration by spraying [2]. In addition, DH-C-BGP systems exhibit shear-thinning behaviour [28], which implies a decrease in viscosity at the applied aerosolisation shear stress.

All DoE samples gelled at the physiological temperature of the nasal mucosa (34 °C) with the gelation time (t_{GEL}) ranging between 0.0 ± 0.0 and 14.9 ± 0.2 min (Table 2), which is below the time of nasal mucus turnover (approximately 20 min) [61]. As expected, the increase in gelation time at 34 °C was coupled with the increase in the temperature of the instant gelation (T_{GEL}), which ranged from 32.2 ± 0.9 to 39.9 ± 0.1 °C within the DoE space. Nonetheless, DoE settings revealed the potential for optimising this crucial formulation property to undergo instant gelation at the temperature of the nasal mucosa.

The spray cone angle (SCA) of the prepared DoE samples was between 15.1 ± 0.3 and 26.6 ± 1.2° (Table 2). The SCA is an important factor that affects nasal deposition and, therefore, the efficacy of a nasally administered drug. The narrow spray cone angles obtained in this study favour targeted nasal deposition [5,57]. The olfactory region of the nasal cavity is a small area (representing ~5–7% of the nasal epithelial surface area) located at the roof of the nasal cavity [62]. It is more likely that the nasal spray will reach the olfactory region if it is concentrated in a narrow plume. Apart from SCA, it is important to note that the deposition in the olfactory region is also affected by the droplet size distribution and the velocity of the applied spray [63].

For all DoE samples, values for D_v10, D_v50, and D_v90 were as follows 23.6 ± 1.4–72.3 ± 3.2 µm, 61.6 ± 4.8–167.6 ± 6.3 µm, and 137.2 ± 7.3–320.6 ± 15.2 µm, respectively (Table 2). The measured DSD values are in accordance with regulatory requirements for nasal sprays (the vast majority of droplets being larger than 10 microns) [31,64]. The span ranged from 1.45 ± 0.06 to 1.89 ± 0.06 (Table 2). A span smaller than 2.0 indicates a monodisperse system with narrow size distribution [65]. Droplets with a narrow size distribution are more likely to deposit uniformly to the targeted area (e.g., olfactory region) in comparison with droplets with a broad size distribution. This could be explained by the fact that droplets with a narrow size distribution have more consistent aerodynamic behaviour and are less likely to undergo deposition by inertial impaction, which can cause uneven deposition in the nasal cavity [56,63,66].

Table 2. Sample sequence from the design of the experiment and the corresponding DC (drug concentration), pH, zero-shear viscosity (η_0), gelation temperature (T_{GEL}), gelation time (t_{GEL}), spray cone angle (SCA), droplet size distribution (D_v10, D_v50, and D_v90) and span, olfactory deposition (OD), and turbinate deposition (TD).

	c_{DH} (mg mL^{-1})	c_C (mg mL^{-1})	IFR * (L min^{-1})	AAH * (°)	DC (mg mL^{-1})	pH	η_0 (mPa s)	T_{GEL} (°)	t_{GEL} (min)	SCA (°)	D_v10 (µm)	D_v50 (µm)	D_v90 (µm)	Span	OD (%)	TD (%)
1	0.30	6.15	0	75	0.30 ± 0.00	7.35 ± 0.00	35.26 ± 1.11	34.2 ± 0.3	1.3 ± 0.7	26.6 ± 1.2	23.6 ± 1.4	61.6 ± 4.8	140.0 ± 7.1	1.9 ± 0.1	65.9 ± 1.6	11.4 ± 1.6
2	0.30	6.15	30	45	0.29 ± 0.00	7.28 ± 0.01	36.49 ± 0.03	33.8 ± 0.4	1.2 ± 0.6	24.9 ± 0.2	26.5 ± 1.3	71.1 ± 9.4	153.5 ± 17.8	1.8 ± 0.0	1.9 ± 1.0	62.7 ± 1.0
3	0.30	6.15	30	75	0.30 ± 0.00	7.24 ± 0.00	35.03 ± 0.82	34.9 ± 0.6	1.0 ± 0.4	25.5 ± 0.7	29.1 ± 2.8	87.0 ± 10.2	184.2 ± 14.9	1.8 ± 0.1	28.3 ± 1.6	60.3 ± 1.6
4	0.30	7.69	0	45	0.31 ± 0.02	7.12 ± 0.02	88.30 ± 1.81	34.2 ± 0.8	1.2 ± 1.0	19.6 ± 0.1	39.2 ± 6.3	120.5 ± 13.2	240.1 ± 19.7	1.7 ± 0.1	3.5 ± 3.3	38.3 ± 3.3
5	0.30	9.23	0	75	0.30 ± 0.00	7.02 ± 0.00	206.37 ± 1.46	33.7 ± 0.1	0.0 ± 0.0	15.5 ± 0.4	69.8 ± 3.7	161.1 ± 5.2	309.7 ± 10.9	1.5 ± 0.0	71.8 ± 0.8	10.5 ± 0.8
6	0.30	9.23	15	45	0.30 ± 0.00	7.06 ± 0.01	194.28 ± 5.27	32.2 ± 0.9	0.0 ± 0.0	16.4 ± 1.6	42.5 ± 4.1	115.2 ± 4.5	226.5 ± 7.1	1.6 ± 0.1	10.6 ± 0.1	63.8 ± 0.1
7	0.30	9.23	30	60	0.30 ± 0.00	7.03 ± 0.01	201.55 ± 0.46	33.4 ± 1.0	0.0 ± 0.0	15.6 ± 0.2	46.8 ± 1.4	129.5 ± 1.5	255.3 ± 1.7	1.6 ± 0.0	21.4 ± 0.3	40.3 ± 0.3
8	0.40	6.15	0	45	0.42 ± 0.02	7.15 ± 0.00	37.08 ± 0.24	36.9 ± 0.2	5.1 ± 0.4	23.1 ± 0.6	25.9 ± 2.3	72.8 ± 9.7	154.8 ± 17.0	1.8 ± 0.0	7.9 ± 3.3	65.1 ± 3.3
9	0.40	7.69	15	60	0.41 ± 0.01	7.09 ± 0.00	90.02 ± 0.38	36.3 ± 0.6	3.2 ± 0.3	19.6 ± 0.3	45.0 ± 8.9	129.3 ± 15.6	250.9 ± 25.9	1.6 ± 0.1	29.4 ± 3.9	49.2 ± 3.9
10	0.40	9.23	30	75	0.40 ± 0.00	7.06 ± 0.01	225.58 ± 3.33	33.7 ± 0.2	0.1 ± 0.2	15.5 ± 0.4	72.0 ± 3.3	166.2 ± 7.6	315.2 ± 17.9	1.5 ± 0.0	35.0 ± 3.4	41.4 ± 3.4
11	0.50	6.15	0	60	0.50 ± 0.00	7.11 ± 0.00	39.70 ± 1.45	39.9 ± 0.1	13.9 ± 0.9	23.3 ± 0.2	23.8 ± 0.9	61.7 ± 4.3	137.2 ± 7.3	1.8 ± 0.0	31.4 ± 5.0	31.7 ± 5.0
12	0.50	6.15	15	75	0.50 ± 0.00	7.21 ± 0.03	39.29 ± 0.59	38.0 ± 0.3	14.3 ± 1.2	23.2 ± 1.1	26.5 ± 1.1	66.3 ± 4.3	141.6 ± 7.3	1.7 ± 0.0	45.6 ± 1.3	26.6 ± 1.3
13	0.50	6.15	30	45	0.49 ± 0.00	7.15 ± 0.00	37.67 ± 0.55	39.2 ± 0.5	14.9 ± 0.2	23.0 ± 0.4	26.7 ± 1.0	68.4 ± 2.6	145.4 ± 4.2	1.7 ± 0.0	6.8 ± 0.3	31.5 ± 0.3
14	0.50	7.69	30	75	0.52 ± 0.02	7.07 ± 0.01	91.15 ± 0.87	38.5 ± 0.1	11.2 ± 0.0	18.7 ± 0.7	47.3 ± 7.3	133.4 ± 11.6	258.2 ± 16.7	1.6 ± 0.1	25.5 ± 5.7	32.9 ± 5.7
15	0.50	9.23	0	45	0.50 ± 0.01	7.03 ± 0.02	209.01 ± 2.98	35.3 ± 0.4	4.4 ± 1.0	16.1 ± 1.0	70.9 ± 14.0	162.3 ± 18.3	306.1 ± 31.0	1.5 ± 0.1	1.9 ± 2.1	60.2 ± 2.1
16	0.50	9.23	0	75	0.50 ± 0.01	7.04 ± 0.00	232.21 ± 2.30	35.7 ± 0.1	2.1 ± 0.4	15.1 ± 0.3	72.3 ± 3.2	167.6 ± 6.3	320.6 ± 15.2	1.5 ± 0.0	22.9 ± 4.7	42.5 ± 4.7
17	0.50	9.23	30	45	0.49 ± 0.00	7.06 ± 0.01	218.45 ± 2.33	35.5 ± 1.6	4.2 ± 0.3	15.6 ± 0.7	61.7 ± 3.8	150.1 ± 7.6	286.6 ± 15.3	1.5 ± 0.0	6.1 ± 1.2	63.9 ± 1.2

c_{DH} = donepezil hydrochloride concentration; c_C = chitosan concentration in the spray-drying solution; IFR = inspiratory flow rate; and AAH = administration angle in relation to horizontal plane. All samples were prepared at a BGP concentration of 188.00 mg mL^{-1}. * Administration parameters related to the deposition studies. Values for the responses are mean ± SD, n = 3, except OD and TD where n = 2.

Regression Modelling

The statistical analysis of the regression models for zero-shear viscosity, gelation time and temperature, spray cone angle, and volume diameters or spray droplets revealed a good fit (Table 3). Each of the aforementioned responses was significantly influenced by DH and CH concentrations (apart or in interaction), confirming the rationale for their consideration as DoE variables.

Impact of Chitosan Concentration

Chitosan concentration revealed linear and/or quadratic impacts on the zero-shear viscosity, gelation time, gelation temperature, spray cone angle, and droplet size distribution (Table 3).

An increase in chitosan concentration led to increased zero-shear viscosity, owing to the entanglement of the polymer chains that led to the limited movement of individual chains and the rise in zero-shear viscosity [67]. At the same time, the increase in C concentration decreased gelation time and temperature, which is in accordance with the literature [41,68]. Namely, due to the entanglements of the polymeric chains, less heat is needed to create a 3D gel network. However, too high a concentration of chitosan can slow down the gelation process. Due to the high chitosan concentration, the solution becomes highly viscous, and the attraction between the chitosan amino groups and the BGP phosphate groups is hindered [51]. In conclusion, setting the right interval of chitosan concentration in the preliminary studies was crucial to obtain valid regression modelling for gelation properties.

The increase in C concentration resulted in a spray cone angle decrease and spray droplet size increase, both of which are related to increased solution viscosity [55,66,69]. Namely, the increased viscosity of the nasal spray led to the decrease in the velocity of the spray droplets as they exited the nozzle. Thereupon, the droplets of the spray spread out less and formed a narrower spray cone angle [69,70]. The increased viscosity resulted in the production of larger droplets in the aerosolisation process [56]. Larger droplets tend to travel in a narrower direction and will ultimately be deposited in the narrower area into which they are directed [66].

Impact of DH Concentration

DH concentration exhibited a significant influence on the monitored rheological thermogelling and spray properties, as a single parameter and/or in combination with the C concentration (Table 3). The increase in DH concentration led to the increase in zero-shear viscosity. This effect can be explained by the presence of DH molecules in the chitosan network that increased the steric repulsion between the polymer chains, increasing the system viscosity [71]. The same reason could be behind the decrease in the spray cone angle that occurred with the increase in DH concentration.

The rising DH concentration in the C-BGP thermosensitive platform increased the gelation time and temperature. As explained above, the addition of the drug in the system increased the viscosity, and the diffusion of the heat was reduced [71]. Moreover, the addition of salt decreased the pKa of the BGP and consequently led to the chitosan's higher degree of ionisation; hence, more heat was needed for gel formation [72].

The interaction between the DH and C concentrations within the derived regression model for the gelation time (Table 3) could be explained by the presumption that the DH affected the steric repulsions between the polymer chains to an extent that was dependent on the C concentration in the system [72–74].

Table 3. The results of the statistical analysis on zero-shear viscosity, gelation time, gelation temperature, spray cone angle, and droplet size distribution within the DoE.

Common DoE Response	Regression Model	Regression Analysis			
		R^2	RMSE	PRESS R^2	PRESS RMSE
Zero-shear viscosity	$\eta_0 = 93.50^* + 5.01 \times c_{DH}{}^* + 87.63 \times c_C{}^* + 3.97 \times c_{DH} \times c_C - 5.52 \times c_{DH}{}^{2\,*} + 36.08 \times c_C{}^{2\,*}$	1.00	6.79	0.99	8.53
Gelation time	$t_{GEL} = 3.60^* + 4.31 \times c_{DH}{}^* - 2.92 \times c_C{}^* - 2.41 \times c_{DH} \times c_C{}^* + 2.41 \times c_{DH}{}^{2\,*} - 1.19 \times c_C{}^{2\,*}$	0.99	0.72	0.97	0.91
Gelation temperature	$T_{GEL}\ (°) = 35.61^* + 1.84 \times c_{DH}{}^* - 1.24 \times c_C{}^*$	0.87	0.86	0.80	0.96
Spray cone angle	$SCA(°) = 19.02^* - 0.65 \times c_{DH}{}^* - 4.27 \times c_C{}^* + 0.57 \times c_{DH} \times c_C{}^* + 0.43 \times c_{DH}{}^2 + 0.58 \times c_C{}^2$	0.99	0.59	0.96	0.76
Droplet size distribution	$D_v10\ (\mu m) = 43.82^* + 3.69 \times c_{DH} + 18.14 \times c_C{}^* + 4.00 \times c_{DH} \times c_C + 0.32 \times c_C{}^2$	0.89	7.25	0.78	8.45
	$D_v50\ (\mu m) = 127.74^* + 4.56 \times c_{DH} + 40.22 \times c_C{}^* + 8.12 \times c_{DH} \times c_C{}^* - 17.69 \times c_C{}^{2\,*}$	0.93	12.70	0.86	14.87
	$D_v90\ (\mu m) = 249.71^* - 6.17 \times c_{DH} + 68.80 \times c_C{}^* + 14.60 \times c_{DH} \times c_C{}^* - 29.94 \times c_C{}^2$	0.92	22.51	0.84	26.41

c_{DH} = donepezil hydrochloride concentration; c_C = chitosan concentration in the spray-drying solution. R^2 = the coefficient of determination; RMSE = root mean square error; and PRESS = predicted residual error sum of squares. * Statistically significant parameters (individual and in interaction; $p < 0.05$).

3.2.2. Nasal Deposition of DH-C-BGP Formulations

A growing number of studies that are tackling nose-to-brain delivery of drugs have emerged over the past decade [2]. However, the question of how to deliver drugs to the small, hindered area of the olfactory zone still remains a major obstacle. For neurological drugs to manifest their optimal therapeutic effect, the goal is to achieve high drug concentrations in the previously mentioned area. Apart from targeting the olfactory region, a direct delivery to the brain is enabled through the trigeminal nerve innervating both the olfactory and respiratory mucosa [75–77].

To ensure the targeted delivery of the nasal drug, deposition studies should be implemented in the early phase of formulation development [2]. In this work, nasal deposition studies were performed using a multi-sectional 3D-printed model based on the CT scan of a patient with healthy airway passages. Inflammatory disorders, such as rhinitis or rhinosinusitis, may influence the nasal deposition pattern [9,78]. However, they are not common for patients with Alzheimer's disease [79]. Hence, a healthy phenotype of the nasal cavity is chosen for this study. The smallest vertical cross-sectional areas (valve region) and the length of the nasal cavity fit into the 'normative range' [32,80]. The model was connected to the respiratory pump to simulate three breathing patterns: no breathing, rest breathing, and deep moderate breathing [81–83]. One nostril was closed during the actuation [55]. For the nasal device, we used an Aptar's VP7 pump, which was previously also used in other studies [56,84].

Deposition in the Olfactory Region

The olfactory region corresponds to the upper turbinate with a small fragment of the middle turbinate and the corresponding part of the nasal septum (Figure 1). The respiratory region is presented by the rest of the turbinates and septum, lined with respiratory epithelium, and innervated by the trigeminal nerve [32].

The olfactory deposition pattern in the 3D-printed nasal cast used in this study was monitored for all DoE samples differing in formulation and administration parameters, and the results ranged from 1.9 ± 2.1 to $71.8 \pm 0.8\%$ (Table 2). Regression modelling produced a model that showed a good fit (R-squared 0.89, RMSE 8.83, Press R-squared 0.59 and Press RMSE 13.25), represented in the following equation:

$$OD\ (\%) = 24.46 - 4.51 \times c_{DH} - 5.74 \times IFR^* + 18.31 \times AAH^* + 4.48 \times c_{DH} \times IFR - 4.38 \times c_{DH} \times AAH - 4.63 \times IFR \times AAH \quad (4)$$

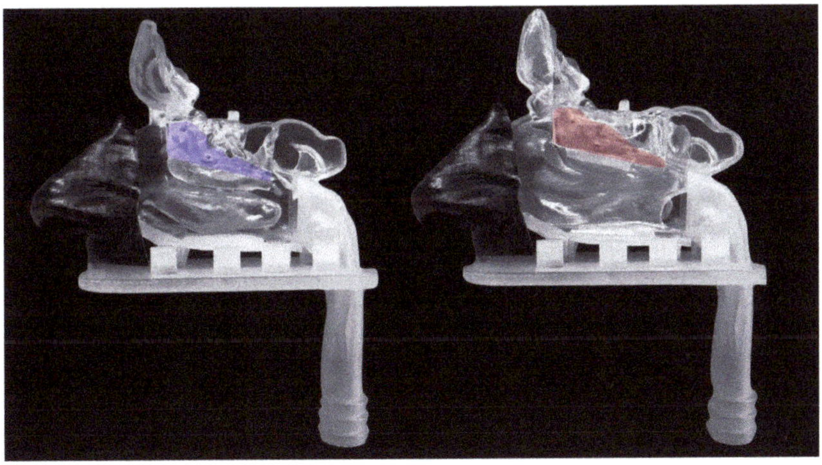

Figure 1. The olfactory region of the 3D-printed nasal cast: superior turbinate with a small portion of the middle turbinate (**left**, in blue) and corresponding segment of the nasal septum (**right**, in red).

The formulation parameters showed no significant influence on the deposition in the olfactory region. However, the equation above indicates that both administration parameters (AAH and IFR) have a significant influence on the olfactory deposition. The increase in the angle of administration from the horizontal plane (from 45° to 75°) increased the fraction of the drug deposited in the olfactory region. For liquid systems, high angles of administration have the potential to pass the nasal valve and aim for the olfactory region [56]. Indeed, in our study, the highest olfactory deposition was achieved at the highest angle of administration (at 75°), which is equal to 71.8 ± 0.8% of the administered dose, proving the assumption that the angle of administration is the critical factor for targeted olfactory deposition of nasal liquid sprays.

The inspiratory flow rate was shown to decrease the olfactory deposition (Equation (4)). This could be due to the pattern of airflow during low to moderate breathing conditions. According to Tian et al. [85], during the moderate breathing flow, most air flows through the turbinate region (middle and inferior meatus), while airflow in the olfactory region stays very low to unchanged. It can be assumed that breathing and airflow steer the formulation from its original direction to the turbinate region and, as a result, a smaller fraction of the drug is deposited in the olfactory region. From the patient's perspective, a 'breath hold' condition is preferred during the administration: less coordination between breathing and actuation leads to lower variability, and thus patient adherence to the therapy is facilitated [12,32].

For nasally administered neurological drugs, 0.01–1% of the orally applied dose needs to be delivered by nose-to-brain direct pathways to achieve its therapeutic potential [47]. In this study, the highest olfactory deposition attained by single-dose actuation represents 0.4% or 0.2% of oral daily dose (5 mg/10 mg) prescribed for the treatment of Alzheimer's patients [86]. It is evident that the drug concentration set by the experimental design, coupled with an appropriate mode of administration, resulted in effective drug dosing. In addition, by nasal administration, the daily dose of donepezil can be reduced, which leads to reduced systemic bioavailability, with the potential to minimise side effects.

Deposition in the Turbinate Region

The fraction of the deposited dose in the turbinate region for all DoE samples ranged between 10.5 ± 0.8 and 65.1 ± 3.3% (Table 2). The model retrieved from the regression modelling showed a good fit (R-squared 0.86, RMSE 9.41, Press R-squared 0.39 and Press RMSE 13.49) and is presented in the following equation:

$$TD\ (\%) = 52.41 + 0.14 \times c_{DH} + 2.38 \times c_C + 5.24 \times IFR - 11.42 \times AAH^* + 8.81 \times c_{DH} \times c_C{}^* - 6.77 \times c_{DH} \times IFR^* - 11.33 \times IFR^2 + 5.18 \times IFR \times AAH \quad (5)$$

The administration angle measured from the horizontal plane had a significant impact on the turbinate deposition. It can be observed that the decrease in AAH led to an increase in the turbinate deposition. This effect has already been described in the literature [10,11,87], and it is explained by the fact that low angles, coupled with appropriate formulation parameters, have a great potential for delivering the formulation to the turbinate region, surpassing the nasal valve.

The inspiratory flow rate exhibited a quadratic effect on the turbinate deposition. A flow rate of 15 L min^{-1} showed a positive influence, which can be explained by the rise in air flow through the turbinate region [85]. The spray is carried by the airflow and the deposition is the result of convection. However, at 30 L min^{-1} airflow, a decrease in turbinate deposition was evident. At high airflows, liquid escapes the streamline and it is deposited by impaction [57]. The observed interaction between the DH concentration and the inspiratory flow rate indicates the combined impact of the formulation and administration parameters on spray aerodynamic properties.

The interaction between the formulation parameters (donepezil and chitosan concentrations) showed a positive effect on the turbinate deposition, which can be related the observed positive effect on solution viscosity and DSD. These characteristics, coupled with appropriate administration parameters, provided a greater potential for deposition beyond the nasal valve [70].

In conclusion, by using QbD methodology, we paved the way for the targeted drug delivery, resulting in an astoundingly high-dose fraction deposited in the olfactory region. So far, to the best of our knowledge, no studies have reported a fractional deposition pattern this high. The precise selection of components and their concentrations, followed by carefully selected administration parameters, resulted in an optimal DH nose-to-brain delivery. DH incorporated into a developed in situ gelling C-BGP platform showed great potential to achieve its therapeutic effect by a simple mode of nasal administration.

3.3. Selection of the Leading DH-C-BGP In Situ Gelling Formulation

The design of the experiments, combining formulation and administration parameters, was used to identify the optimal DH-C-BGP in situ gelling formulation for nasal DH delivery. Guided by QbD principles and based on the identified quality target product profile (QTPP—development of thermosensitive DH-C-BGP platform for safe and efficient nose-to-brain delivery) during the formulation development, we assessed: the quality target product profile, critical quality attributes (CQA—spray characteristics: zero-shear viscosity, DSD, and plume geometry), thermogelling properties (gelation time and temperature), and nasal deposition profile and critical material attributes (CMA—concentration and type of compounds) [46].

The applied approach enabled the identification of the leading formulation, consisting of 0.3 mg mL^{-1} DH, 9.23 mg mL^{-1} C, and 188 mg mL^{-1} BGP (denoted as LF). The LF exhibited immediate gelling at the temperature of the nasal mucosa, and combined with a 75° administration angle measured from the horizontal plane at breath hold, resulted in the highest olfactory deposition (71.8 ± 0.8% of the applied dose). The selected formulation was characterised by a zero-shear viscosity of 206.37 ± 1.46 mPa s, a narrow plume angle (15.5 ± 0.4°), and an appropriate range of droplet sizes; all characteristics that are preferred for targeted olfactory deposition. The LF was further subjected to thorough biopharmaceutical characterisation to account for its performance in contact with the nasal mucosa.

3.4. In-Depth Characterisation of the Leading DH-C-BGP Formulation (LF)

3.4.1. DH In Vitro Release Profile

In vitro release studies were performed under sink conditions using an automated Franz diffusion system. The DH release profile from the LF was compared with two control samples: (i) the DH-C-BGP in situ gelling system differing from the LF in C concentration (control formulation—CF; chitosan concentrations in the leading and control samples were 9.23 and 6.15 mg mL^{-1}, respectively) and (ii) the corresponding aqueous DH solution. SNF was used as a physiologically relevant acceptor medium. In order to stimulate the conditions at the nasal mucosa, the membranes placed between the donor and acceptor compartments were soaked in SNF for 15 min prior to the experiment, at 34 °C [88]. In vitro release profiles of the tested samples are presented in Figure 2.

The drug release behaviour was studied over a 5 h period. It was observed that the DH release rate decreased in the following order: DH solution > CF > LF. The dissimilarity of all compared DH release profiles was confirmed using an f_2 similarity criteria (f_2 = 36.3 for the LF vs. the CF, f_2 = 21.4 for the LF vs. the DH solution, and f_2 = 35.4 for the CF vs. the DH solution).

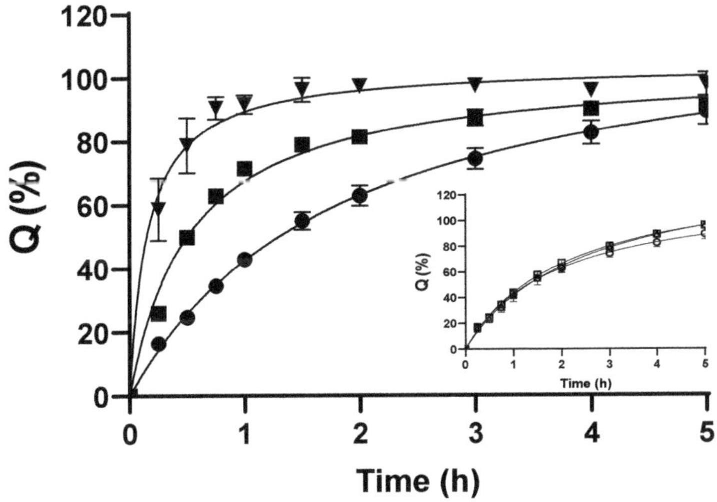

Figure 2. In vitro release profiles from the leading DH-C-BGP formulation (LF—circle) and the corresponding DH-C-BGP control formulation (CF—square) compared with the dissolution of the DH solution (reverse triangle). Graph insert: in vitro release profile of the LF immediately after preparation (empty circle), upon 30 days of storage (empty triangle), and upon 90 days of storage (empty square). Data are expressed as the mean ± SD, n = 3.

Both the LF and the CF formed a gel at 34 °C. During the formation of the gel, its structure and viscosity determine the drug diffusion rate through the gel matrix and its release from the formulation [88,89]. Indeed, both thermosensitive formulations showed prolonged release (32.5 ± 4.0% and 62.9 ± 1.0% in 45 min for the LF and the CF, respectively) in comparison with the DH solution (90.6 ± 3.5% of the drug released in 45 min).

Due to different C concentrations and, consequently, different gelling times and viscosities, distinct release profiles for the LF and the CF were observed. The lower initial burst of DH from the LF can be explained by the fact that it exhibited instant gelation at 34 °C (i.e., the drug is entrapped in the gel from the beginning of the experiment), while the CF turned to gel after 1.0–1.3 min of exposure to 34 °C (Table 2). The overall slower drug release profile observed for the LF can be ascribed to higher viscosity and diffusion resistance of the gel prepared at higher chitosan concentrations [6,43,90]. The resultant sustained and efficient drug release, when coupled with prolonged residence time at the deposition site, bears the potential to increase drug absorption and bioavailability at the action site.

3.4.2. Mucoadhesion

Increasing nasal residence time is a crucial task for an efficient nasal drug delivery. It can be achieved by the sol–gel transition of the formulation in contact with the nasal mucosa and is also promoted by the use of mucoadhesive agents. These agents interact with mucins in the mucus layer, decreasing mucociliary clearance and improving formulation mucosal affinity [91].

A mucoadhesion study of the LF was carried out using nasal porcine mucosa, on account of its physiological and histological similarity to human mucosa [92]. The following control samples were employed: (i) control formulation—CF (gelation time at 34 °C of the CF is 1.0–1.3 min (Table 2); and (ii) corresponding aqueous DH solution (DH). Mucoadhesion of the CF was determined: (i) under the described test conditions applied for all samples (sol–gel transition of the CF appeared in the last third of the testing time), and employing longer thermostating (2 min) to ensure gelation before the start of the test (CF_{gel}). Filter paper served as a negative control (NC). The obtained results are presented in Figure 3.

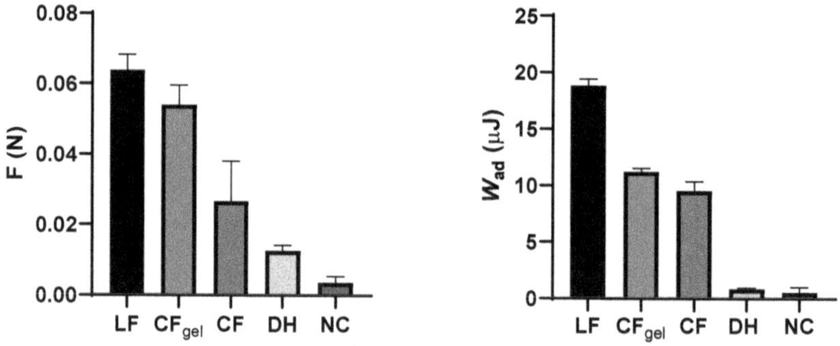

Figure 3. Maximum detachment force (*F*; **left**) and work of adhesion (W_{ad}; **right**) of the leading DH-C-BGP formulation (LF), the control DH-C-BGP formulation (CF), the control DH-C-BGP formulation after gelation (CF_{gel}), the DH aqueous solution (DH), and filter paper as the negative control (NC). Data are expressed as the mean ± SD, n = 3.

The LF showed prominent mucoadhesive properties, with a five-fold higher maximum detachment force and a 20-fold higher work of adhesion in relation to the drug solution. The LF presented a 2.4-fold higher maximum detachment force and 2.0-fold higher work of adhesion in relation to the CF formulation. The obtained results indicate a largely improved nasal retention potential of the LF in relation to the DH simple solution and an impact of gelation time and chitosan concentration on its mucoadhesive performance. To differentiate between these two effects, CF_{gel} was also analysed for its mucoadhesive properties. Comparing the results for the CF and the CF_{gel}, it was observed that the sol–gel transition contributed significantly to the detachment force ($p = 0.019$). At the same time, the comparison of the leading and control gelled formulations (LF and CF_{gel}) suggested a significant influence of chitosan concentration on the work of adhesion ($p < 0.001$).

The chitosan's mechanism of mucoadhesion is a result of alectrostatic interaction between positively charged amino groups of chitosan and negatively charged mucins of the nasal mucosa [93]. It is important to note that the pH of the leading formulation is about neutral (pH = 7.02). At this pH, amino groups of chitosan are not fully protonated and the percentage of chitosan ionisation at the pH of the formulation can be calculated according to the Henderson–Hasselbalch equation [94]. Considering the pKa of chitosan (pKa = 6.5 [95]), the percentage of ionisation of chitosan in the DH-C-BGP is 23.1%. Nonetheless, a moderate electrostatic interaction might contribute to a better mucosal tolerability of chitosan [42,96].

Chitosan also interacts with mucin through other attractive forces—hydrogen bonding and hydrophobic interaction [97]. Higher values of detachment force and work of adhesion for formulations with higher chitosan concentrations can be explained by all the above-mentioned mechanisms of chitosan mucoadhesivness.

3.4.3. In Vitro Biocompatibility

Excipients used in the formulation of DH thermosensitive gelling systems are known to be safe—applied individually or in combination [27,29,43]. As stated earlier, chitosan is a non-toxic and biocompatible polymer [98] and BGP is a substance naturally present in the human body that is also approved by the Food and Drug Administration (FDA) as a parenteral phosphate supplement [51].

The human airway epithelial Calu-3 cell line was used to evaluate the biocompatibility of the LF. The LF was diluted with HBSS/HEPES (pH = 7.0) in a 1:1 volume ratio, resulting in DH, C, and BGP concentrations of 0.15 mg mL^{-1}, 4.62 mg mL^{-1}, and 94.00 mg mL^{-1}, respectively. The DH solution (0.05 and 0.25 mg mL^{-1}) and BGP solution (94.00 mg mL^{-1}) served as controls. Pure HBSS/HEPES (pH = 7.0) served as a negative control. The cells' incubation temperature (37 °C) induced the gel formation of the leading formulation. No cytotoxic effect was observed in any of the tested formulations. The viability of the Calu-3 cells was above 80% in relation to the control (86.0 ± 1.4% for the LF; 86.4 ± 2.5% and 99.1 ± 9.9% for 0.05 mg mL^{-1} and 0.25 mg mL^{-1} for the DH solutions, respectively; and 95.7 ± 9.7% for the BGP solution). At the pH of the leading formulation, chitosan is not fully protonated, as discussed in Section 3.4.2. Positive amino groups of chitosan interact with negatively charged cell membranes and this interaction can lead to a reduction in cell viability. However, a lower extent of chitosan protonation at a higher pH, or shielding the positive charges on the chitosan molecule, can result in a decreased chitosan cytotoxicity [96,99]. The obtained results showed appropriate biocompatibility of the LF at the Calu-3 cell model. The selected compound concentrations are recognised to be optimal for further permeability studies.

3.4.4. In Vitro DH Permeability

Permeability studies were performed using Calu-3 cells grown at an air–liquid interface. Calu-3 cells form monolayers that adequately simulate the nasal epithelial barrier considering its ultrastructure, mucus production, and barrier properties [100], while providing benefits of immortalised cell lines including high reproducibility and genetic homogeneity [101]. Recently, the Calu-3 cell model was successfully used by our group to screen chitosan-based powder formulations intended for DH nose-to-brain delivery [12].

In this work, the permeability study was designed to screen the permeation enhancing potential of the LF compared with the DH solution and to differentiate between the effect of chitosan and hyperosmotic conditions on monolayer integrity and the DH permeation profile. Thus, the following samples were tested on Calu-3 cell monolayers: (i) the LF mixed with HBSS/HEPES (pH = 7.0) in a ratio of 1:1, v/v (final DH concentration 0.15 mg mL^{-1}; osmolality 750 ± 3 mOsm/kg), and (ii) the DH solution in hyperosmolar HBSS/HEPES (pH = 7.0) (DH concentration 0.15 mg mL^{-1}; osmolality 745 ± 9 mOsm/kg) and DH solution in HBSS/HEPES (pH = 7.0) (DH concentration 0.25 mg mL^{-1}; osmolality 340 ± 1 mOsm/kg). The permeability study was performed under sink conditions, and assuming predominant passive paracellular transport of the hydrophilic drug, no influence of DH concentration in the donor/receiver compartment on DH permeation could be expected [102,103]. Transepithelial electric resistance (TEER) was monitored over the experiment and up to 24 h upon the start of the experiment, as an indicator of the monolayer integrity.

The results of permeability studies of DH from the tested samples across the Calu-3 cell monolayer are given in Table 4. The P_{app} value of the DH from the solution in

HBSS/HEPES (pH 7.0) (DH concentration 0.25 mg mL^{-1}; P_{app} = 3.38 × 10^{-5} cm s^{-1}) evaluated in this study is in line with the previously obtained P_{app} value for the DH solution in HBSS-Ca^{2+}/HEPES (pH = 6.0) (DH concentration 0.008 mg mL^{-1}; osmolality 321 ± 1 mOsm/kg; P_{app} = 3.59 × 10^{-5} cm s^{-1}) using the same cell model [12].

Table 4. Osmolality and DH apparent permeability coefficients (P_{app}) across the Calu-3 monolayer of the LF, the DH solution in hyperosmolar HBSS/HEPES (pH = 7.0), and the DH solution in HBSS/HEPES (pH = 7.0).

Sample	Osmolality (mOsm kg^{-1})	P_{app} (10^{-5} cm s^{-1})	Attenuation Factor
Leading DH-C-BGP formulation (LF)	750 ± 3	4.96 ± 0.84	1.47
DH solution in hyperosmolar HBSS/HEPES (pH = 7.0)	745 ± 9	3.31 ± 2.60	0.98
DH solution in HBSS/HEPES (pH = 7.0)	340 ± 1	3.38 ± 3.23	-
HBSS/HEPES (pH = 7.0)	312 ± 2	-	-

The attenuation factor was calculated as the ratio between the P_{app} value of the LF or DH solution in hyperosmolar HBSS/HEPES (pH = 7.0) and the P_{app} value of the DH solution in HBSS/HEPES (pH = 7.0). Values are the mean ± SD, n = 3.

The P_{app} value of the DH from the LF was 1.47-fold higher than that of the DH solution, confirming the formulation's permeation-enhancing effect. Considering the prolonged DH release observed in in vitro release studies, it may be concluded that the permeation-enhancing effect was even higher than described with the calculated attenuation factor. Namely, in the case of the LF, only the released fraction of the drug was available for permeation at each time point, while in the case of drug solution, the total dose of dissolved drug is instantly available for permeating the cell monolayer [12,104]. The permeation-enhancing effect of the LF can be explained by the observed decrease in the TEER value of the cell monolayer (Figure 4), indicating the loosening of the barrier properties and favouring paracellular transport of a hydrophilic drug.

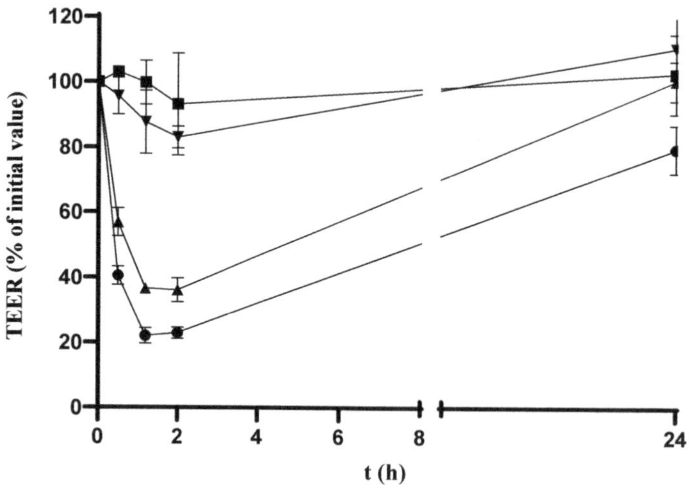

Figure 4. Trans-epithelial electric resistance (TEER) values of the Calu-3 cell monolayer during the study of DH permeability from the LF (circle), the DH solution in hyperosmolar HBSS/HEPES (pH = 7.0) (triangle), the DH solution in HBSS/HEPES (pH = 7.0) (square), and HBSS/HEPES (pH = 7.0) (reverse triangle). Data are expressed as the mean ± SD, n = 3.

The reversible nature of the LF effect on the barrier integrity was confirmed by the TEER increase to 80 ± 7% of the initial value 22 h after the formulation was washed off the cell monolayer. The observed TEER decrease was ascribed to the reversible opening of the tight junctions resulting from a combined effect of the chitosan and the hyperosmolality of the formulation. Such a conclusion was supported by a more pronounced TEER decrease observed for the leading hyperosmolar chitosan-based formulation than for the chitosan-free hyperosmolar DH solution (Figure 4). Interestingly, the hyperosmolar DH solution showed no permeation-enhancing effect compared with the isoosmolar DH solution (attenuation factor = 0.98), stressing the role of chitosan in promoting DH permeation across the cell monolayer barrier.

3.4.5. Slug Mucosal Irritation Assay

Due to the intense contact of the applied nasal formulation and the sensitive nasal mucosa, certain nasal discomfort, described as stinging, itching, and burning (SIB) sensations, may occur. These adverse effects affect patient compliance, and consequently the outcome of the treatment [105]. For this reason, it is very important to assess the formulation's potential for irritation in the early stage of formulation development. Adriaens and Remon [106] developed a simple and inexpensive method to predict the formulation's potential irritancy on the mucosal surfaces. The slug mucosal irritation (SMI) assay uses slugs of species *Arion lusitanicus* as a test organism to assess the irritation potency. Slugs are placed on a tested substance. If the formulation causes irritation, the slug produces mucus as a protective mechanism [107]. Based on the total amount of the produced mucus, and in relation to the positive and negative controls, it is possible to assess the irritation potential of the formulation and predict the discomfort the formulation may cause to the patient [37].

We performed the SMI assay as described earlier [37]. The mucus production after exposing the slug to the LF was compared with the results of the SMI assay performed on the positive control (maximum irritation) and the negative control (no irritation). The results of the performed SMI assay are presented in Table 5.

Table 5. Total mucus production from the three contact periods in the SMI assay expressed as a percentage of the initial body weight of the slugs. The results are expressed as the mean ± SD, n = 3.

Sample	Total Mucus Production (%)
Leading DH-C-BGP formulation (LF)	6.64 ± 1.04
PBS—negative control	0.48 ± 1.50
BAC 1% (*w*/*v*)—positive control	17.64 ± 4.33

The mucus production for the LF was 2.7 times lower compared with the BAC 1% (*w*/*v*), which is used as a marker for severe discomfort [108]. The observed LF-induced mucus production was comparable to a previously reported result obtained for mannitol (sieved fraction 32–90 µm; 6.30 ± 0.61%), employing the same SMI assay. The observed mucus production was ascribed to a size-related dissolution rate and osmotic effect [37].

The tolerability and formulation potential to cause irritation can be ascribed to formulation pH, constituents, and osmolality [105]. Considering the relatively high mucus production previously observed for carboxymethyl chitosan powder [37], it may be assumed that the neutral pH of the LF contributed to its tolerability, as a neutral pH renders the chitosan charge density to a moderately low value.

The hypertonic nature of thermosensitive chitosan/polyol-phosphate in situ gelling systems has already been reported [43,51,109]. Lenoir et al. tested a hypertonic NaCl solution (2.6%, *w*/*v*), characterised by similar osmolality to the LF, employing a human nose irritation test [105]. After 5 min of the nasal exposure, 54% of the participants did not feel discomfort, while 41.5% experienced mild discomfort. Ten minutes after the exposure, 79% of the participants did not feel discomfort anymore.

It can be concluded that the LF in the SMI assay showed an acceptable irritability profile, demonstrating its potential for safe nasal delivery.

3.4.6. Stability Profile

The physicochemical stability of the LF was monitored over a period of 3 months. The formulation was stored in an impermeable container at 5 ± 3 °C and inspected for drug concentration, rheological and gelling properties (zero-shear viscosity, and gelation temperature and time), spray characteristics, and drug release profile. Stability studies revealed no significant change in any of the tested characteristics, confirming the suitability of the formulation stability profile (Table 6). The f_2 criteria for similarity estimation revealed no significant difference between release profiles of the LF determined after 0, 30, and 90 days of storage at described conditions (Table 6; Figure 2, insert).

Table 6. Three-month stability data for the leading DH-C-BGP in situ gelling formulation.

Inspected Property	Immediately after Preparation	After 30 Days	After 90 Days
DC (mg mL^{-1})	0.30 ± 0.00	0.30 ± 0.00	0.30 ± 0.01
η_0 (mPa s)	206.37 ± 1.46	192.28 ± 11.57	211.02 ± 6.53
T_{GEL} (°)	33.7 ± 0.1	33.9 ± 0.3	34.9 ± 0.1
t_{GEL} (min)	0.0 ± 0.0	0.0 ± 0.0	0.0 ± 0.0
D_v10 (μm)	69.8 ± 3.7	74.6 ± 6.0	70.2 ± 1.4
D_v50 (μm)	161.1 ± 5.2	167.2 ± 4.5	166.5 ± 2.6
D_v90 (μm)	309.7 ± 10.9	313.1 ± 3.9	317.4 ± 7.7
Span	1.5 ± 0.0	1.4 ± 0.1	1.5 ± 0.0
SCA (°)	15.5 ± 0.4	15.6 ± 0.2	15.8 ± 0.1
f_2	-	72.7	70.2

DC = drug concentration; η_0 = zero-shear viscosity; T_{GEL} = gelation temperature; t_{GEL} = gelation time; D_v10; D_v50 and D_v90 = droplet size distribution; SCA = spray cone angle; and f_2 = similarity factor of in vitro release profiles after 30 and 90 days compared with the release profile immediately after preparation.

3.5. Discussing the Potential of the Developed DH Liquid Formulation in Comparison with the DH Powder Formulation

In this study, a thermoresponsive chitosan-based in situ gelling system was proven to be a promising platform for an efficient nasal DH delivery. Recently, our research group developed a comparable nasal spray-dried DH formulation, embedding the well-known advantages of a dry nasal form [12]. The applied complementary approach, including the development of both powder and liquid DH delivery platforms, is beneficial considering the patient perspective, as patients still prefer liquid formulations over nasal powders [110, 111]. This aspect is particularly important in the targeted patient population since the adherence of AD patients is linked to the tolerability of drug therapy [112].

The comparison between powder and liquid formulations, based on their advantages and disadvantages, is presented in the literature [2,5]. However, to the best of our knowledge, there are no reports in which the comparability between powder and liquid platforms of the same active substance has been discussed, particularly in terms of nasal deposition profiles.

Both technological platforms, apart from being of simple production and acceptable stability profile, allowed for the optimisation of physicochemical, biopharmaceutical, and nasal deposition properties, which are crucial for an efficient DH nose-to-brain delivery. Indeed, a high olfactory deposition was obtained with both liquid (71.8% of the applied dose) and powder (65.5% of the applied dose) formulations [12], despite distinct aerodynamic properties of dispersed droplets and dried particles. The direct comparison of deposition profiles is feasible since the same 3D-printed model of the nasal cavity was used for the evaluation of both types of formulations. The high olfactory deposition was achieved by a fine-tuning of administration parameters in relation to formulation-specific properties. Generally, different administration angles from the horizontal plane were found to favour an olfactory deposition of aerosolised droplets and dry particles, while inspiratory airflow reduced the olfactory deposition of both formulations. Complex regression models for olfactory deposition efficiency, coupling formulation properties, and mode of administration stress the need for deposition considerations in the early phase of the formulation development.

Finally, the comparison of distinct liquid and powder DH formulations using an animal model is needed to rate their in vivo performance in terms of potentiating DH brain bioavailability.

4. Conclusions

A thermogelling chitosan-based donepezil formulation was prepared by a fast, single-step method applicable in industrial settings. The manufacturing process enabled the fine-tuning of the formulation parameters that resulted in a final product of desirable characteristics. Droplet size, rheology, and sprayability were optimised features of the nasal product that, coupled with appropriate administration parameters, resulted in an efficient olfactory deposition (71.8% of the applied dose), which is crucial for the therapeutic outcome of nasally applied donepezil. The optimised formulation proved to be stable at the observed period of time and showed biopharmaceutical properties, suggesting the potential for safe nasal administration, prolonged retention at the nasal mucosa, sustained DH release, and increased permeability across the epithelial barrier. The obtained results indicate the formulation potential to promote DH brain bioavailability and support the continuation of studies aimed at gaining in vivo proof-of-concept and comparison of distinct liquid and powder DH formulations.

Supplementary Materials: The following supporting information can be downloaded at: https://www.mdpi.com/article/10.3390/pharmaceutics15061660/s1.

Author Contributions: Conceptualization, A.H., M.P., L.N.N. and D.Š.; methodology, A.H., M.P., L.N.N., D.Š., I.U., C.J.B., I.P., J.L., M.S.K., M.T., R.S., D.Z. and L.K.; validation, M.P., C.J.B. and A.H.; formal analysis, M.P., L.N.N., D.Š., I.U., C.J.B., M.T., R.S. and A.H.; investigation, M.P., L.N.N., C.J.B., I.P., J.L., M.T., R.S. and A.H.; resources, A.H., J.L., M.S.K., R.S., D.Z. and L.K.; data curation, M.P., I.P., J.L., D.Š., I.U. and A.H.; writing—original draft, A.H., M.P., L.N.N., D.Š. and I.U.; writing—review and editing, M.P., L.N.N., D.Š., I.U., C.J.B., I.P., J.L., M.S.K., M.T., R.S., D.Z., L.K. and A.H.; visualization, M.P., L.N.N. and A.H.; supervision, A.H. and R.S.; project administration, A.H.; and funding acquisition, A.H. All authors have read and agreed to the published version of the manuscript.

Funding: This work was supported in part by the Croatian Science Foundation under the project UIP-2017-05-4592, the European Social Fund under the Croatian Science Foundation project DOK-2020-01-2473, and by the project FarmInova (KK.01.1.1.02.0021) funded by the European Regional Development Fund.

Institutional Review Board Statement: The development of the nasal cavity model based on a CT scan of a patient was carried out following the rules of the Declaration of Helsinki. The protocol was approved by the Ethics Committee of the Sisters of Charity Hospital (project identification code: EP-9941/19-3) and the Ethics Committee of the University of Zagreb Faculty of Pharmacy and Biochemistry (class: 643-02/19-01/02; registry number: 251-62-03-19-43).

Informed Consent Statement: The patient gave informed consent for inclusion before exporting data for the reconstruction of the nasal cavity and 3D printing.

Data Availability Statement: Not applicable.

Acknowledgments: The authors thank Miodrag Katalenić and Mladen Šercer (Cateh d.o.o., Zagreb) for help in the production of the 3D nasal cavity model and AptarGroup Inc. for providing us with the VP7 device used for nasal deposition studies.

Conflicts of Interest: The authors declare no conflict of interest.

References

1. Giunchedi, P.; Gavini, E.; Bonferoni, M.C. Nose-to-Brain Delivery. *Pharmaceutics* **2020**, *12*, 138. [CrossRef] [PubMed]
2. Deruyver, L.; Rigaut, C.; Lambert, P.; Haut, B.; Goole, J. The Importance of Pre-Formulation Studies and of 3D-Printed Nasal Casts in the Success of a Pharmaceutical Product Intended for Nose-to-Brain Delivery. *Adv. Drug Deliv. Rev.* **2021**, *175*, 113826. [CrossRef] [PubMed]

3. Laffleur, F.; Bauer, B. Progress in Nasal Drug Delivery Systems. *Int. J. Pharm.* **2021**, *607*, 120994. [CrossRef] [PubMed]
4. Scherließ, R. Nasal Formulations for Drug Administration and Characterization of Nasal Preparations in Drug Delivery. *Ther. Deliv.* **2020**, *11*, 183–191. [CrossRef] [PubMed]
5. Salade, L.; Wauthoz, N.; Goole, J.; Amighi, K. How to Characterize a Nasal Product. The State of the Art of in Vitro and Ex Vivo Specific Methods. *Int. J. Pharm.* **2019**, *561*, 47–65. [CrossRef] [PubMed]
6. Agrawal, M.; Saraf, S.; Saraf, S.; Dubey, S.K.; Puri, A.; Gupta, U.; Kesharwani, P.; Ravichandiran, V.; Kumar, P.; Naidu, V.G.M.; et al. Stimuli-Responsive In Situ Gelling System for Nose-to-Brain Drug Delivery. *J. Control. Release* **2020**, *327*, 235–265. [CrossRef]
7. Formica, M.L.; Real, D.A.; Picchio, M.L.; Catlin, E.; Donnelly, R.F.; Paredes, A.J. On a Highway to the Brain: A Review on Nose-to-Brain Drug Delivery Using Nanoparticles. *Appl. Mater. Today* **2022**, *29*, 101631. [CrossRef]
8. Pandey, V.; Gadeval, A.; Asati, S.; Jain, P.; Jain, N.; Roy, R.K.; Tekade, M.; Soni, V.; Tekade, R.K. Formulation Strategies for Nose-to-Brain Delivery of Therapeutic Molecules. In *Drug Delivery Systems*; Tekade, R.K., Ed.; Elsevier: Amsterdam, The Netherlands, 2020; pp. 291–332.
9. Le Guellec, S.; Ehrmann, S.; Vecellio, L. In Vitro–in Vivo Correlation of Intranasal Drug Deposition. *Adv. Drug Deliv. Rev.* **2021**, *170*, 340–352. [CrossRef]
10. Nižić, L.; Ugrina, I.; Špoljarić, D.; Saršon, V.; Kučuk, M.S.; Pepić, I.; Hafner, A. Innovative Sprayable in Situ Gelling Fluticasone Suspension: Development and Optimization of Nasal Deposition. *Int. J. Pharm.* **2019**, *563*, 445–456. [CrossRef]
11. Nižić Nodilo, L.; Perkušić, M.; Ugrina, I.; Špoljarić, D.; Jakobušić Brala, C.; Amidžić Klarić, D.; Lovrić, J.; Saršon, V.; Safundžić Kučuk, M.; Zadravec, D.; et al. In Situ Gelling Nanosuspension as an Advanced Platform for Fluticasone Propionate Nasal Delivery. *Eur. J. Pharm. Biopharm.* **2022**, *175*, 27–42. [CrossRef]
12. Perkušić, M.; Nižić Nodilo, L.; Ugrina, I.; Špoljarić, D.; Jakobušić Brala, C.; Pepić, I.; Lovrić, J.; Matijašić, G.; Gretić, M.; Zadravec, D.; et al. Tailoring Functional Spray-Dried Powder Platform for Efficient Donepezil Nose-to-Brain Delivery. *Int. J. Pharm.* **2022**, *624*, 122038. [CrossRef]
13. Agrawal, M.; Saraf, S.; Saraf, S.; Antimisiaris, S.G.; Chougule, M.B.; Shoyele, S.A.; Alexander, A. Nose-to-Brain Drug Delivery: An Update on Clinical Challenges and Progress towards Approval of Anti-Alzheimer Drugs. *J. Control. Release* **2018**, *281*, 139–177. [CrossRef]
14. Knopman, D.S.; Amieva, H.; Petersen, R.C.; Chételat, G.; Holtzman, D.M.; Hyman, B.T.; Nixon, R.A.; Jones, D.T. Alzheimer Disease. *Nat. Rev. Dis. Prim.* **2021**, *7*, 33. [CrossRef]
15. Prabakaran, A.; Agrawal, M.; Dethe, M.R.; Ahmed, H.; Yadav, A.; Gupta, U.; Alexander, A. Nose-to-Brain Drug Delivery for the Treatment of Alzheimer's Disease: Current Advancements and Challenges. *Expert Opin. Drug Deliv.* **2022**, *19*, 87–102. [CrossRef]
16. Adlimoghaddam, A.; Neuendorff, M.; Roy, B.; Albensi, B.C. A Review of Clinical Treatment Considerations of Donepezil in Severe Alzheimer's Disease. *CNS Neurosci. Ther.* **2018**, *24*, 876–888. [CrossRef]
17. Gu, F.; Fan, H.; Cong, Z.; Li, S.; Wang, Y.; Wu, C. Preparation, Characterization, and in Vivo Pharmacokinetics of Thermosensitive in Situ Nasal Gel of Donepezil Hydrochloride. *Acta Pharm.* **2020**, *70*, 411–422. [CrossRef]
18. Espinoza, L.C.; Guaya, D.; Calpena, A.C.; Perotti, R.M.; Halbaut, L.; Sosa, L.; Brito-Llera, A.; Mallandrich, M. Comparative Study of Donepezil-Loaded Formulations for the Treatment of Alzheimer's Disease by Nasal Administration. *Gels* **2022**, *8*, 715. [CrossRef]
19. Bhavna; Md, S.; Ali, M.; Ali, R.; Bhatnagar, A.; Baboota, S.; Ali, J. Donepezil Nanosuspension Intended for Nose to Brain Targeting: In Vitro and in Vivo Safety Evaluation. *Int. J. Biol. Macromol.* **2014**, *67*, 418–425. [CrossRef]
20. Al Asmari, A.K.; Ullah, Z.; Tariq, M.; Fatani, A. Preparation, Characterization, and in Vivo Evaluation of Intranasally Administered Liposomal Formulation of Donepezil. *Drug Des. Dev. Ther.* **2016**, *10*, 205–215. [CrossRef]
21. de Souza, I.F.F.; Dos Santos, T.Q.; Placido, R.V.; Mangerona, B.A.; Carvalho, F.C.; Boralli, V.B.; Ruela, A.L.M.; Pereira, G.R. The Liquid Crystalline Phase Behaviour of a Nasal Formulation Modifies the Brain Disposition of Donepezil in Rats in the Treatment of Alzheimer's Disease. *Colloids Surf. B Biointerfaces* **2021**, *203*, 111721. [CrossRef]
22. Espinoza, L.C.; Silva-Abreu, M.; Clares, B.; Rodríguez-Lagunas, M.J.; Halbaut, L.; Cañas, M.-A.; Calpena, A.C. Formulation Strategies to Improve Nose-to-Brain Delivery of Donepezil. *Pharmaceutics* **2019**, *11*, 64. [CrossRef]
23. Akel, H.; Csóka, I.; Ambrus, R.; Bocsik, A.; Gróf, I.; Mészáros, M.; Szecskó, A.; Kozma, G.; Veszelka, S.; Deli, M.A.; et al. In Vitro Comparative Study of Solid Lipid and PLGA Nanoparticles Designed to Facilitate Nose-to-Brain Delivery of Insulin. *Int. J. Mol. Sci.* **2021**, *22*, 13258. [CrossRef] [PubMed]
24. Espinoza, L.C.; Vacacela, M.; Clares, B.; García, M.L.; Fabrega, M.-J.; Calpena, A.C. Development of a Nasal Donepezil-Loaded Microemulsion for the Treatment of Alzheimer's Disease: In Vitro and Ex Vivo Characterization. *CNS Neurol. Disord. Drug Targets* **2018**, *17*, 43–53. [CrossRef] [PubMed]
25. Kaur, P.; Garg, T.; Rath, G.; Goyal, A.K. In Situ Nasal Gel Drug Delivery: A Novel Approach for Brain Targeting through the Mucosal Membrane. *Artif. Cells Nanomed. Biotechnol.* **2016**, *44*, 1167–1176. [CrossRef] [PubMed]
26. Casettari, L.; Illum, L. Chitosan in Nasal Delivery Systems for Therapeutic Drugs. *J. Control. Release* **2014**, *190*, 189–200. [CrossRef]
27. Kolawole, O.M.; Cook, M.T. In Situ Gelling Drug Delivery Systems for Topical Drug Delivery. *Eur. J. Pharm. Biopharm.* **2023**, *184*, 36–49. [CrossRef]
28. Gholizadeh, H.; Cheng, S.; Pozzoli, M.; Messerotti, E.; Traini, D.; Young, P.; Kourmatzis, A.; Ong, H.X. Smart Thermosensitive Chitosan Hydrogel for Nasal Delivery of Ibuprofen to Treat Neurological Disorders. *Expert Opin. Drug Deliv.* **2019**, *16*, 453–466. [CrossRef]

29. Kolawole, O.M.; Lau, W.M.; Khutoryanskiy, V.V. Chitosan/β-Glycerophosphate in Situ Gelling Mucoadhesive Systems for Intravesical Delivery of Mitomycin-C. *Int. J. Pharm. X* **2019**, *1*, 100007. [CrossRef]
30. Supper, S.; Anton, N.; Seidel, N.; Riemenschnitter, M.; Schoch, C.; Vandamme, T. Rheological Study of Chitosan/Polyol-Phosphate Systems: Influence of the Polyol Part on the Thermo-Induced Gelation Mechanism. *Langmuir* **2013**, *29*, 10229–10237. [CrossRef]
31. Center for Drug Evaluation and Research. Bioavailability and Bioequivalence Studies for Nasal Aerosols and Nasal Sprays for Local Action. Available online: https://www.fda.gov/regulatory-information/search-fda-guidance-documents/bioavailability-and-bioequivalence-studies-nasal-aerosols-and-nasal-sprays-local-action (accessed on 15 March 2023).
32. Nižić Nodilo, L.; Ugrina, I.; Špoljarić, D.; Amidžić Klarić, D.; Jakobušić Brala, C.; Perkušić, M.; Pepić, I.; Lovrić, J.; Saršon, V.; Safundžić Kučuk, M.; et al. A Dry Powder Platform for Nose-to-Brain Delivery of Dexamethasone: Formulation Development and Nasal Deposition Studies. *Pharmaceutics* **2021**, *13*, 795. [CrossRef]
33. Pappa, H.; Farrú, R.; Vilanova, P.O.; Palacios, M.; Pizzorno, M.T. A New HPLC Method to Determine Donepezil Hydrochloride in Tablets. *J. Pharm. Biomed. Anal.* **2002**, *27*, 177–182. [CrossRef]
34. EMA ICH Q2(R2) Validation of Analytical Procedures—Scientific Guideline. Available online: https://www.ema.europa.eu/en/ich-q2r2-validation-analytical-procedures-scientific-guideline (accessed on 1 April 2023).
35. Fachel, F.N.S.; Medeiros-Neves, B.; Dal Prá, M.; Schuh, R.S.; Veras, K.S.; Bassani, V.L.; Koester, L.S.; Henriques, A.T.; Braganhol, E.; Teixeira, H.F. Box-Behnken Design Optimization of Mucoadhesive Chitosan-Coated Nanoemulsions for Rosmarinic Acid Nasal Delivery–In Vitro Studies. *Carbohydr. Polym.* **2018**, *199*, 572–582. [CrossRef]
36. Soni, V.; Pandey, V.; Tiwari, R.; Asati, S.; Tekade, R.K. Chapter 13—Design and Evaluation of Ophthalmic Delivery Formulations. In *Basic Fundamentals of Drug Delivery*; Tekade, R.K., Ed.; Advances in Pharmaceutical Product Development and Research; Academic Press: Cambridge, MA, USA, 2019; pp. 473–538. ISBN 978-0-12-817909-3.
37. Trenkel, M.; Scherließ, R. Nasal Powder Formulations: In-Vitro Characterisation of the Impact of Powders on Nasal Residence Time and Sensory Effects. *Pharmaceutics* **2021**, *13*, 385. [CrossRef]
38. Nippe, S.; Preuße, C.; General, S. Evaluation of the in Vitro Release and Pharmacokinetics of Parenteral Injectable Formulations for Steroids. *Eur. J. Pharm. Biopharm.* **2013**, *83*, 253–265. [CrossRef]
39. Blažević, F.; Milekić, T.; Romić, M.D.; Juretić, M.; Pepić, I.; Filipović-Grčić, J.; Lovrić, J.; Hafner, A. Nanoparticle-Mediated Interplay of Chitosan and Melatonin for Improved Wound Epithelialisation. *Carbohydr. Polym.* **2016**, *146*, 445–454. [CrossRef]
40. Ghasemi Tahrir, F.; Ganji, F.; Mani, A.R.; Khodaverdi, E. In Vitro and in Vivo Evaluation of Thermosensitive Chitosan Hydrogel for Sustained Release of Insulin. *Drug Deliv.* **2016**, *23*, 1038–1046. [CrossRef]
41. Zhou, H.Y.; Jiang, L.J.; Cao, P.P.; Li, J.B.; Chen, X.G. Glycerophosphate-Based Chitosan Thermosensitive Hydrogels and Their Biomedical Applications. *Carbohydr. Polym.* **2015**, *117*, 524–536. [CrossRef]
42. Szymańska, E.; Sosnowska, K.; Miltyk, W.; Rusak, M.; Basa, A.; Winnicka, K. The Effect of β-Glycerophosphate Crosslinking on Chitosan Cytotoxicity and Properties of Hydrogels for Vaginal Application. *Polymers* **2015**, *7*, 2223–2244. [CrossRef]
43. Naik, A.; Nair, H. Formulation and Evaluation of Thermosensitive Biogels for Nose to Brain Delivery of Doxepin. *BioMed Res. Int.* **2014**, *2014*, 847547. [CrossRef]
44. Foxman, E.F.; Storer, J.A.; Fitzgerald, M.E.; Wasik, B.R.; Hou, L.; Zhao, H.; Turner, P.E.; Pyle, A.M.; Iwasaki, A. Temperature-Dependent Innate Defense against the Common Cold Virus Limits Viral Replication at Warm Temperature in Mouse Airway Cells. *Proc. Natl. Acad. Sci. USA* **2015**, *112*, 827–832. [CrossRef]
45. Karavasili, C.; Fatouros, D.G. Smart Materials: In Situ Gel-Forming Systems for Nasal Delivery. *Drug Discov. Today* **2016**, *21*, 157–166. [CrossRef] [PubMed]
46. Grangeia, H.B.; Silva, C.; Simões, S.P.; Reis, M.S. Quality by Design in Pharmaceutical Manufacturing: A Systematic Review of Current Status, Challenges and Future Perspectives. *Eur. J. Pharm. Biopharm.* **2020**, *147*, 19–37. [CrossRef] [PubMed]
47. Erdő, F.; Bors, L.A.; Farkas, D.; Bajza, Á.; Gizurarson, S. Evaluation of Intranasal Delivery Route of Drug Administration for Brain Targeting. *Brain Res. Bull.* **2018**, *143*, 155–170. [CrossRef] [PubMed]
48. Gholizadeh, H.; Messerotti, E.; Pozzoli, M.; Cheng, S.; Traini, D.; Young, P.; Kourmatzis, A.; Caramella, C.; Ong, H.X. Application of a Thermosensitive In Situ Gel of Chitosan-Based Nasal Spray Loaded with Tranexamic Acid for Localised Treatment of Nasal Wounds. *AAPS PharmSciTech* **2019**, *20*, 299. [CrossRef] [PubMed]
49. Aliaghaie, M.; Mirzadeh, H.; Dashtimoghadam, E.; Taranejoo, S. Investigation of Gelation Mechanism of an Injectable Hydrogel Based on Chitosan by Rheological Measurements for a Drug Delivery Application. *Soft Matter* **2012**, *8*, 7128–7137. [CrossRef]
50. Zhou, H.Y.; Chen, X.G.; Kong, M.; Liu, C.S.; Cha, D.S.; Kennedy, J.F. Effect of Molecular Weight and Degree of Chitosan Deacetylation on the Preparation and Characteristics of Chitosan Thermosensitive Hydrogel as a Delivery System. *Carbohydr. Polym.* **2008**, *73*, 265–273. [CrossRef]
51. Supper, S.; Anton, N.; Seidel, N.; Riemenschnitter, M.; Curdy, C.; Vandamme, T. Thermosensitive Chitosan/Glycerophosphate-Based Hydrogel and Its Derivatives in Pharmaceutical and Biomedical Applications. *Expert Opin. Drug Deliv.* **2014**, *11*, 249–267. [CrossRef]
52. Zhou, J.-F.; Duan, L.; Wang, Y.-X.; Wang, C.-L.; Tian, M.-L.; Qi, X.-J.; Qiu, F. Design, Characterization of Resveratrol-Thermosensitive Hydrogel System (Res-THS) and Evaluation of Its Anti-Depressant Effect v Intranasal Administration. *Mater. Des.* **2022**, *216*, 110597. [CrossRef]
53. Peng, Y.; Li, J.; Li, J.; Fei, Y.; Dong, J.; Pan, W. Optimization of Thermosensitive Chitosan Hydrogels for the Sustained Delivery of Venlafaxine Hydrochloride. *Int. J. Pharm.* **2013**, *441*, 482–490. [CrossRef]

54. Warnken, Z.N.; Smyth, H.D.C.; Davis, D.A.; Weitman, S.; Kuhn, J.G.; Williams, R.O. Personalized Medicine in Nasal Delivery: The Use of Patient-Specific Administration Parameters To Improve Nasal Drug Targeting Using 3D-Printed Nasal Replica Casts. *Mol. Pharm.* **2018**, *15*, 1392–1402. [CrossRef]
55. Moraga-Espinoza, D.; Warnken, Z.; Moore, A.; Williams, R.O.; Smyth, H.D.C. A Modified USP Induction Port to Characterize Nasal Spray Plume Geometry and Predict Turbinate Deposition under Flow. *Int. J. Pharm.* **2018**, *548*, 305–313. [CrossRef]
56. Kundoor, V.; Dalby, R.N. Effect of Formulation- and Administration-Related Variables on Deposition Pattern of Nasal Spray Pumps Evaluated Using a Nasal Cast. *Pharm. Res.* **2011**, *28*, 1895–1904. [CrossRef]
57. Xi, J.; Yuan, J.E.; Zhang, Y.; Nevorski, D.; Wang, Z.; Zhou, Y. Visualization and Quantification of Nasal and Olfactory Deposition in a Sectional Adult Nasal Airway Cast. *Pharm. Res.* **2016**, *33*, 1527–1541. [CrossRef]
58. Needham, D. The PH Dependence of Niclosamide Solubility, Dissolution, and Morphology: Motivation for Potentially Universal Mucin-Penetrating Nasal and Throat Sprays for COVID19, Its Variants and Other Viral Infections. *Pharm. Res.* **2022**, *39*, 115–141. [CrossRef]
59. Chusakul, S.; Warathanasin, S.; Suksangpanya, N.; Phannaso, C.; Ruxrungtham, S.; Snidvongs, K.; Aeumjaturapat, S. Comparison of Buffered and Nonbuffered Nasal Saline Irrigations in Treating Allergic Rhinitis. *Laryngoscope* **2013**, *123*, 53–56. [CrossRef]
60. Optimal Design of Experiments: A Case Study Approach. Available online: https://www.wiley.com/en-us/Optimal+Design+of+Experiments%3A+A+Case+Study+Approach-p-9780470744611 (accessed on 15 March 2023).
61. Ghadiri, M.; Young, P.M.; Traini, D. Strategies to Enhance Drug Absorption via Nasal and Pulmonary Routes. *Pharmaceutics* **2019**, *11*, 113. [CrossRef]
62. Maaz, A.; Blagbrough, I.S.; De Bank, P.A. In Vitro Evaluation of Nasal Aerosol Depositions: An Insight for Direct Nose to Brain Drug Delivery. *Pharmaceutics* **2021**, *13*, 1079. [CrossRef]
63. Gao, M.; Shen, X.; Mao, S. Factors Influencing Drug Deposition in The Nasal Cavity upon Delivery via Nasal Sprays. *J. Pharm. Investig.* **2020**, *50*, 251–259. [CrossRef]
64. Trows, S.; Wuchner, K.; Spycher, R.; Steckel, H. Analytical Challenges and Regulatory Requirements for Nasal Drug Products in Europe and the U.S. *Pharmaceutics* **2014**, *6*, 195–219. [CrossRef]
65. Party, P.; Bartos, C.; Farkas, Á.; Szabó-Révész, P.; Ambrus, R. Formulation and In Vitro and In Silico Characterization of "Nano-in-Micro" Dry Powder Inhalers Containing Meloxicam. *Pharmaceutics* **2021**, *13*, 211. [CrossRef]
66. Guo, Y.; Laube, B.; Dalby, R. The Effect of Formulation Variables and Breathing Patterns on the Site of Nasal Deposition in an Anatomically Correct Model. *Pharm. Res.* **2005**, *22*, 1871–1878. [CrossRef] [PubMed]
67. do Amaral Sobral, P.J.; Gebremariam, G.; Drudi, F.; De Aguiar Saldanha Pinheiro, A.C.; Romani, S.; Rocculi, P.; Dalla Rosa, M. Rheological and Viscoelastic Properties of Chitosan Solutions Prepared with Different Chitosan or Acetic Acid Concentrations. *Foods* **2022**, *11*, 2692. [CrossRef] [PubMed]
68. Cho, J.; Heuzey, M.-C.; Bégin, A.; Carreau, P.J. Chitosan and Glycerophosphate Concentration Dependence of Solution Behaviour and Gel Point Using Small Amplitude Oscillatory Rheometry. *Food Hydrocoll.* **2006**, *20*, 936–945. [CrossRef]
69. Pu, Y.; Goodey, A.P.; Fang, X.; Jacob, K. A Comparison of the Deposition Patterns of Different Nasal Spray Formulations Using a Nasal Cast. *Aerosol Sci. Technol.* **2014**, *48*, 930–938. [CrossRef]
70. Foo, M.Y.; Cheng, Y.-S.; Su, W.-C.; Donovan, M.D. The Influence of Spray Properties on Intranasal Deposition. *J. Aerosol Med.* **2007**, *20*, 495–508. [CrossRef] [PubMed]
71. Coutu, J.-M.; Fatimi, A.; Berrahmoune, S.; Soulez, G.; Lerouge, S. A New Radiopaque Embolizing Agent for the Treatment of Endoleaks after Endovascular Repair: Influence of Contrast Agent on Chitosan Thermogel Properties. *J. Biomed. Mater. Res. B Appl. Biomater.* **2013**, *101*, 153–161. [CrossRef]
72. Lavertu, M.; Filion, D.; Buschmann, M.D. Heat-Induced Transfer of Protons from Chitosan to Glycerol Phosphate Produces Chitosan Precipitation and Gelation. *Biomacromolecules* **2008**, *9*, 640–650. [CrossRef]
73. Filion, D.; Lavertu, M.; Buschmann, M.D. Ionization and Solubility of Chitosan Solutions Related to Thermosensitive Chitosan/Glycerol-Phosphate Systems. *Biomacromolecules* **2007**, *8*, 3224–3234. [CrossRef]
74. Sandri, G.; Bonferoni, M.C.; Rossi, S.; Ferrari, F.; Mori, M.; Del Fante, C.; Perotti, C.; Caramella, C. Thermosensitive Eyedrops Containing Platelet Lysate for the Treatment of Corneal Ulcers. *Int. J. Pharm.* **2012**, *426*, 1–6. [CrossRef]
75. Johnson, N.J.; Hanson, L.R.; Frey, W.H., II. Trigeminal Pathways Deliver a Low Molecular Weight Drug from the Nose to the Brain and Orofacial Structures. *Mol. Pharm.* **2010**, *7*, 884–893. [CrossRef]
76. Martins, P.P.; Smyth, H.D.C.; Cui, Z. Strategies to Facilitate or Block Nose-to-Brain Drug Delivery. *Int. J. Pharm.* **2019**, *570*, 118635. [CrossRef]
77. Djupesland, P.G.; Messina, J.C.; Mahmoud, R.A. The Nasal Approach to Delivering Treatment for Brain Diseases: An Anatomic, Physiologic, and Delivery Technology Overview. *Ther. Deliv.* **2014**, *5*, 709–733. [CrossRef]
78. Möller, W.; Schuschnig, U.; Celik, G.; Münzing, W.; Bartenstein, P.; Häussinger, K.; Kreyling, W.G.; Knoch, M.; Canis, M.; Becker, S. Topical Drug Delivery in Chronic Rhinosinusitis Patients before and after Sinus Surgery Using Pulsating Aerosols. *PLoS ONE* **2013**, *8*, e74991. [CrossRef]
79. Yasue, M.; Sugiura, S.; Uchida, Y.; Otake, H.; Teranishi, M.; Sakurai, T.; Toba, K.; Shimokata, H.; Ando, F.; Otsuka, R.; et al. Prevalence of Sinusitis Detected by Magnetic Resonance Imaging in Subjects with Dementia or Alzheimer's Disease. *Curr. Alzheimer Res.* **2015**, *12*, 1006–1011. [CrossRef]

80. Djupesland, P.G.; Messina, J.C.; Mahmoud, R.A. Role of Nasal Casts for in Vitro Evaluation of Nasal Drug Delivery and Quantitative Evaluation of Various Nasal Casts. *Ther. Deliv.* **2020**, *11*, 485–495. [CrossRef]
81. Issakhov, A.; Mardieyeva, A.; Zhandaulet, Y.; Abylkassymova, A. Numerical Study of Air Flow in the Human Respiratory System with Rhinitis. *Case Stud. Therm. Eng.* **2021**, *26*, 101079. [CrossRef]
82. Xi, J.; Si, X.; Kim, J.W.; Berlinski, A. Simulation of Airflow and Aerosol Deposition in the Nasal Cavity of a 5-Year-Old Child. *J. Aerosol Sci.* **2011**, *42*, 156–173. [CrossRef]
83. Schroeter, J.D.; Tewksbury, E.W.; Wong, B.A.; Kimbell, J.S. Experimental Measurements and Computational Predictions of Regional Particle Deposition in a Sectional Nasal Model. *J. Aerosol Med. Pulm. Drug Deliv.* **2015**, *28*, 20–29. [CrossRef]
84. Grmaš, J.; Stare, K.; Božič, D.; Injac, R.; Dreu, R. Elucidation of Formulation and Delivery Device-Related Effects on In Vitro Performance of Nasal Spray with Implication to Rational Product Specification Identification. *J. Aerosol Med. Pulm. Drug Deliv.* **2017**, *30*, 230–246. [CrossRef]
85. Tian, L.; Shang, Y.; Chen, R.; Bai, R.; Chen, C.; Inthavong, K.; Tu, J. Correlation of Regional Deposition Dosage for Inhaled Nanoparticles in Human and Rat Olfactory. *Part. Fibre Toxicol.* **2019**, *16*, 6. [CrossRef]
86. Sutthapitaksakul, L.; Dass, C.R.; Sriamornsak, P. Donepezil—An Updated Review of Challenges in Dosage Form Design. *J. Drug Deliv. Sci. Technol.* **2021**, *63*, 102549. [CrossRef]
87. Chen, J.Z.; Kiaee, M.; Martin, A.R.; Finlay, W.H. In Vitro Assessment of an Idealized Nose for Nasal Spray Testing: Comparison with Regional Deposition in Realistic Nasal Replicas. *Int. J. Pharm.* **2020**, *582*, 119341. [CrossRef] [PubMed]
88. Patel, S.; Koradia, H.; Parikh, R. Design and Development of Intranasal in Situ Gelling System of Midazolam Hydrochloride Using 32 Full Factorial Design. *J. Drug Deliv. Sci. Technol.* **2015**, *30*, 154–162. [CrossRef]
89. Jug, M.; Hafner, A.; Lovrić, J.; Kregar, M.L.; Pepić, I.; Vanić, Ž.; Cetina-Čižmek, B.; Filipović-Grčić, J. An Overview of in Vitro Dissolution/Release Methods for Novel Mucosal Drug Delivery Systems. *J. Pharm. Biomed. Anal.* **2018**, *147*, 350–366. [CrossRef] [PubMed]
90. Shelke, S.; Shahi, S.; Jalalpure, S.; Dhamecha, D. Poloxamer 407-Based Intranasal Thermoreversible Gel of Zolmitriptan-Loaded Nanoethosomes: Formulation, Optimization, Evaluation and Permeation Studies. *J. Liposome Res.* **2016**, *26*, 313–323. [CrossRef] [PubMed]
91. Patil, M. Chapter 7—Mucoadhesion as a Strategy to Enhance the Direct Nose-to-Brain Drug Delivery. In *Direct Nose-to-Brain Drug Delivery*; Pardeshi, C.V., Souto, E.B., Eds.; Academic Press: Cambridge, MA, USA, 2021; pp. 115–156, ISBN 978-0-12-822522-6.
92. Yang, J.; Dai, L.; Yu, Q.; Yang, Q. Histological and Anatomical Structure of the Nasal Cavity of Bama Minipigs. *PLoS ONE* **2017**, *12*, e0173902. [CrossRef]
93. Popescu, R.; Ghica, M.V.; Dinu-Pîrvu, C.-E.; Anuța, V.; Lupuliasa, D.; Popa, L. New Opportunity to Formulate Intranasal Vaccines and Drug Delivery Systems Based on Chitosan. *Int. J. Mol. Sci.* **2020**, *21*, 5016. [CrossRef]
94. Dowd, F.J. 2—Pharmacokinetics: The Absorption, Distribution, and Fate of Drugs. In *Pharmacology and Therapeutics for Dentistry*, 7th ed.; Dowd, F.J., Johnson, B.S., Mariotti, A.J., Eds.; Mosby: Maryland Heights, MO, USA, 2017; pp. 15–43, ISBN 978-0-323-39307-2.
95. Abouelmagd, S.A.; Ku, Y.J.; Yeo, Y. Low Molecular Weight Chitosan-Coated Polymeric Nanoparticles for Sustained and PH-Sensitive Delivery of Paclitaxel. *J. Drug Target.* **2015**, *23*, 725–735. [CrossRef]
96. Kudsiova, L.; Lawrence, M.J. A Comparison of the Effect of Chitosan and Chitosan-Coated Vesicles on Monolayer Integrity and Permeability across Caco-2 and 16HBE14o-Cells. *J. Pharm. Sci.* **2008**, *97*, 3998–4010. [CrossRef]
97. M. Ways, T.M.; Lau, W.M.; Khutoryanskiy, V.V. Chitosan and Its Derivatives for Application in Mucoadhesive Drug Delivery Systems. *Polymers* **2018**, *10*, 267. [CrossRef]
98. Kou, S.G.; Peters, L.; Mucalo, M. Chitosan: A Review of Molecular Structure, Bioactivities and Interactions with the Human Body and Micro-Organisms. *Carbohydr. Polym.* **2022**, *282*, 119132. [CrossRef]
99. Casettari, L.; Vllasaliu, D.; Mantovani, G.; Howdle, S.M.; Stolnik, S.; Illum, L. Effect of PEGylation on the Toxicity and Permeability Enhancement of Chitosan. *Biomacromolecules* **2010**, *11*, 2854–2865. [CrossRef]
100. Sibinovska, N.; Žakelj, S.; Trontelj, J.; Kristan, K. Applicability of RPMI 2650 and Calu-3 Cell Models for Evaluation of Nasal Formulations. *Pharmaceutics* **2022**, *14*, 369. [CrossRef]
101. Sibinovska, N.; Žakelj, S.; Roškar, R.; Kristan, K. Suitability and Functional Characterization of Two Calu-3 Cell Models for Prediction of Drug Permeability across the Airway Epithelial Barrier. *Int. J. Pharm.* **2020**, *585*, 119484. [CrossRef]
102. Fredlund, L.; Winiwarter, S.; Hilgendorf, C. In Vitro Intrinsic Permeability: A Transporter-Independent Measure of Caco-2 Cell Permeability in Drug Design and Development. *Mol. Pharm.* **2017**, *14*, 1601–1609. [CrossRef]
103. Flaten, G.E.; Dhanikula, A.B.; Luthman, K.; Brandl, M. Drug Permeability across a Phospholipid Vesicle Based Barrier: A Novel Approach for Studying Passive Diffusion. *Eur. J. Pharm. Sci.* **2006**, *27*, 80–90. [CrossRef]
104. Ventura, C.A.; Tommasini, S.; Crupi, E.; Giannone, I.; Cardile, V.; Musumeci, T.; Puglisi, G. Chitosan Microspheres for Intrapulmonary Administration of Moxifloxacin: Interaction with Biomembrane Models and In Vitro Permeation Studies. *Eur. J. Pharm. Biopharm.* **2008**, *68*, 235–244. [CrossRef]
105. Lenoir, J.; Bachert, C.; Remon, J.-P.; Adriaens, E. The Slug Mucosal Irritation (SMI) Assay: A Tool for the Evaluation of Nasal Discomfort. *Toxicol. Vitr.* **2013**, *27*, 1954–1961. [CrossRef]
106. Adriaens, E.; Remon, J.P. Gastropods as an Evaluation Tool for Screening the Irritating Potency of Absorption Enhancers and Drugs. *Pharm. Res.* **1999**, *16*, 1240–1244. [CrossRef]

107. Adriaens, E.; Remon, J.P. Mucosal Irritation Potential of Personal Lubricants Relates to Product Osmolality as Detected by the Slug Mucosal Irritation Assay. *Sex. Transm. Dis.* **2008**, *35*, 512–516. [CrossRef]
108. Lenoir, J.; Adriaens, E.; Remon, J.-P. New Aspects of the Slug Mucosal Irritation Assay: Predicting Nasal Stinging, Itching and Burning Sensations. *J. Appl. Toxicol.* **2011**, *31*, 640–648. [CrossRef] [PubMed]
109. Ahmadi, R.; de Bruijn, J.D. Biocompatibility and Gelation of Chitosan–Glycerol Phosphate Hydrogels. *J. Biomed. Mater. Res. A* **2008**, *86*, 824–832. [CrossRef] [PubMed]
110. Henriques, P.; Fortuna, A.; Doktorovová, S. Spray Dried Powders for Nasal Delivery: Process and Formulation Considerations. *Eur. J. Pharm. Biopharm.* **2022**, *176*, 1–20. [CrossRef] [PubMed]
111. Tiozzo Fasiolo, L.; Manniello, M.D.; Tratta, E.; Buttini, F.; Rossi, A.; Sonvico, F.; Bortolotti, F.; Russo, P.; Colombo, G. Opportunity and Challenges of Nasal Powders: Drug Formulation and Delivery. *Eur. J. Pharm. Sci.* **2018**, *113*, 2–17. [CrossRef]
112. Borah, B.; Sacco, P.; Zarotsky, V. Predictors of Adherence among Alzheimer's Disease Patients Receiving Oral Therapy. *Curr. Med. Res. Opin.* **2010**, *26*, 1957–1965. [CrossRef]

pharmaceutics

MDPI

Review

The Upper Nasal Space: Option for Systemic Drug Delivery, Mucosal Vaccines and "Nose-to-Brain"

Stephen B. Shrewsbury

Formerly of Impel Pharmaceuticals, 201 Elliott Ave West, Seattle, WA 98119, USA; steve.shrewsbury@me.com; Tel.: +1-(415)-250-1169

Abstract: Sino-nasal disease is appropriately treated with topical treatment, where the nasal mucosa acts as a barrier to systemic absorption. Non-invasive nasal delivery of drugs has produced some small molecule products with good bioavailability. With the recent COVID pandemic and the need for nasal mucosal immunity becoming more appreciated, more interest has become focused on the nasal cavity for vaccine delivery. In parallel, it has been recognized that drug delivery to different parts of the nose can have different results and for "nose-to-brain" delivery, deposition on the olfactory epithelium of the upper nasal space is desirable. Here the non-motile cilia and reduced mucociliary clearance lead to longer residence time that permits enhanced absorption, either into the systemic circulation or directly into the CNS. Many of the developments in nasal delivery have been to add bioadhesives and absorption/permeation enhancers, creating more complicated formulations and development pathways, but other projects have shown that the delivery device itself may allow more differential targeting of the upper nasal space without these additions and that could allow faster and more efficient programs to bring a wider range of drugs—and vaccines—to market.

Keywords: nasal delivery; intranasal delivery; upper nasal space; olfactory epithelium; blood-brain barrier (BBB); central nervous system (CNS); ViaNase®; OptiNose®; Precision Olfactory Delivery (POD®); nose-to-brain (N2B)

1. Introduction

Deliberate nasal administration of drugs for medicinal purposes has a long history, was well documented in traditional Chinese medical practice [1], and is more extensively discussed in many Persian texts dating from the 9th to 18th centuries [2]. In recent history, it has been used primarily for treating local sino-nasal disease where systemic absorption was neither needed nor desired [3].

As more large molecule drugs were developed, especially the biological drugs in the last 10 years [4] and acute situations requiring self-administration and diseases with associated or comorbid gastrointestinal dysmotility were tackled, so non-invasive, non-oral delivery of drugs have become a more pressing need.

Nasal delivery started to gather more attention, however, as animal experiments demonstrated direct delivery of drugs to the brain [5–9], so-called "Nose-to-Brain" (or N2B) delivery, and it was speculated for humans [10], thus avoiding the difficulty that systemically administered drugs encounter of crossing the protective Blood Brain Barrier (BBB). This barrier effectively blocks high molecular weight (MW) substances, such as proteins and peptides [11] and even 98% of small molecular weight drugs [12] from access to the brain from the systemic circulation. There is emerging promising data bypassing the BBB with insulin, leptin, oxytocin and orexin A, but also hydrophilic molecules and charged molecules [13]. Indeed, even cells may be able to cross from the upper nasal space directly to the brain, as has already been shown in animals [11,14].

The data and opportunity were nicely summarized in a 2022 review [15], which reiterated many of the points made in a 2014 review [16], highlighting the slow progress, at least in clinical application, in the intervening 8 years. Indeed, one statement from the 2014 review, "evidence of direct N2B transport in man may still be considered lacking," remains true, although differential delivery to the olfactory epithelium remains an important step in that direction which has now been achieved. The 2022 review nicely summarized the BBB and suggested how direct N2B delivery may be possible along branches of the trigeminal nerve, but most research indicates the olfactory nerve is the more promising access point. Both nerves may involve extracellular convective flow [17], transcellular [16], perivascular/paracellular [16,18], or perineuronal [16] routes. This 2022 review focused on the N2B delivery of insulin (and some other products) rather than the benefits of delivering to the olfactory epithelium of the UNS per se. Nanoparticles have been detected in the olfactory bulb 5 min after dosing [19], making N2B delivery potentially suitable even for acute indications. This interest in N2B has grown as more large MW drugs are developed for CNS indications, although low MW drugs can also benefit from rapid entry into the CNS. Parkinson's disease (off episodes), epilepsy [20], migraine and acute agitation are all indications where drug penetration into the brain may be time-sensitive, and Alzheimer's disease, multiple sclerosis and stroke have large MW candidates in development. For glioblastoma (direct access of cytotoxic drugs to the tumor may avoid undesired systemic toxicity. A comprehensively researched 2020 review [21] dealt with some of the device options being considered, specifically for N2B delivery, and those devices are summarized herein.

While interest in nasal delivery has gathered pace for high MW compounds, the COVID pandemic has shown that nasal mucosal immunity may not be sufficient with systemic vaccine administration to avoid mild disease or asymptomatic carriage and transmission. In addition to viral disease, the concept of being able to induce immunity to certain cancers with vaccination is also stimulating research [22]. There are now multiple nasal vaccine programs in development with the additional advantage that these vaccines may be more suitable for widespread use, where healthcare is less accessible or cold storage less available, and they may induce immunity at other distant mucosal surfaces [23]—e.g., the gastrointestinal and urogenital tracts.

Different approaches have been taken to target systemic disease by nasal drug delivery, with much interest and development focused on the addition of bioadhesives and absorption/permeation enhancers to formulations (especially liquid) delivered as a cloud to the lower nasal space. There are several excellent reviews of the range of excipients that have been investigated for these purposes [24,25], while others have focused on the drug-delivery systems more broadly [26–28]. An alternative approach has been to identify areas within the nose where absorption may be enhanced and deliver drugs to that area. This complimentary area of research has received much less attention, but with N2B delivery requiring non-invasive delivery to the olfactory epithelium of the upper nasal space, that interest is now growing and is the focus of this review.

2. Local Delivery

Local delivery within the nose has tended to deliver a cloud of liquid droplets (or powder particles) to the inside of the nostril. Much of the plume from most traditional options is actually deposited on the impermeable squamous epithelium of the nasal vestibule, with varying amounts penetrating to the mucus-covered respiratory epithelium of the lower nasal space.

2.1. Local Nasal and Sinus Disease

Many local sino-nasal diseases, specifically allergic rhinitis and rhinosinusitis with or without nasal polyps, have responded to the development of numerous topical corticosteroid sprays, starting with triamcinolone in 1957 but followed by beclomethasone, budesonide, flunisolide, fluticasone, mometasone and ciclesonide. All were delivered with either a pressurized metered-dose inhaler (pMDI) that was originally chlorofluorocarbon

(CFC)-propelled but later changed to hydrofluoroalkane (HFA) or an aqueous product delivered by a "traditional" pump-spray.

Although many cases of chronic rhinosinusitis, especially with the additional pathology of nasal polyposis, are perennial, many patients have seasonal allergy problems making year-round administration of potent corticosteroids unnecessary. The target of the respiratory epithelium on the turbinates (conchae) of the LNS has been effectively reached by the traditional nasal spray delivering a diffuse cloud of droplets. In addition, systemic absorption is not desired, allowing for simpler formulations and delivery systems. Most recently, fluticasone has been approved for delivery by the OptiNose bidirectional Exhalation Delivery System (EDS) specifically for the treatment of chronic rhinosinusitis with nasal polyps (CRSwNP) [29] and is able to deliver more of the potent steroid "higher and deeper" into the nasal cavity (compared to traditional sprays) where many polyps originate [30]. The OptiNose device generally distributes better throughout the nasal cavity (than traditional nasal sprays) with its bidirectional design and is propelled by the patient's own exhalation, which also elevates the vellum (soft palate), thus closing off the nose from the rest of the respiratory tract (Table 1). The nose piece directs the exhaled breath to push the drug product into one nostril, allowing it to reach the back of the nose, pass behind the septum and exit from the other nostril, hence creating the "bi-directional flow path" [16].

Table 1. Examples of Different Nasal Delivery Systems (in development or approved). The bottom four devices are basically syringes with different nozzles attached so that as a Healthcare Practitioner pushes the plunger of the syringe in, the liquid vaccine is forced out of the various tips creating a local mist or broad plume of particles 30–100 μm in diameter (in the case of the MAD).

Manufacturer	Device	Propellant	No. Doses	[Drug/Other Programs]	Pros	Cons	Reference/ Website
Aptar (Crystal Lake, IL, USA) (Device only) Multiple programs with drug companies	Unidose (UDS) Liquid Nasal Spray	None No spring. Finger squeeze pressure.	1 of up to 100 μL	Zomig® [zolmitriptan] Zavzpret® [zavegepant] Valtoco® [diazepam] Tosymra® [DHE] [+ several others + multiple partnered programs	One-handed operation. Low actuation force. No priming. No shaking. Multiple approved FDA/EMA products—for migraine (and other indications).	No distinction between UNS and LNS deposition. Diffuse "cloud" of droplets/particles.	[31]
	Bidose (BDS) Liquid Nasal Spray	None Spring	2 × 100 μL	Spravato® [esketamine]			[32]
	Unidose (UDS) Powder Nasal Spray	None No spring. Finger squeeze pressure	1	Baqsimi® [glucagon]	Ideal for low solubility molecules, minimizes excipient requirements, allows for larger dose administration, improves bioavailability and enhances drug diffusion/absorption. No shaking/priming.	No distinction between UNS and LNS deposition. Complex formulation and may increase irritability.	[33]
	Multi-Dose (preservative-free) VP3 Nasal Spray Systems	None	Multiple	Tyrvaya® [varenicline]	The "traditional" nasal spray for >40 years. Mechanical system. Reference pump for originator anti-allergy brands and their generic alternatives.	No distinction between UNS and LNS deposition.	[34]
Bausch Health (Laval, Canada) (Drug device combination product)	Traditional Nasal Spray	None	1	Migranal® [DHE]	Approved (>20 years) for delivery of 2.0 mg liquid DHE for acute treatment of migraines. Has a "traditional" pump spray.	Requires assembly and priming. No distinction between UNS and LNS deposition. Diffuse "cloud" of droplets/particles.	[35,36]

Table 1. *Cont.*

Manufacturer	Device	Propellant	No. Doses	[Drug/Other Programs]	Pros	Cons	Reference/ Website
Haleon (Weybridge, UK)	Sensimist (liquid)	None	60 doses	Flonase® [fluticasone] (generics and OTC focus)	Now OTC product. Designed to deliver a cloud of liquid fluticasone droplets to the LNS for allergic rhinitis. Systemic absorption is NOT desired.	Typical systemic corticosteroid effects are seen with long-term use and absorption.	[37]
Impel (Seattle, WA, USA) (Drug-device combination products)	Precision Olfactory Delivery (POD®) (Liquid)	HFA134a	1	Trudhesa® [DHE] INP102 [insulin]	Focus on UNS for N2B.Device adapted for each product. Approved for delivery of 1.45 mg liquid DHE formulation for acute treatment of migraine	First Generation device—requires assembly and priming.	[38]
	POD (Powder)	HFA134a	Multiple exchangeable tips	INP103 [levodopa] INP107 [carbidopa/levodopa combination]	Several iterations of the device; research (which uses drug powder products in capsules) and single (no assembly) or multiple (changeable tip) dose design	Although delivering to UNS, there are no data on N2B delivery.Remains "in development."	[39]
	POD (Powder)	Nitrogen	1	INP105 [olanzapine]	Single-use, preloaded device (no priming or assembly)	Research and development halted Q1 2023 (for business reasons)	[40]
Kurve (Lynnwood, WA, USA) (Device only)	ViaNase™ (liquid)	None	1	N/A [insulin]	Focus on UNS for N2B. Device adapted for each product. Sixteen programs, fourteen in-clinic. Battery powered.	Unreliable performance in large NIH AD-insulin trial	[41,42]
OptiNose (Yardley, PA, USA) Drug-device combination products	Xhance® (OptiMist®) Bi-directional	None (breath powered)	120 sprays	Xhance® [fluticasone]	Approved for CRSwNP. Broader dispersion around the nasal cavity. The soft palate closes during use preventing the drug from entering the pharynx (or lungs).	Patient unfamiliarity with blowing into own nose. Initial priming is needed, and shaking before every dose. Focus on nasal disease—not systemic or N2B delivery.	[43]
	Bi-directional Exhalation Delivery System (EDS)—Onzetra® Xsail®		1	Onzetra® Xsail® [sumatriptan]	More of the drug reaches UNS. Approved for the delivery of sumatriptan powder (for migraine).	Patient unfamiliarity with blowing into own nose.	[44]

Table 1. *Cont.*

Manufacturer	Device	Propellant	No. Doses	[Drug/Other Programs]	Pros	Cons	Reference/ Website
Satsuma (Durham, NC, USA) (Drug-device combination product)	STS101—a manually squeezed plastic bottle	None	1	N/A [DHE]	Small, portable, and no assembly or priming, delivering 6.0 mg DHE powder	Two failed phase 3 studies, with device modifications in between to improve delivery. No distinction between UNS and LNS delivery	[45]
AeroPump (Hochheim am Main, Germany) (Device only)	AeroPump	None		N/A [insulin] (adaptable for use by OTC and generic drugs)	Requires priming. Simple. Easy to use.	Non-targeted, LNS delivery	[46]
PharmaSystems (Markham, ON, Canada) (Device only)	Metered Nasal Dispenser	None	Multiple	N/A [insulin] (Canadian pharmacy supplier)	Requires priming. Simple. Easy to use. Programs showed benefits in postoperative delirium and postoperative cognitive function	Non-targeted, LNS delivery	[47]
MeadWestvaco (Richmond, VA, USA)/Silgan (Richmond, VA, USA) (Device only)	Mistette MkII Pump	None	Single/Multiple?	N/A [insulin] (provide bottles/pumps for liquid formulation delivery)	Requires priming. Simple. Easy to use.	Non-targeted, LNS delivery.	[48]
Nemera (La Verpillière, France) (Device only)	SP270+	None	Single/Multiple	N/A [insulin]	Requires priming. Simple. Easy to use.	Program was discontinued due to variations in viscosity.	[49]
SipNose (Yokneam, Israel) (Drug-device combination products)	Sipnose	Compressed air	Single and Multiple dose	N/A [insulin] (seven programs; five in-clinic, three of their own, and two partnered)	Performed well in Patient-Centered Care Impact Analysis [50] compared to two invasive ROAs (intrathecal and intracerebroventricular injection. Liquid and powder formulations. Targeted for UNS delivery.	Clinical data awaited	[51]

Table 1. *Cont.*

Manufacturer	Device	Propellant	No. Doses	[Drug/Other Programs]	Pros	Cons	Reference/ Website
Teleflex (Wayne, PA, USA) (Device only)	Mucosal Atomisation Device (MAD)	None	1	N/A [vaccines] (Astra Zeneca: ChAdOx1nCoV-19 vaccine)	Fitted to the tip of a standard syringe in clinical trials of vaccines	Liquid (vaccines or drugs) administration by HCP	[52,53]
BD (Franklin Lakes, NJ, USA) (Device only)	Accuspray™	None	1	N/A [vaccines] 510(k) cleared	Fitted to the tip of a standard syringe in clinical trials of vaccines	Liquid (vaccines or drugs) administration by HCP	[54,55]
Aptar	BiVax	None	1 (either 200 µL or 500 µL—split across 2 nostrils)	N/A [vaccines]	The liquid vaccine can be transferred directly from vial to applicator.	Liquid (vaccines or drugs) administration by HCP	[56,57]
Aptar	LuerVax (nozzle only)	None	1	N/A [vaccines]	Fitted to the tip of a standard syringe in clinical trials of vaccines.	For HCP liquid administration	

AD = Alzheimer's disease; CRSwNP = chronic rhinosinusitis with nasal polyps; DHE = dihydroergotamine (for migraine); EMA = European Medicines Agency; FDA = Food and Drug Administration; HCP = healthcare practitioner; HFA = hydrofluoroalkane; LNS = lower nasal space; N/A = not applicable (no approved product); N2B = nose-to-brain delivery; NIH = National Institutes of Health; OTC = over the counter; POD = Precision Olfactory Delivery; UNS = upper nasal space.

2.2. Nasal Vaccination

The emergence in 2020 of COVID-19 as a global pandemic stretched public health systems globally but led to accelerated vaccine development programs. SARS-CoV-2, the novel coronavirus that causes COVID, as with all other airborne viruses, enters the body through the nose. Entry of the virus via the nose and, specifically, the olfactory mucosa of the nasal cavity is thought to be responsible for a number of the symptoms of COVID, including anosmia [58] and central nervous system effects [59]. Many vaccine development programs are now looking at nasal administration of vaccines to ensure mucosal, as well as humoral, immunity and appreciating that mass vaccination campaigns, especially in rural communities will benefit from vaccines that do not require refrigeration and/or administration by healthcare personnel using a needle. The rationale for nasal delivery of vaccines and the range of options now being considered is covered in Supplementary Material.

Nasal delivery of vaccines is not new, with three influenza (live attenuated) vaccines having received market approval in the US (Table 2) and a similar number in Europe, while another, Nasalflu (using an inactivated virosome), had to be withdrawn from the Swiss market [60]. However, the US Center for Disease Control reviewed data in 2016 and recommended the nasal Flumist vaccine (popular with children) not be used the following season due to poor results in the previous flu season, despite good results in previous years [61]. This highlights one of the issues with any vaccine for a seasonal disease, such as flu. Each year a new strain (or strains) emerge, usually in the Far East. Scientists must predict which will be the prevalent strain(s) in Europe/US the following season, and the vaccine must then be updated to deliver antigen from that strain or those strains. Sometimes those predictions turn out to be incorrect, and even the IM-administered vaccine can provide disappointing levels of protection.

Table 2. Currently US-approved nasally administered vaccines (US).

Vaccine	Approved	Manufacturer	Target	Antigen	Adjuvant & Excipients
Influenza A (2009) Monovalent	2009	MedImmune (Gaithersburg, MD, USA)	H1N1 Influenza	Cold-adapted, live attenuated virus: A/California/7/2009 H1N1v	Monosodium glutamate; porcine gelatin; arginine; sucrose; potassium phosphate; gentamicin.
FluMist® (Trivalent)	2003	MedImmune	3 Influenza strains	Cold adapted, live attenuated virus: A/California/7/2009(H1N1); A/Perth/16/2009(H3N2); B/Brisbane/60/2008	Monosodium glutamate; porcine gelatin; arginine; sucrose; potassium phosphate; gentamicin.
FluMist® Quadrivalent	2003	MedImmune	2 Influenza A strains and 2 B strains	Cold adapted, live attenuated virus: A/Victoria/1/2020(H1N1); A/Norway/16606/2021(H3N2); B/Phuket/3073/2013; B/Austria/13599417/2021	Monosodium glutamate; porcine gelatin; arginine; sucrose; potassium phosphate; ovalbumin; gentamicin; ethylenediaminetetraacetic acid (EDTA).

A comprehensive summary of the nasal vaccines in development was recently published [62], citing nine ongoing programs against SARS-CoV-2, six against influenza, four against Respiratory Syncytial Virus (RSV), three against *Shigella sonnei*, two against *Bordetella pertussis* (whooping cough), with others against parainfluenza, norovirus, *Neisseria*, Ebola, anthrax, tuberculosis and HIV. In total, 36 current nasal vaccine development programs were registered, the vast majority, 31, were in phase 1 clinical development, three were in phase 2, one was in phase 4, and one was undisclosed. Details of the nasal delivery devices were minimal but suggested that 21 were simple nasal drops delivered by pipette or atomized from the tip of a syringe. A further eight used the term "nasal spray" but also appeared (according to the sponsoring organization's website) to use a syringe with an atomizer tip (e.g., the Teleflex Mucosal Atomization Device, MAD Nasal™ [52], BD Accuspray™ [55] or Aptar's LuerVax™) (Table 1); one program compared the results obtained between vaccine delivered by "sprayer" and "pipette." It was not possible to determine the delivery device in the remaining six programs, only that nasal delivery was planned for the vaccine. With intranasal delivery of vaccines already approved [63] and the knowledge that mucosal immunization drives CD8+ and CD4+ T cell responses [64] and leads to mucosal immunity, a better understanding of where in the nose vaccine payloads are delivered and then processed, is overdue. Aptar's LuerVax delivered water droplets ranging in size from a Dv10 of 20 μm to Dv90 of 65 μm (meaning 10% of particles were smaller than 20 μm and 90% were smaller than 65 μm with a Dv50 of 35 μm [57] according to laser diffraction. This size range may be good for targeting the nasal turbinate, but for optimal delivery to the nasopharynx (where the Nasal Associated Lymphoid Tissue (NALT) is located, smaller droplets in the range of 7–17 μm are considered optimal [65]. For further information, see Supplementary Material.

3. Systemic Delivery

Most drugs, especially small molecules, are given orally, and this remains the most popular and widely used method of administration. When those drugs are peptides or proteins that will not survive transit through the gut; are largely metabolized on the first pass through the liver; are needed for situations where gastrointestinal absorption is delayed, such as in Parkinson's disease [66] or migraine [67]; or if the drug is needed acutely, such as for seizure or anaphylaxis, then a non-oral route of administration is necessary—and preferably one that leads to rapid and reliable systemic drug concentrations. By avoiding oral administration, nasal delivery (to either the UNS or LNS) or pulmonary delivery with formulations of good bioavailability can often deliver microgram doses of a drug that access the systemic circulation, thus avoiding some of the adverse effects reported with milligram doses when administered orally. Intravenous injection is the gold standard, especially for acute situations, but when those situations occur in the community without immediate access to healthcare personnel, other options are required. Much focus has been on formulation changes that increase absorption (e.g., a powder desmopressin formulation improved on the liquid nasal formulation [68]) rather than where in the nose the drug is deposited. As such, many excipients and formulations have been tried; some with success, such as a dry-powder, chitosan-coated, liposome formulation loaded with ghrelin delivered with the Aptar UDS, which showed >50% deposition in the UNS using a 3D printed nasal cast model that was also better than the liquid formulation [69]. Further work has been conducted with thyrotrophin-releasing hormone [70], selective opioid agonist [19] and a chitosan-enhanced formulation of a modified peptide calcitonin gene-related (CGRP) antagonist [71]. Some of these programs look to explore N2B rather than systemic absorption and subsequent distribution to the brain.

3.1. Lower Nasal Space (LNS) Delivery

The delivery of drugs to the LNS can provide good bioavailability (BAV), i.e., access to the systemic circulation, with products such as Valtoco® (diazepam) through the Aptar Unit Dose System (UDS) reported at 97% [72], although this good bioavailability was obtained with the help of dodecyl maltoside (DDM) as an absorption/permeation enhancer and Vitamin E to increase solubility. Another product with good nasal bioavailability is Nayzilam® (midazolam), also delivered by Aptar's UDS. Section 12.3 of the Prescribing Information states the absolute bioavailability to be approximately 44%. However, other intranasal midazolam formulations have been independently investigated [73], delivered by a different unit dose device obtained from Ing. Erich Pfeiffer GmbH, demonstrating better bioavailability ranging from 76 to 92%. These different formulations contained different concentrations of randomly methylated-β5-cyclodextrin (0, 2, 4, or 12%); different concentrations of saline and with or without 0.5% chitosan added as an absorption enhancer. In contrast, a very recent approval of Zavzpret™ (vazegepant), also given by the Aptar UDS device [74], only reported ~5% bioavailability. The liquid formulation has the additional inactive ingredients: dextrose, hydrochloric acid, sodium hydroxide, succinic acid and water. In these examples, the same basic Aptar UDS delivery was used, presumably delivering to the same part of the nose (the LNS) with a diffuse nasal spray, showing that the addition of absorption enhancers was required to increase bioavailability. That, in turn, increases the complexity of the development program but does illustrate the extremes of the level of bioavailability that can be achieved through LNS delivery.

3.2. Upper Nasal Space (UNS) Delivery

There is now a greater appreciation that drugs delivered to the upper nasal space (UNS) may experience faster and more extensive absorption than when delivered to the LNS. Data were initially generated with the OptiNose® bi-directional system and then, more recently, by several clinical programs using the Precision Olfactory Delivery (or POD®) system (Table 1), which specifically targets the upper nasal space (UNS). These programs have served as important steps as they highlighted the complex nasal architecture (Figure 1a) and showed one of the potential benefits of delivering drugs to the olfactory epithelium lining in the UNS. As can be appreciated, a cloud or broad plume of droplets delivered into the nose by a mechanical pump will coat the surfaces of the septum, inferior turbinate and lateral wall, with some penetrating to the middle turbinate but little to the superior turbinate and even less to the upper nasal space lying mostly above the superior turbinate. The nose is designed to convey volatile molecules to the olfactory epithelium in the UNS carried by inhaled air but not to allow a broad plume of droplets/particles to reach it. The olfactory epithelium has distinct differences from the respiratory epithelium of the nose's humidification and filtering system covering the three turbinates (or conchae), mostly located in the lower nasal space (Figure 1b). These differences lead to very different absorption profiles for drugs landing on different mucosae [75]. Few data have historically been generated looking at where nasal devices deliver their payloads, with options being to investigate in cadavers, nasal cavity replicas, nasal casts or by using in vivo gamma camera imaging [76].

Investigating the novel breath-actuated, bi-directional system, Djupesland and colleagues compared the systemic levels of midazolam with those obtained after traditional nasal spray delivery and IV delivery [77]. The 100 μL of bespoke formulation, including cyclodextrin, HPMC, EDTA and benzalkonium chloride, to 12 healthy adult subjects showed similar serum concentration curves for the two nasal devices, both with rapid T_{max} of 15 min and a geometric mean ratio (OptiMist/Traditional spray) of 97.6%, suggesting no difference in systemic delivery between the two devices. However, this group went on to deliver ^{99m}Technetium-labelled aerosol [78] to nine healthy subjects and showed increased delivery to the UNS, of 32%, versus 11% with a traditional spray. Subsequent work with the OptiNose® system reported 53.6% of the formulation reaching the UNS (upper and middle posterior regions) versus only 15.7% with the traditional liquid spray [79] with no lung deposition.

Hoekman and colleagues generated data supporting the differential delivery systems to the UNS with Precision Olfactory Delivery (POD®) using MAG-3 (^{99m}Technetium-labelled peptide) as determined by SPECT imaging in seven healthy subjects [80]. For this assessment, the nasal cavity was divided into four sections (Figure 1c): (1) vestibule, (2) lower nasal space, (3) UNS and (4) nasopharynx, determined from MRI imaging [81]. The UNS is where the olfactory epithelium is confined, which will be further discussed in the context of N2B delivery below—although there is also an approximately equal area of respiratory epithelium in the UNS, as it covers the superior turbinate. POD delivered substantially more (approaching 50%) to the UNS and less to the vestibule than the traditional spray (Figure 1d). The olfactory epithelium covers ~5 cm^2, representing ~3% of the total surface area of the nasal cavity [82]. The enhanced delivery of radioisotopes to the UNS then led to several clinical programs being launched with the POD system. The STOP 101 [83] clinical study specifically looked at the delivery of the same liquid formulation through an approved, traditional spray to the lower nasal space and compared it with POD (using the same device that was subsequently used in the phase 3 study [84] and thereafter approved and commercialized) delivering it to the UNS and showed a four-fold increase in (C_{max}), an almost four-fold increase in absolute bioavailability (59% vs. 15%) and an almost three-fold increase in $AUC_{0\text{-}inf}$ (Figure 2a). To accomplish this, the POD system has a novel design for the nozzle (dosing tip), which focuses the plume of emitted liquid droplets into a narrow plume [85], which is pictured in the publication. The differences in plume and aerosol characteristics between the two systems, with the same formulation of dihydroergotamine (DHE) mesylate, were further explained in a technical manuscript [86] as well as the Anderson Cascade Impactor data and using Spraytec technology, with a particle size distribution of Dv10 ranging from ~290 µm, Dv50 ranging from 402–472 µm across 10 samples from two lots and Dv90 ranging from 561–734 µm—all well above the respirable range. In addition, the novel nozzle of the POD device allows patients to position the device in the correct orientation if they follow the Instructions for Use and insert the device up to the "shoulder" of the actuator arm, which was confirmed to be easy to achieve in human factor testing.

To complete the clinical development for this INP104 program, the FDA required safety assessments of the UNS over 24 weeks with repeat dosing [84], which seemingly no other nasal delivery program had been asked to perform. This required the development of specific tools to assess the mucosal integrity of the olfactory epithelium and olfactory function, which detected no significant adverse effects over 24 and even 52 weeks [87].

A subsequent program, INP105, with a spray-dried powder formulation of olanzapine [88], showed in phase 1 a similar C_{max} and AUC as the same dose administered by intramuscular injection but with a faster T_{max}; however with no approved IV formulation of olanzapine to compare against, absolute bioavailability could not be determined in this study (Figure 2b). The POD powder programs (both INP105 and INP103/107 with levodopa/carbidopa) [89] benefited from the previous development of both rodent and primate versions of the POD which expedited formulation development and pharmacokinetic characterization before, or even during, human trials [90], with the structure and function of the non-human primate nose being most similar to that of humans [91].

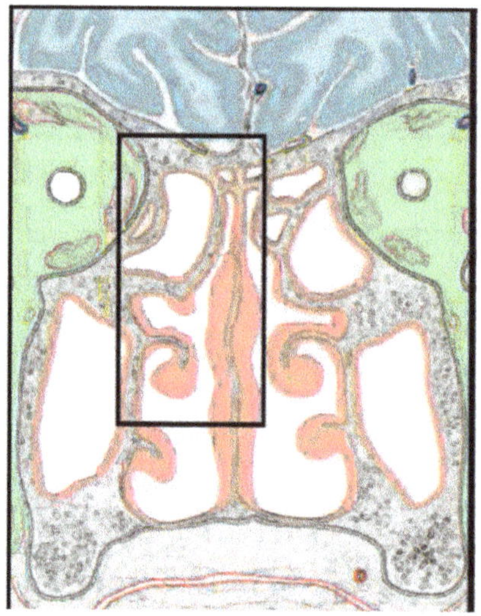

(**a**)

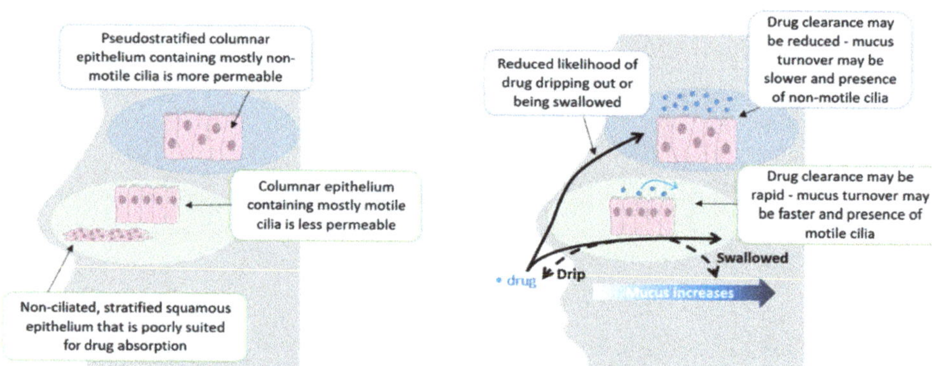

(**b**)

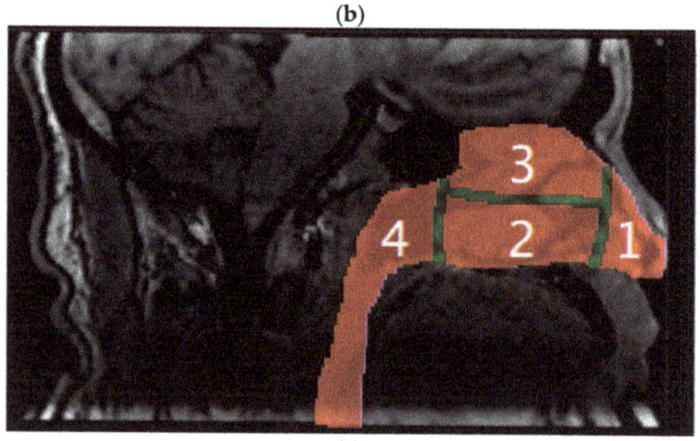

(**c**)

Figure 1. *Cont.*

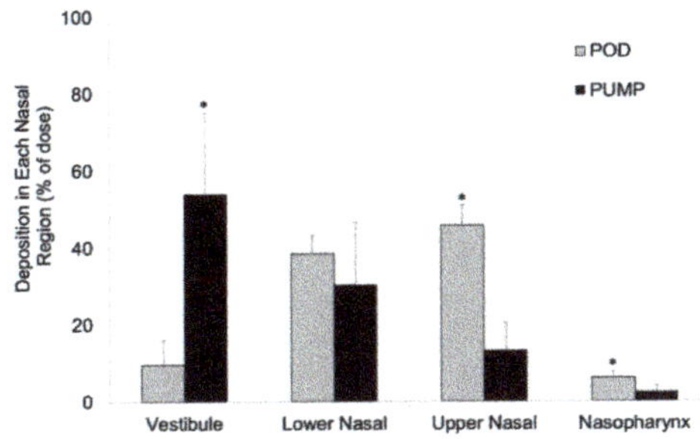

(d)

Figure 1. (**a**) Cross-section of the frontal portion of the human head, representing the posterior third of the nasal cavity, with outlined region (black box) highlighting areas commonly enriched with olfactory epithelium. Adapted from Salazar, I.; Sanchez-Quinteiro, P.; Barrios, A.W.; López Amado, M.; Vega, J.A. *Handb. Clin. Neurol.* **2019**, *164*, 47–65, with original adaptation from Schünke, M.; Schulte, E.; Schumacher, U. et al. *Prometheus: Texto y Atlas de Anatomía.* 3ª edición, vol. 3. Madrid: Panamericana; 2014 [19]. (**b**) Diagram showing the different epithelium (left panel) and clearance mechanisms (right panel) of the nose [75]. Reproduced with permission from the publisher. (**c**) SPECT Imaging data of nasal delivery of MAG-3 (^{99m}Technetium-labeled peptide) by POD vs. a traditional nasal spray in 7 Healthy Volunteers. To determine nasal deposition, the nasal cavity was divided into four regions: (1) Vestibule, (2) Lower nasal space, (3) UNS and (4) Nasopharynx based on MRI imaging [58]. (**d**) POD delivery led to significantly (* $p < 0.05$) greater deposition in the UNS (and nasopharynx) and less deposition in the vestibule (than the traditional spray) [81]. Regions defined in (**c**).

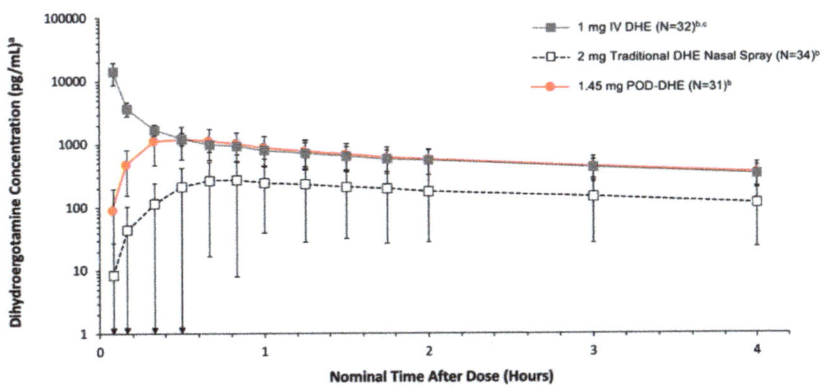

(a)

Figure 2. *Cont.*

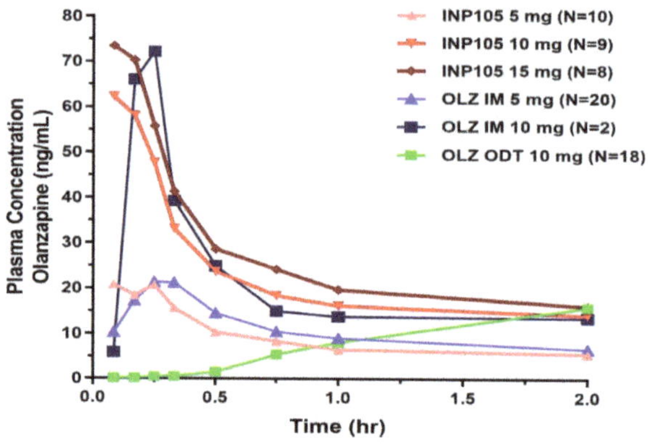

(b)

Figure 2. (a) STOP 101: Mean plasma DHE concentrations 0 to 4 Hours postdose (Safety Population) [61]. [a] Measures dihydroergotamine free base on a semi-log scale; [b] Doses represent dihydroergotamine mesylate; [c] N = 31 for time points of 5, 10, 30, and 40 min. Note: Dihydroergotamine concentration measurements begin at the 5-min timepoint. Represented as mean (SD). For the calculation of mean values, individual BLQ values were set to zero before determining the mean. BLQ = below the limit of quantitation data; IV = intravenous; SD = standard deviation. (**b**) SNAP 101: Plasma olanzapine concentrations 0 to 2 h post-dose [86]. INP105 = POD OLZ.

4. Nose-to-Brain (N2B) Delivery

In the last decade, some big companies exited drug development for neurological indications [92], but research and development in CNS indications has seemingly now picked up again [93] as CNS diseases are increasingly recognized as the leading cause of disability globally [94]. The challenge remains that at least two approved new therapies, both antisense oligonucleotides developed by Ionis Pharmaceuticals for devastating neurological diseases—spinal muscular atrophy [95] and amyotrophic lateral sclerosis [96], have to be delivered by intrathecal injection. So, the search continues for a less invasive way to circumvent or breach the Blood Brain Barrier (BBB). A comprehensive review of the direct N2B delivery of therapeutic peptides was published in 2022 [97]. To summarize that work: The therapeutic peptide market is large (US$39.3 Billion in 2021) but is expanding rapidly and is due to reach nearly $91.25 Billion in 2031 [98], while the nasal delivery market is also rapidly expanding (from $7.8 Billion in 2018 to $12 Billion by 2026 [99]. The article listed 14 approved small molecule products delivered nasally and 21 large molecular weight (MW) products (of which 9 were various versions of desmopressin), including one attenuated live virus vaccine (Flumist®). Of those large MW products, only three have received approval in the last 10 years, and only 1 of those, glucagon (Baqsimi™) in the last 5 years. This slow pace of translating the exciting preclinical data into clinical programs is disappointing, but at last, that situation may be changing with ongoing research programs in several indications where interesting data has been generated: insulin in cognitive impairment/Alzheimer's disease [100] in 2017; oxytocin to improve social communication in autism spectrum disorders [101] 2018; orexin-A in narcolepsy [102] 2011; basic fibroblast growth factor in Parkinsonism [103] 2021; leptin in obesity [104] in 2018, and there remains vigorous activity in oligonucleotide development for neurological disease [95,96]. However, clinical progress still remains slow, with direct injection of growth factor protein into the brain proposed as remaining the most promising option [103], with the development of protective biomaterials and device selection still required to better deliver these peptides across the BBB in a less invasive manner.

In his 2014 paper [16], Djupesland reviewed many of the articles claiming N2B transport, commenting then that encouraging data had been generated with both insulin and orexin, based on MRI imaging and/or clinical response, but that "convincing, unequivocal proof of N2B transport was still missing in humans, largely due to methodological and ethical considerations". Sadly, 9 years later, we are really no further forward.

Insulin N2B has been the most studied large molecular weight (5808 Da) peptide [100,105–110], perhaps not surprising since the discovery of specific insulin receptors in the olfactory bulb, hippocampus, hypothalamus and lower brainstem [111].

A 2018 study [109] looked at data from 38 clinical studies of acute nasal insulin administration that had dosed 1092 individuals and a further 18 studies in 832 individuals for periods between 21 days and 9.7 years and found no evidence of symptomatic hypoglycemia or serious adverse events, while 10 of the acute studies reported minor, temporary reductions in blood glucose and one report of minor glucose reduction in the chronic study. Overall blood glucose fell by 0.2–0.5 mmol/L (4–9 mg/dL) and lasted longer than the temporary rise in circulating insulin [110]

Another review from 2021 similarly looked at the growing number of clinical trials investigating N2B delivery [111]. One such device claiming UNS delivery and showing promising results with the delivery of insulin is the Kurve ViaNase® device leading to the Study of Nasal Insulin to Fight Forgetfulness (SNIFF) study, a large phase 3 NIH trial [42]. Kurve's ViaNase technology incorporates an electronic atomizer that creates a vortex of nebulized particles, their Controlled Particle Dispersion (CPD®) nasal delivery technology to "create a precisely-controlled turbulent flow" appropriate for monoclonal antibodies and larger peptides, maximize distribution to the UNS and minimize pharyngeal deposition. Several publications have featured Kurve's technologies, with one of those publications [112] reporting, in 2015, an exploratory study delivering a single dose of 2-PMPA (a blocker of the brain metallopeptidase, glutamate carboxypeptidase II, thought to be responsible for excess glutamate in neurodegenerative diseases) to a single non-human primate. At 30 min post-dosing, 2-PMPA was undetectable in the plasma (lower limit of quantitation being 50 nM), while the concentration in the CSF was 0.32 μg/mL (~1.5 μM) determined by LC/MS/MS. Several ^{99}Technetium labeled scintigraphic images on their website (kurvetx.com/research/peer-review-deposition comparison, dated 2005) show the widespread distribution of isotope throughout the nasal cavity, but it is not clear that this data was, in fact, peer-reviewed or if it has ever been published.

Kurve technology was selected for the NIH SNIFF trial, but the device suffered from frequent malfunctions and after 49 patients were dosed, it was replaced with the POD device for the remaining 240 patients with mild cognitive impairment [42]. The trial failed to show clinical benefit compared to placebo, but there were no reports of hypoglycemia, suggesting a lack of significant systemic absorption of the insulin. Kurve's ViaNase technology is still being advanced for treating psychiatric conditions, post-stroke and cognitive impairment in multiple sclerosis, with six separate programs delivering insulin in mild cognitive impairment, five programs delivering polyclonal antibodies in neurodegenerative disease, and five other programs featured on their corporate website. Other N2B delivery projects have looked at cholecystokinin [113], erythropoietin [114], melanocortin [115], glutathione [116], perillyl alcohol [117], angiotensin II [118] and neurotrophic factors [119] all with promising preclinical, or clinical case study results but have yet to be subjected to large scale, randomized clinical trial investigation.

While the importance of delivery of these drugs and peptides to the olfactory epithelium for N2B was stressed, there is little data comparing UNS delivery to LNS delivery to demonstrate this. Neither is there clarity about what device was actually used to generate the data. This highlights one of the important questions still to be addressed in clinical development: how to demonstrate N2B delivery in humans before investing in and conducting long-term clinical studies.

4.1. Olfactory Delivery

Millions of Olfactory Sensory Neurons (OSNs) are embedded in the olfactory epithelium and have long, non-motile cilia extending into the UNS. This is the only place in the body where the CNS is in direct contact with the environment [16,120]. These OSNs die and regenerate—perhaps the best-known neurons with that ability likely resulting from their exposure to inhaled chemicals—with a lifecycle of 30–60 days [15], although much of the research showing this comes from mice [121]. Once drugs are delivered onto the UNS, they may be transported across the olfactory epithelium inside the nerve axon (intracellularly), between the epithelial cells (paracellularly) or through the epithelial cells (transcellularly) [16], and thereafter the drug enters the olfactory bulb and then may distribute to other areas of the brain. Uptake by the OSN is by either non-specific or receptor-mediated endocytosis, predominantly the former [111]. The endocytosed drug is then transported to the olfactory bulb, taking an estimated 0.74–2.67 h [15,122]. Data from mice has shown drug in the CNS by 5 min post administration [123], peaks in the olfactory bulb by ~10 min [15] and distributes to distant brain regions such as the hypothalamus and midbrain by 30 min [124]. As the OSNs apoptose, so there are temporary gaps between the sustentacular cells of the epithelium, through which drug can pass—the paracellular route—and enter the perineural space that surround the OSNs as they traverse the cribriform plate [125]. Once in the brain, distribution may be by continued intracellular transport, although considered more likely is ongoing extracellular transport by convective bulk flow and a putative "perivascular pump" [15]. It is important to remember that many of the experimental studies conducted in rodents (whose olfactory epithelium may cover 50% of their nasal cavity [126] rather than the ~5% in humans) will be conducted by highly trained and familiar technicians applying drugs to anesthetized animals lying on their backs. The olfactory epithelial surface area to body weight ratio in humans is very different from those found in other animal species [127] (Table 3), and unanesthetized humans will be physiologically different from anesthetized animals. These considerations make it challenging to extrapolate animal data to humans, and the usual allometric scaling conventions applied when moving from preclinical to clinical experiments may not apply. Hence knowing both the surface area of an animal's olfactory mucosa and its surface area to weight ratio may need to be considered prior to clinical studies. As yet, there is no consensus on how to measure the direct CNS uptake of drugs in humans, short of the longer-term efficacy benefits that all drugs seek. What is known, however, is that cerebrospinal fluid levels obtained by lumbar puncture may not accurately reflect tissue levels in the brain [12,128]. As the route of administration of intrathecal drugs, such as the oligonucleotides Spinraza® [95] and Qalsody® [96], is also through a lumbar puncture, there may be other excellent therapeutics that, even with intrathecal delivery, show disappointing clinical results due to the failure to get from the CSF into the CNS tissue due to the protective arachnoid membrane and its tight junctions [129] with only ~5% of the CSF reaching and circulating around the olfactory region [12]. It is estimated that the dose delivered by this route may only need to be 0.01–1% of an oral dose [125].

Table 3. Olfactory epithelium surface area:Body weight ratio (cm^2/kg) of different species. Adapted from [130].

Species	Olfactory Epithelium Surface Area (cm^2)	Olfactory Epithelium Surface Area:Body Weight Ratio (cm^2/kg)
Mouse	1.25–1.40	31.0–35.0
Rat	4.20–6.80	12.0–19.0
Dog	170.0–380.0	17.0–38.0
Small primate	0.25–0.55	2.30–2.75
Human	10.0	0.14

4.2. Trigeminal Delivery

The trigeminal nerve provides sensory innervation to the LNS through its ophthalmic (V1) and maxillary (V2) branches. These supply upper anterior segments of the nasal space (i.e., also supply areas that the olfactory nerve serves, through its OSNs) and lower parts of the nasal space, respectively, and provide the respiratory epithelium with both sensory and parasympathetic innervation, projecting back to the pons. Unlike the OSN, the trigeminal nerve endings do not project above the epithelial surface; thus, any trigeminal transport first has to cross this respiratory epithelium or pass between the tight junctions of the mucosal cells to reach the underlying neurons. This results in transport via the trigeminal nerve being slower than via the olfactory nerve, estimated at 17–56 h [15] from mucosa to brain, with the axonal transport component alone also being slower (than olfactory transport) at 3.7–13.3 h [120]. However, even some drugs delivered to the LNS may be taken up by these neurons and transported directly to the brain. That could be the reason why one traditional nasal spray administered vaccine containing a neurotoxin resulted in dozens of cases of Bell's palsy and had to be withdrawn from the (Swiss) market [60]. Whether this route will be able to supplement or supplant olfactory delivery remains unknown at this time, and similarly unknown is whether future imaging technology will be able to differentiate between the two neuronal routes.

4.3. Vomeronasal Terminalis

The vomeronasal organ (VNO) [130] is present in newborn infants in the soft tissue at the base of the nasal septum just above the hard palate and is the termination of the vomeronasal terminalis nerve [79]. The VNO (or Jacobson's organ) is fully functional in the macrosmotic rodents and canines, sensing not only compounds emanating from prey and predators but sex pheromones [131] too, but is vestigial in human adults. It is unknown how much, if any, drug may reach the olfactory bulb via this nerve.

5. Discussion

As medicine advances, and especially as many CNS diseases are now receiving much greater attention, so focus on how to deliver these new medicines has increased. Drug delivery has to address the inability of these medicines to be delivered orally and how to cross the BBB. Only ~2% of small molecule drugs cross the BBB from the bloodstream, and maybe only 0.1% reach the CNS [132], so it is only suitable for potent molecules, especially peptides and proteins. With advances in bioadhesives, absorption/permeation enhancers and other Drug-Delivery Solutions (such as the addition of alkylsaccharides [133]—as used in Valtoco—see Table 1) and new devices, the non-invasive delivery of more of these future medicines has become possible.

Emerging infectious diseases, such as COVID that enter the body through the nose—can still cause illness and be transmitted in subjects who have received systemic vaccination, making nasal vaccine delivery and mucosal immunity a higher priority [134]. So far, vaccine programs have not further investigated where in the nose their payload is delivered or whether delivering to different parts of the nose affects the immunological response. If a vaccine were to be delivered to the olfactory epithelium, depending on its components, it too could gain direct access to the CNS, which could be detrimental, although allowing a vaccine to dwell longer on the epithelium could aid uptake into the Nasal Associated Lymphoid Tissue (NALT) and thus confer greater mucosal protection for the whole nasal mucosa. To date, most vaccine programs have utilized traditional nasal aerosol sprays or "nose drops," which deposit most of their contents in the non-absorptive (squamous epithelium lined) vestibule or respiratory epithelium lined lower nasal space [135].

The UNS is also the target for drugs seeking N2B delivery, and while imaging (MRI, PET, SPECT and gamma scintigraphy [21] can provide some supportive data and all show promise, none have yet to be fully validated as a way to measure deposition into the UNS, let alone absorption into the CNS although PET/MRI is considered most sensitive at quantifying N2B delivery [135]. Current options to assay the drug levels remain HPLC, high sensitivity mass spectrometry and immunoassay [127], while other methods to determine direct N2B delivery are also being considered, such as changes in brain metabolism [108], selective insulin impairment [136], changes in brain blood flow [137] and neuromodulation [138]. These options need to be vigorously explored so that the requisite evidence of direct N2B delivery in humans can be convincingly demonstrated.

Previous nasal delivery systems have not proven to be very popular for a variety of cultural or clinical reasons: unfamiliarity, local intolerability (e.g., drug dripping down the back of the throat, bad taste and swallowing), drug loss as it drips out of the front of the nose (requiring lying head hanging to combat gravity), or lack of consistency of absorption and thus effect. Patient adherence is critical, and thus formulation for taste should be considered early in development with patient input to the design of devices, their instructions for use and important Human Factor work undertaken prior to commercialization. Different strategies have been employed to try and overcome these difficulties, with varying degrees of success, but only recently has attention shifted to delivering drugs to different parts of the nose, specifically to land on the olfactory epithelium of the UNS for drugs requiring rapid and extensive absorption, or potentially N2B.

Targeting the olfactory epithelium may, by virtue of its non-motile cilia and high vascularity, also provide potentially highly differentiated systemic PK profiles for drugs compared to traditional nasal delivery and may be better than intramuscular injection and only surpassed in efficiency by intravenous injection, at least for some, maybe simpler nasal formulations. Conditions where acute treatment is required, such as seizures, migraine, agitation, off episodes in Parkinson's disease and anaphylaxis, could well benefit from drugs redirected to this epithelium when access to a healthcare practitioner and the requisite equipment for IV injection or infusion are not available. Delivery to the UNS may be the optimal target within the nose for small- and large-molecule drugs and perhaps for some vaccines. Further information about mucosal immunity and vaccine adjuvant and excipients, nanotechnology and the surge of nasal vaccine delivery clinical trials [139–159] can be found in the Supplementary Materials.

6. Conclusions

Nasal delivery of drugs and vaccines using small, portable, easily operated (by patients themselves, caregivers or healthcare professionals) devices will likely never replace oral pills, capsules and tablets. But where rapid drug levels are required, oral drugs are prone to gut or liver degradation, disease-related gastrointestinal dysfunction or comorbidity delay absorption, large molecules need to be delivered, delivery of drugs N2B for CNS disease is being contemplated, or induction of nasal (or distant) mucosal immunity by vaccinations is required, there are compelling reasons to consider nasal delivery and as we understand more about the complex anatomy and physiology of this organ, perhaps targeting the UNS within the nose. I believe that in the years to come, nasal delivery will become much more popular for all three situations: non-invasive systemic delivery, N2B delivery, and ensuring broad mucosal immunity. Regional deposition within the nose will thus become a standard part of development programs, along with an array of formulations to ensure safe, effective and consistent delivery of their large molecule and even future cellular cargo.

Supplementary Materials: The following supporting information can be downloaded at: https://www.mdpi.com/article/10.3390/pharmaceutics15061720/s1. The Supplementary Material provides a short summary of mucosal immunity; recent vaccine, adjuvant, excipient, nanotechnology and attenuated viral developments, and the surge in nasal delivery in clinical trials [139–159]. Table S1: Different vaccine platforms (with some examples, advantages and disadvantages).

Funding: Initial draft prepared while a full time employee of Impel Pharmaceuticals; but three rounds of revision prepared and submitted post Impel employment.

Institutional Review Board Statement: Not applicable.

Informed Consent Statement: Not applicable.

Data Availability Statement: Not applicable.

Conflicts of Interest: SBS was a full-time employee of Impel Pharmaceuticals when this article was conceived. He was fully responsible for the design and execution of Studies STOP 101, SNAP 101 and STOP 301 which were designed, conducted and analyzed while he was a full time employee of Impel Pharmaceuticals. The company had no role in the development of the manuscript, and in the decision to publish the results.

Abbreviations

AD	Alzheimer's disease
APC	Antigen Presenting Cell
AUC	Area Under Curve (of concentration against time)
BBB	Blood-Brain Barrier
CNS	Central Nervous System
CRSwNP	Chronic Rhinosinusitis with Nasal Polyps
CSF	Cerebrospinal Fluid
DDM	Dodecyl maltoside
Dv10/50/90	Volume Diameter: 10%, 50%, or 90% of particles less than these diameters, respectively
EDS	Exhalation Delivery System
EDTA	Ethylenediaminetetracetic Acid
EMA	European Medicines Agency
FDA	Food and Drug Administration
HFA	Hydrofluoroalkane
HPLC	High-Performance Liquid Chromatography
HPMC	Hydroxypropyl methylcellulose
IM	Intramuscular
LC/MS/MS	Liquid chromatography-tandem mass spectrometry
LNS	Lower Nasal Space
MAG-3	Mercaptuacetyltriglycerine
MCC	Mucociliary Clearance
MRI	Magnetic Resonance Imaging
MW	Molecular Weight
N2B	Nose-to-Brain
NALT	Nasal Associate Lymphoid Tissue
NIH	National Institutes of Health
OSN	Olfactory Sensory Neuron
OTC2-PMPA	Over the Counter 2-(Phosphonomethyl)pentanedioic acid
PET	Positron Emission Tomography
POD	Precision Olfactory Delivery
SC	Subcutaneous
SPECT	Single Photon Emission Computerized Tomography
UDS	Unit Dose Spray
UNS	Upper Nasal Space
VLP	Virus-Like Particle
VNO	Vomeronasal organ

References

1. Hou, H.; Li, Y.; Xu, Z.; Yu, Z.; Peng, B.; Wang, C.; Liu, W.; Li, W.; Ye, Z.; Zhang, G. Applications and research progress of Traditional Chinese medicine delivered via nasal administration. *Biomed. Pharmacother.* **2013**, *157*, 113933. [CrossRef] [PubMed]
2. Zarshenas, M.M.; Zargaran, A.; Müller, J.; Mohagheghzadeh, A. Nasal Drug Delivery in Traditional Persian Medicine. *Jundishapur. J. Nat. Pharm. Prod.* **2013**, *8*, 144–148. [CrossRef] [PubMed]
3. Ilum, L. Nasal Drug Delivery—Recent developments and future prospects. *J. Con. Rel.* **2012**, *161*, 254–263. [CrossRef]
4. De la Torre, B.G.; Albericio, F. The Pharmaceutical Industry in 2022: An Analysis of FDA Drug Approvals from the Perspective of Molecules. *Molecules* **2023**, *28*, 1038. [CrossRef] [PubMed]
5. Hanson, L.R.; Frey, W.H., 2nd. Strategies for intranasal delivery of therapeutics for the prevention and treatment of neuroAIDS. *J. Neuroimmune Pharmacol.* **2007**, *2*, 81–86. [CrossRef]

6. Dhuria, S.V.; Hanson, L.R.; Frey, W.H., 2nd. Intranasal drug targeting of hypocretin-1 (orexin-A) to the central nervous system. *J. Pharm. Sci.* **2009**, *98*, 2501–2515. [CrossRef] [PubMed]
7. Gomez, D.; Martinez, J.A.; Hanson, L.R.; Frey, W.H., 2nd; Toth, C.C. Intranasal treatment of neurodegenerative diseases and stroke. *Front. Biosci. Schol. Ed.* **2012**, *4*, 74–89. [CrossRef]
8. Johnson, N.J.; Hanson, L.R.; Frey, W.H. Trigeminal pathways deliver a low molecular weight drug from the nose to the brain and orofacial structures. *Mol. Pharm.* **2010**, *7*, 884–893. [CrossRef]
9. Correa, D.; Scheuber, M.I.; Shan, H.; Weinmann, O.W.; Baumgartner, Y.A.; Harten, A.; Wahl, A.-S.; Skaar, K.L.; Schwab, M.E. Intranasal delivery of full-length anti-Nogo-A antibody: A potential alternative route for therapeutic antibodies to central nervous system target. *Proc. Natl. Acad. Sci. USA* **2023**, *120*, e2200057120. [CrossRef]
10. Pardeshi, C.V.; Belgamwar, V.S. Direct nose to brain drug delivery via integrated nerve pathways bypassing the blood-brain barrier: An excellent platform for brain targeting. *Expert. Opin. Drug Deliv.* **2013**, *10*, 957–972. [CrossRef]
11. Chapman, C.D.; Frey, W.H.; Craft, S.; Danielyan, L.; Hallschmid, M.; Schioth, H.B.; Benedict, C. Intranasal Treatment of Central Nervous System Dysfunction in Humans. *Pharm. Res.* **2013**, *30*, 2475–2484. [CrossRef] [PubMed]
12. Pardridge, W.M. Drug Transport across the Blood-Brain Barrier. *J. Cerebr. Blood Flow Met.* **2012**, *32*, 1959–1972. [CrossRef] [PubMed]
13. Kashyap, K.; Shukla, R. Drug Delivery and Targeting to the Brain Through the Nasal Route: Mechanisms, Applications and Challenges. *Curr. Drug Deliv.* **2019**, *16*, 887–901. [CrossRef] [PubMed]
14. van Velthoven, C.T.J.; Kavelaars, A.; van Bel, F.; Heijnen, C.J. Nasal Administration of Stem Cells: A Promising Novel Route to Treat Neonatal Ischemic Brain Damage. *Pediatr. Res.* **2010**, *68*, 419–422. [CrossRef]
15. Crowe, T.P.; Hsu, W.H. Evaluation of Recent Intranasal Drug Delivery Systems to the Central Nervous System. *Pharmaceutics* **2022**, *14*, 629. [CrossRef] [PubMed]
16. Djupesland, P.G.; Messina, J.C.; Mahmoud, R.A. The Nasal Approach to Delivering Treatment for Brain Diseases: An Anatomic, Physiologic, and Delivery Technology Overview. *Ther. Deliv.* **2014**, *5*, 709–733. [CrossRef]
17. Lockhead, J.J.; Thorne, R.G. Intranasal Delivery of Biologics to the Central Nervous System. *Adv. Drug Deliv. Rev.* **2012**, *64*, 614–628. [CrossRef]
18. Lockhead, J.J.; Wolak, D.J.; Pizzo, M.E.; Thorne, R.G. Rapid Transport within Perivascular Spaces Underlies Widespread Tracer Distribution in the Brain after Intranasal Administration. *J. Cereb. Blood Flow Metab.* **2015**, *35*, 371–381. [CrossRef]
19. Godfrey, L.; Iannitelli, A.; Garrett, N.L.; Moger, J.; Imbert, I.; King, T.; Porreca, F.; Soundararajan, R.; Lalatsa, A.; Schatzlein, A.G.; et al. Nanoparticulate Peptide Delivery Exclusivity to the Brain Produces Tolerance Free Analgesia. *J. Control. Release* **2018**, *270*, 135–144. [CrossRef]
20. Ul Islam, S.; Shehzad, A.; Ahmed, M.B.; Lee, Y.S. Intranasal Delivery of Nanoformulations: A Potential Way of Treatment for Neurological Disorders. *Molecules* **2020**, *25*, 1929. [CrossRef]
21. Trevino, J.T.; Quispe, R.C.; Khan, F.; Novak, V. Non-Invasive Stategies for Nose-to-Brain Drug Delivery. *J. Clin. Trials* **2020**, *10*, 439. [PubMed]
22. Scott, B.A.; Yarchoan, M.; Jaffee, E.M. Prophylactic Vaccines for Nonviral Cancers. *Ann. Rev. Cancer Biol.* **2018**, *2*, 195–211. [CrossRef]
23. Mato, Y.L. Nasal Route for Vaccine and Drug Delivery: Features and Current Opportunities. *Int. J. Pharm.* **2019**, *572*, 118813. [CrossRef]
24. Keller, L.-A.; Merkel, O.; Popp, A. Intranasal Drug Delivery: Opportunities and Toxicologic Challenges During Drug Development. *Drug Deliv. Transl. Res.* **2022**, *12*, 735–757. [CrossRef]
25. Rabinowicz, A.L.; Carrazana, E.; Maggio, E.T. Improvement of Intranasal Delivery with Intravail® Alkylsaccharide Excipient as a Mucosal Absorption Enhancer Aiding in the Treatment of Conditions of the Central Nervous System. *Drug RD* **2021**, *21*, 361–369. [CrossRef]
26. Suman, J. How Evolving Patient Needs Have Fueled the Development of Nasal Drug Delivery. *ONdrugDelivery*, 17 May 2021; 18–22.
27. Alnasser, S. A Review on Nasal Drug Delivery System and its Contribution in Therapeutic Management. *Asian J. Pharm. Clin. Res.* **2019**, *12*, 40–45. [CrossRef]
28. Wang, Z.; Xiong, G.; Tsang, W.C.; Schatzlein, A.G.; Uchegbu, I.F. Nose-to-Brain Delivery. *J. Pharmacol. Exp. Therapeut.* **2019**, *370*, 593–601. [CrossRef]
29. Leopold, D.A.; Elkayam, D.; Messina, J.C.; Kosik-Gonzalez, C.; Djupesland, P.G.; Mahmoud, R.A. NAVIGATE II: Randomized Double-blind Trial of the Exhalation Delivery System with Fluticasone for Nasal Polyposis. *J. Allergy Clin. Immunol.* **2019**, *143*, 126–134. [CrossRef]
30. Larsen, P.L.; Tos, M. Origin of Nasal Polyps: An Endoscopic Autopsy Study. *Laryngoscope* **2004**, *114*, 710–719. [CrossRef]
31. Unidose (UDS) Liquid Nasal Spray System. Available online: https://aptar.com/products/pharmaceutical/uds-unidose-liquid-nasal-spray-system/ (accessed on 9 June 2023).
32. Bidose (BDS) Liquid Nasal Spray System. Available online: https://aptar.com/products/pharmaceutical/bds-bidose-nasal-spray-system-manufacturer/ (accessed on 9 June 2023).

33. Unidose (UDS) Powder Nasal Spray System. Available online: https://aptar.com/products/pharmaceutical/unidose-nasal-powder-system-manufacturer/#:~:text=Aptar%20Pharma%E2%80%99s%20Unidose%20(UDS)%20Nasal,precise%20dose%20quickly%20and%20easily (accessed on 9 June 2023).
34. VP3 Multi-Dose Spray Pump. Available online: https://aptar.com/products/pharmaceutical/vp3-technology-platform/ (accessed on 9 June 2023).
35. Dihydroergotamine Mesylate. Available online: https://pi.bauschhealth.com/globalassets/BHC/PI/Migranal-PI.pdf (accessed on 9 June 2023).
36. Migranal. Available online: https://www.pdr.net/drug-summary/?drugLabelId=Migranal-dihydroergota-mine-mesylate-771 (accessed on 9 June 2023).
37. Flonase Allergy Relief Nasal Spray. Available online: https://www.flonase.com/products/flonase-allergy-relief/?gclid=CjwKCAi-Att2tBhBDEiwALZuhAEB-kI6eRoGWy2L-7zrmgp5zkSAX4ZcmpbvWvYIPwoRMvP0lijEufshoCvo8QAvD_BwE&gclsrc=aw.ds (accessed on 9 June 2023).
38. Trudhesa®. Available online: https://www.trudhesa.com/ (accessed on 9 June 2023).
39. Impel Pharmaceuticals. Available online: https://impelpharma.com/our-science/ (accessed on 9 June 2023).
40. INP105 Proof-of-concept Study for the Acute Treatment of Agitation in Adolescents and Young Adults With ASD (CALM 201). Available online: https://clinicaltrials.gov/study/NCT05163717?cond=Autism&term=NCT05163717&rank=1 (accessed on 9 June 2023).
41. The Future of Systemic and Central Nervous System (CNS) Therapies. Available online: https://kurvetx.com/ (accessed on 9 June 2023).
42. Craft, S.; Raman, R.; Chow, T.W.; Rafii, M.S.; Sun, C.K.; Rissman, R.A.; Rissman, R.A.; Donohue, M.C.; Brewer, J.B.; Jenkins, C.; et al. Safety, Efficacy, and Feasibility of Intranasal Insulin for the Treatment of Mild Cognitive Impairment and Alzheimer Disease Dementia: A Randomized Clinical Trial. *JAMA Neurol.* **2020**, *77*, 1099–1109. [CrossRef]
43. XHANCE® (Fluticasone Propionate). Available online: https://www.optinose.com/products/xhance-fluticasone-propionate/ (accessed on 9 June 2023).
44. ONZETRA Xsail. Available online: https://www.onzetra.com/ (accessed on 9 June 2023).
45. STS101 (DHE Nasal Powder). Available online: https://www.satsumarx.com/our-research/sts101/ (accessed on 9 June 2023).
46. Aero Pump. Available online: https://www.aeropump.de/en/products/nasal (accessed on 9 June 2023).
47. Metered Pump Nasal Spray Bottles, 1 oz. Available online: https://pharmasystems.com/metered-pump-nasal-spray-bottles-1-oz-10271 (accessed on 9 June 2023).
48. Healthcare Mark II™. Available online: https://silgandispensing.com/products/mark-ii (accessed on 9 June 2023).
49. Nemera Ear, Nose, Throat. Available online: https://www.nemera.net/wp-content/uploads/2021/11/Nemera-ENT-brochure-digital.pdf (accessed on 9 June 2023).
50. Kobo-Greenhut, A.; Frankenthal, H.; Darawsha, A.; Karasik, A.; Beja, A.Z.; Ben Hur, T.; Ekstien, D.; Amir, L.; Shahaf, D.; Ben Shlomo, I.; et al. A Non-Invasive Direct Nose to Brain Drug Delivery Platform vs. Invasive Brain Delivery Approach: Patient-Centered Care Impact Analysis. *Drug Deliv.* **2022**, *29*, 1754–1763. [CrossRef] [PubMed]
51. SipNose Nasal Delivery System. Available online: https://sipnose.com/products/ (accessed on 9 June 2023).
52. MAD Nasal™ Intranasal Mucosal Atomization Device. Available online: https://www.teleflex.com/usa/en/product-areas/anesthesia/atomization/mad-nasal-device/ (accessed on 9 June 2023).
53. Teleflex Intranasal Drug Delivery. 2023. Available online: https://teleflex.com/usa/en/product-areas/emergency-medicine/intranasal-drug-delivery/mad-nasal-intranasal-device/index.html (accessed on 24 March 2023).
54. BD Accuspray™ Nasal Spray System. Available online: https://www.bd.com/en-us/products-and-solutions/products/product-families/accuspray-nasal-spray-system (accessed on 9 June 2023).
55. Becton Dickinson. BD AccusprayTM Nasal Spray System. 2023. Available online: https://drugdeliverysystems.bd.com/products/prefillable-syringe-systems/vaccine-syringes/accuspray-nasal-spray-system (accessed on 24 March 2023).
56. The Potential and the Challenges of Nasal Vaccination. Available online: https://www.ondrugdelivery.com/the-potential-and-the-challenges-of-nasal-vaccination/ (accessed on 9 June 2023).
57. Suman, J. Intranasal Vaccination: Rationale, Progress and Challenges. RDD Online 2023. In Proceedings of the RDD 2023, Antibes (Nice), France, 2–5 May 2023.
58. Butowt, R.; von Bartheld, C.S. Anosmia in COVID-19: Underlying Mechanisms and Assessment of an Olfactory Route to Brain Infection. *Neuroscientist* **2021**, *27*, 582–603. [CrossRef]
59. Meinhardt, J.; Radke, J.; Dittmayer, C.; Franz, J.; Thomas, C.; Mothes, R.; Laue, M.; Schneider, J.; Brünink, S.; Greuel, S.; et al. Olfactory Transmucosal SARS-CoV-2 Invasion as a Port of Central Nervous System Entry in Individuals with COVID-19. *Nat. Neurosci.* **2021**, *24*, 168–175. [CrossRef]
60. Mutsch, M.; Zhou, W.; Rhodes, P.; Bopp, M.; Chen, R.T.; Linder, T.; Spyr, C.; Steffen, R. Use of the Inactivated Intranasal Influenza Vaccine and the Risk of Bell's Palsy in Switzerland. *NEJM* **2004**, *350*, 896–903. [CrossRef]
61. Scutti, S. *CDC Panel Recommends against Using FluMist Vaccine*; CNN Health: Atlanta, GA, USA, 2016.
62. Xu, H.; Cai, L.; Hufnagel, S.; Cui, Z. Intranasal vaccine: Factors to consider in research and development. *Int. J. Pharm.* **2021**, *609*, 121180. [CrossRef]

63. Peace, R.M. Mucosal Immunization for Cancer: Opportunities and Challenges. Master's Thesis, Dept of Pathology, Duke University, Durham, NC, USA, 2015.
64. Nizard, M.; Diniz, M.O.; Roussel, H.; Tran, T.; Ferreira, L.C.S.; Badoual, C.; Tartour, E. Novel Strategies and Applications for the Control of Pathogens and Tumors at Mucosal Sites. *Hum. Vacc. Immunother.* **2014**, *10*, 2175–2187. [CrossRef]
65. Akash, M.M.H.; Lao, Y.; Balivada, P.A.; Ato, P.; Ka, N.K.; Mituniewicz, A.; Silfen, Z.; Suman, J.D.; Chakravarty, A.; Joseph-McCarthy, D.; et al. On a Model-based Approach to Improve Intranasal Spray Targeting for Respiratory Viral Infections. *Front. Drug Deliv.* **2023**, *3*, 4671. [CrossRef]
66. Soliman, H.; Coffin, B.; Gourcerol, G. Gastroparesis in Parkinsons Disease: Pathophysiology and Clinical Management. *Brain. Sci.* **2021**, *11*, 831. [CrossRef]
67. Aurora, S.K.; Papapetropoulos, S.; Kori, S.H.; Kedar, A.; Abell, T.L. Gastric Stasis in Migraineurs: Etiology, Characteristics and Clinical and Therapeutic Implications. *Cephalalgia* **2013**, *33*, 408–415. [CrossRef] [PubMed]
68. Fransen, N.; Bredenberg, S.; Bjork, E. Clincial Study Shows Improved Absorption of Desmopressin with Novel Formulation. *Pharm. Res.* **2009**, *26*, 1618–1625. [CrossRef] [PubMed]
69. Salade, L.; Wuathoz, N.; Vermeersch, M.; Amighi, K.; Goole, J. Chitosan-Coated Liposome Dry-Powder Formulations Loaded with Ghrelin for Nose-to-Brain Delivery. *Eur. J. Pharm. Biopharm.* **2018**, *129*, 257–266. [CrossRef] [PubMed]
70. Zada, M.H.; Kubek, M.; Khan, W.; Kumar, A.; Domb, A. Dispersable Hydrolytically Sensitive Nanoparticles for Nasal Delivery of Thyrotrophin Releasing Hormone (TRH). *J. Control. Release* **2019**, *295*, 278–289. [CrossRef] [PubMed]
71. Von Mentzer, B.; Russo, A.F.; Zhang, Z.; Kuburas, A.; Killoran, P.M.; D'Aloisio, V.; Nizic, L.; Capel, V.; Kendall, D.A.; Coxon, C.R.; et al. A CGRP Receptor Antagonist Peptide Formulated for Nasal Administration to Treat Migraine. *J. Pharm. Pharmacol.* **2020**, *72*, 1352–1360. [CrossRef] [PubMed]
72. Cloyd, J.; Haut, S.; Carrazana, E.; Rabinowicz, A.L. Overcoming the Challenges of Developing an Intranasal Diazepam Rescue Therapy for the Treatment of Seizure Clusters. *Epilepsia* **2021**, 62. [CrossRef] [PubMed]
73. Haschke, M.; Suter, K.; Hofman, S.; Witschi, R.; Frohlich, J.; Imanidis, G.; Drewe, J.; Briellmann, T.A.; Dussy, F.E.; Krahenbuhl, S.; et al. Pharmacokinetics and Pharmacodynamics of Nasally Delivered Midazolam. *Br. J. Clin. Pharmacol.* **2010**, *69*, 607–616. [CrossRef] [PubMed]
74. ZAVZPRET^{TM} (zavegepant) Nasal Spray. Prescribing Information. Available online: https://www.accessdata.fda.gov/drugsatfda_docs/label/2023/216386s000lbl.pdf (accessed on 5 April 2023).
75. Martin, V.; Hoekman, J.; Aurora, S.K.; Shrewsbury, S.B. Nasal Delivery of Acute Medications for Migraine: The Upper Versus Lower Nasal Space. *J. Clin. Med.* **2021**, *10*, 2468. [CrossRef] [PubMed]
76. Moffa, A.; Costantino, A.; Rinaldi, V.; Sabatino, L.; Trecca, E.M.C.; Baptista, P.; Campisi, P.; Cassano, M.; Casale, M. Nasal Delivery Devices: A comparative Study on Cadaver Model. *BioMed. Res. Int.* **2019**, *2019*, 4602651. [CrossRef] [PubMed]
77. Dale, O.; Nilsen, T.; Loftsson, T.; Tonnesen, H.H.; Klepstad, P.; Kaasa, S.; Holand, T.; Djupesland, P.G. Intranasal Midazolam: A Comparison of Two Delivery Devices in Human Volunteers. *J. Pharm. Pharmacol.* **2006**, *58*, 1311–1318. [CrossRef] [PubMed]
78. Djupesland, P.G.; Skretting, A.; Winderen, M.; Holand, T. Breath Actuated Device Improves Delivery to Target Sites Beyond the Nasal Valve. *Laryngoscope* **2006**, *116*, 466–472. [CrossRef]
79. Djupesland, P.G.; Skretting, A. Nasal Deposition and Clearance in Man: Comparison of a Bidirectional Powder Device and a Traditional Liquid Nasal Spray. *J. Aerosol. Med. Pul. Drug Deliv.* **2012**, *25*, 280–289. [CrossRef]
80. Hoekman, J.; Brunelle, A.; Hite, M.; Kim, P.; Fuller, C. SPECT Imaging of Direct Nose-to-Brain Transfer of MAG-3 in Man. In Proceedings of the Am Assoc Pharm Scientist Annual Meeting, San Antonio, TX, USA, 10–14 November 2013.
81. Hoekman, J.; Brunelle, A.; Hite, M.; Kim, P.; Fuller, C. Usability and Tolerability Study in Human Subjects with a Novel Precision Olfactory Delivery (POD) Device. Poster (M1050). In Proceedings of the Am Assoc Pharm Scientist Annual Meeting, San Antonio, TX, USA, 10–14 November 2013.
82. Gizurarson, S. Anatomical and Histological Factors Affecting Intranasal Drug and Vaccine Delivery. *Curr. Drug Deliv.* **2012**, *9*, 566–582. [CrossRef] [PubMed]
83. Shrewsbury, S.B.; Jeleva, M.; Satterly, K.H.; Lickliter, J.; Hoekman, J. STOP 101: A Phase 1, Randomized, Open-Label, Comparative Bioavailability Study of INP104, Dihydroergotamine Mesylate (DHE) Administered Intranasally by a I123 Precision Olfactory Delivery (POD®) Device, in Healthy Adult Subjects. *Headache* **2019**, *59*, 394–409. [CrossRef]
84. Smith, T.R.; Winner, P.; Aurora, S.K.; Jeleva, M.D.; Hocevar-Trnka, J.; Shrewsbury, S.B. STOP 301: A Phase 3, Open-label Study of Safety, Tolerability and Exploratory Efficacy of INP104, Precision Olfactory Delivery (POD®) of Dihydroergotamine Mesylate over 24/52 Weeks in Acute Treatment of Migraine Attacks in Adult patients. *Headache* **2021**, *61*, 1214–1226. [CrossRef]
85. Silberstein, S.D.; Shrewsbury, S.B.; Hoekman, J. Dihydroergotamine (DHE)—Then and Now: A Narrative Review. *Headache* **2020**, *60*, 40–57. [CrossRef] [PubMed]
86. Cooper, W.; Ray, S.; Aurora, S.K.; Shrewsbury, S.B.; Fuller, C.; Davies, G.; Hoekman, J. Delivery of Dihydroergotamine Mesylate to the Upper Nasal Space for the Acute Treatment of Migraine: Technology in Action. *J. Aerosol. Med.* **2022**, *35*, 321–332. [CrossRef] [PubMed]
87. Davis, G.; Pransky, S.; Fatakia, A.; Shrewsbury, S.B. The Upper Nasal Space as a Promising New Route for Drug Administration: Implications for Nasal Safety Assessments from the Pivotal STOP 301 Study of INP104. *Ann. Otolaryngol Rhinol.* **2022**, *9*, 1303.

88. Shrewsbury, S.B.; Hocevar-Trnka, J.; Satterly, K.H.; Craig, K.L.; Lickliter, J.D.; Hoekman, J. SNAP 101: Double-Blind, Placebo/Active-Controlled, Safety, Pharmacokinetic (PK), and Pharmacodynamic (PD) Study of INP105 (nasal olanzapine) in Healthy Adults. *J. Clin. Psych.* **2020**, *81*, 12–20. [CrossRef] [PubMed]
89. Hoekman, J.; Ray, S.; Aurora, S.K.; Shrewsbury, S.B. The Upper Nasal Space—A Novel Delivery Route Ideal for Central Nervous System Drugs. *US Neurol.* **2020**, *16*, 25–31. [CrossRef]
90. Shrewsbury, S.B.; Davies, G.; McConnachie, L.; Hoekman, J. The Pharmacokinetics of Drug Delivery to the Upper Nasal Space: A Review of INP105 Development. *Med. Res. Arch.* **2022**, *10*, 9. [CrossRef]
91. Smith, T.D.; Bhanagar, K.P.; Tuladhar, P.; Burrows, A.M. Distribution of Olfactory Epithelium in the Primate Nasal Cavity: Are Microsmia and Macrosmia Valid Morphological Concepts? *Anat. Rec.* **2004**, *281A*, 1173–1181. [CrossRef]
92. Mullard, A. Pfizer Exits Neuroscience. *Nat. Rev. Drug Discov.* **2018**, *17*, 86. [CrossRef]
93. Special Report: 2022 Neurology Drug & Device Approvals. *Pract. Neurol.* **2023**. Available online: https://practicalneurology.com/articles/2023-jan-feb/special-report-2022-neurology-drug-device-approvals (accessed on 24 March 2023).
94. GBD 2016 neurology collaborators. Global, regional, and national burden of neurological disorders, 1990–2016: A systematic analysis for the global burden of disease study 2016. *Lancet Neurol.* **2019**, *18*, 459–480. [CrossRef]
95. FDA Approves First Drug for Spinal Muscular Atrophy. *FDA News Release 23 December 2016*; FDA: Silver Spring, MD, USA, 2016.
96. *FDA Approves Treatment of Amyotrophic Lateral Sclerosis Associated with a Mutation in the SOD1 Gene*; FDA News Release 25 April 2023; FDA: Silver Spring, MD, USA, 2023.
97. Alabsi, W.; Eedara, B.B.; Encinas-Basurto, D.; Polt, R.; Mansour, H.M. Nose-to-Brain Delivery of Therapeutic Peptides as Nasal Aerosols. *Pharmaceutics* **2022**, *14*, 1870. [CrossRef] [PubMed]
98. Peptide Therapeutics Market to Reach US$91.25bn by 2031. Available online: https://www.transparencymarketresearch.com/peptide-therapeutics-market.html (accessed on 9 March 2023).
99. Nasal Drug Formulation: A Guide to Successful Drug Product Development. LLS Health CDMO. 17 February 2021. Available online: https://lubrizolcdmo.com/blog/a-guide-to-the-successful-development-of-nasal-drug-formulations/ (accessed on 9 March 2023).
100. Craft, S.; Claxton, A.; Baker, L.D.; Hanson, A.J.; Cholerton, B.; Trittschuh, E.H.; Dahl, D.; Caulder, E.; Neth, B.; Montine, T.J.; et al. Effects of Regular and Long-acting Insulin on Cognition and Alzheimer's Disease Biomarkers: A Pilot Clinical Trial. *J. Alzheimers. Dis.* **2017**, *57*, 1325–1334. [CrossRef] [PubMed]
101. Yamasue, H.; Domes, G. Oxytocin and Autism Spectrum Disorders. *Curr. Top Behav. Neurosci.* **2018**, *35*, 449–465.
102. De la Herran-Arita, A.K.; Guerra-Crespo, M.; Drucker-Colin, R. Narcolepsy and Orexins: An Example of Progress in Sleep Research. *Front. Neurol.* **2011**, *2*, 26. [CrossRef] [PubMed]
103. Liu, Y.; Deng, J.; Liu, Y.; Li, W.; Nie, X. FGF, Mechanism of Action, Role in Parkinson's Disease and Therapeutics. *Front. Pharmacol.* **2021**, *12*, 675725. [CrossRef] [PubMed]
104. Berger, S.; Pho, H.; Fleury-Curado, T.; Bevans-Fonti, S.; Younas, H.; Shin, M.-K.; Jun, J.C.; Anokye-Danso, F.; Ahima, R.S.; Enquist, L.W.; et al. Intranasal Leptin Relieves Sleep-disordered Breathing in Mice with Diet-induced Obesity. *Am. J. Resp. Crit. Care Med.* **2018**, *199*, 6. [CrossRef]
105. Zhang, H.; Hao, Y.; Manor, B.; Novak, P.; Milberg, W.; Novak, Z.J. Intranasal Insulin Enhanced Resting-state Functional Connectivity of Hippocampal Regions in Type 2 Diabetes. *Diabetes* **2015**, *64*, 1025–1034. [CrossRef]
106. Akintola, A.A.; Van Opstal, A.M.; Westendorp, R.G.; Postmus, I.; Van der Grond, J.; Van Heemst, D. Effect of Intranasally Administered Insulin on Cerebral Blood Flow and Perfusion: A Randomized Experiment in Young and Older Adults. *Aging (Albany NY)* **2017**, *9*, 790. [CrossRef]
107. Novak, V.; Milberg, W.; Hao, Y.; Munshi, M.; Novak, P.; Galica, A.; Manor, B.; Roberson, P.; Craft, S.; Abduljalil, A. Enhancement of Vasoreactivity and Cognition by Intranasal Insulin in Type 2 Diabetes. *Diabetes Care.* **2014**, *37*, 751–759. [CrossRef]
108. Reger, M.A.; Watson, G.; Green, P.S.; Baker, L.D.; Cholerton, B.; Fishel, M.A.; Plymate, S.R.; Cherrier, M.M.; Schellenberg, G.D.; Frey, W.H.; et al. Intranasal Insulin Administration Dose-dependently Modulates Verbal Memory and Plasma Amyloid-ß in Memory-impaired Older Adults. *J. Alzheimers Dis.* **2008**, *13*, 323–331. [CrossRef]
109. Schmid, V.; Kullmann, S.; Gfrörer, W.; Hund, V.; Hallschmid, M.; Lipp, H.P.; Häring, H.U.; Preissl, H.; Fritsche, A.; Heni, M. Safety of intranasal human insulin: A review. *Diabetes Obes. Metab.* **2018**, *20*, 1563–1577. [CrossRef] [PubMed]
110. Stockhorst, U.; de Fries, D.; Steingrueber, H.J.; Scherbaum, W.A. Insulin and the CNS: Effects on food intake, memory, and endocrine parameters and the role of intranasal insulin administration in humans. *Physiol. Behav.* **2004**, *83*, 47–54. [CrossRef] [PubMed]
111. Pandey, A.; Nikam, A.; Basavraj, S.; Mutalik, S.; Gopalan, D.; Kulkarni, S.; Padya, B.; Fernandes, G.; Mutalik, S. *Nose-To-Brain Drug Delivery: Regulatory Aspects, Clinical Trials, Patents, and Future Perspectives*; Elsevier Inc.: Amsterdam, The Netherlands, 2021.
112. Rais, R.; Wozniak, K.; Wu, Y.; Niwa, M.; Stathis, M.; Alt, J.; Giroux, M.; Sawa, A.; Rojas, C.; Slusher, B.S. Selective CNS Uptake of the GCP-II Inhibitor 2-PMPA Following Intranasal Administration. *PLoS ONE* **2015**, *10*, e0131861. [CrossRef]
113. Schneider, R.; Osterburg, J.; Buchner, A.; Pietrowsky, R. Effect of Intranasally Administered Cholecystokinin on Encoding of Controlled and Automatic Memory Processes. *Psychopharmacology.* **2009**, *202*, 559–567. [CrossRef]
114. Pedroso, I.; Garcia, M.; Casabona, E.; Morales, L.; Bringas, M.L.; Pérez, L.; Rodriguez, T.; Sosa, I.; Ricardo, Y.; Padron, A.; et al. Protective Activity of Erythropoyetine in the Cognition of Patients with Parkinson's Disease. *Behav. Sci.* **2018**, *8*, 51. [CrossRef] [PubMed]

115. Wellhöner, P.; Hörster, R.; Jacobs, F.; Sayk, F.; Lehnert, H.; Dodt, C. Intranasal Application of the Melanocortin 4 Receptor Agonist MSH/ACTH(4–10) in Humans Causes Lipolysis in White Adipose Tissue. *Int. J. Obes.* **2012**, *36*, 703–708. [CrossRef] [PubMed]
116. Mischley, L.K.; Lau, R.C.; Shankland, E.G.; Wilbur, T.K.; Padowski, J.M. Phase IIb Study of Intranasal Glutathione in Parkinson's Disease. *J. Parkinsons. Dis.* **2017**, *7*, 289–299. [CrossRef]
117. Faria, G.M.; Soares, I.D.P.; D'Alincourt Salazar, M.; Amorim, M.R.; Pessoa, B.L.; Da Fonseca, C.O.; Quirico-Santos, T. Intranasal Perillyl Alcohol Therapy Improves Survival of Patients with Recurrent Glioblastoma Harboring Mutant Variant for MTHFR rs1801133 Polymorphism. *BMC Cancer* **2020**, *20*, 294. [CrossRef]
118. Derad, I.; Sayk, F.; Lehnert, H.; Marshall, L.; Born, J.; Nitschke, M. Intranasal Angiotensin II in Humans Reduces Blood Pressure When Angiotensin II Type 1 Receptors are Blocked. *Hypertension* **2014**, *63*, 762–767. [CrossRef] [PubMed]
119. Bellis, A.; Bellis, M.; Aloe, L. Long-term Non-invasive Treatment via Intranasal Administration of Nerve Growth Factor Protects the Human Brain in Frontotemporal Dementia Associated with Corticobasal Syndrome: A Pilot Study. *J. Alzheimers. Dis. Rep.* **2018**, *2*, 67–77. [CrossRef]
120. Crowe, T.P.; Greenlee, M.H.W.; Kanthasamy, A.G.; Hsu, W.H. Mechanism of Intranasal Drug Delivery Directly to the Brain. *Life Sci.* **2018**, *195*, 44–52. [CrossRef] [PubMed]
121. McClintock, T.S.; Khan, N.; Xie, C.; Martens, J.R. Maturation of the Olfactory Sensory Neuron and its Cilia. *Chem. Senses* **2020**, *45*, 805–822. [CrossRef] [PubMed]
122. Broadwell, R.D.; Balin, B.J. Endocytic and Exocytic Pathways of the Neuronal Secretory Process and Trans Synaptic Transfer of Wheat Germ Agglutinin-Horseradish Peroxidase in vivo. *J. Comp. Neuro* **1985**, *242*, 632–650. [CrossRef] [PubMed]
123. Falcone, J.A.; Salameh, T.S.; Yi, X.; Cordy, B.J.; Mortell, W.G.; Kabanov, A.V.; Banks, W.A. Intranasal Administration as a Route for Drug Delivery to the Brain: Evidence for a Unique Pathway for Albumin. *J. Pharmacol. Exp. Ther.* **2014**, *351*, 54–60. [CrossRef] [PubMed]
124. Salameh, T.S.; Bullock, K.M.; Hujoel, I.A.; Niehoff, M.L.; Wolden-Hanson, T.; Kim, J.; Morley, J.E.; Farr, S.A.; Banks, W.A. Central Nervous System Delivery on Intranasal Insulin: Mechanisms of Uptake and Effects on Cognition. *J. Alzheimer's Dis.* **2015**, *47*, 715–728. [CrossRef] [PubMed]
125. Erdo, F.; Bors, L.A.; Farkas, D.; Bajza, A.; Gizurarson, S. Evaluation of Intranasal Delivery Route of Drug Administration for Brain Targeting. *Brain Res. Bull.* **2018**, *143*, 155–170. [CrossRef]
126. Wu, H.; Hu, K.; Jiang, X. From Nose to Brain: Understanding Transport Capacity and Transport Rate of Drugs. *Expert. Opin. Drug Deliv.* **2008**, *5*, 1159–1168. [CrossRef]
127. Landis, M.S.; Boyden, T.; Pegg, S. Nasal-to-CNS Drug Delivery: Where are we Now and Where are we Heading? An Industrial perspective. *Ther. Deliv.* **2012**, *3*, 195–220. [CrossRef]
128. De Lange, E.C.; Danhof, M. Considerations in the Use of Cerebrospinal Fluid Pharmacokinetics to Predict Brain Target Concentrations in the Clinical Setting: Implications of the Barriers Between Blood and Brain. *Clin. Pharmacokinet.* **2002**, *41*, 691–703. [CrossRef] [PubMed]
129. Derk, J.; Jones, H.E.; Como, C.; Pawlikowski, B.; Siegenthaler, J.A. Living on the Edge of the CNS: Meninges Cell Diversity in Health and Disease. *Front. Cell. Neurosci.* **2021**, *15*, 703944. [CrossRef] [PubMed]
130. Nakamuta, S.; Nakamuta, N.; Taniguchi, K.; Taniguchi, K. Histological and Ultrastructural Characteristics of the Primordial Vomeronasal Organ in Lungfish. *Anat. Rec.* **2012**, *295*, 481–491. [CrossRef] [PubMed]
131. Ryba, N.J.; Tirindelli, R. A New Multigene Family of Putative Pheromone Receptors. *Neuron* **1997**, *19*, 371–379. [CrossRef] [PubMed]
132. Mistry, A.; Stolnik, S.; Ilum, L. Nanoparticles for Direct-to-Brain Delivery of Drugs. *Int. J. Pharm.* **2009**, *379*, 146–157. [CrossRef] [PubMed]
133. Maggio, E.T. Intravail^{TM}: Highly Effective intranasal Delivery of Peptide and Protein Drugs. *Expert. Opin. Drug Deliv.* **2006**, *3*, 529–539. [CrossRef]
134. Riese, P.; Sakthivel, P.; Trittel, S.; Guzman, C.A. Intranasal Formulations: Promising Strategy to Deliver Vaccines. *Expert. Opin. Drug Deliv.* **2014**, *11*, 1619–1634. [CrossRef] [PubMed]
135. Veronesi, M.C.; Alhamami, M.; Miedema, S.B.; Yun, Y.; Ruiz-Cardozo, M.; Vannier, M.W. Imaging of intranasal drug delivery to the brain. *Am. J. Nucl. Med. Mol. Imaging.* **2020**, *10*, 1. [PubMed]
136. Kullmann, S.; Heni, M.; Veit, R.; Scheffler, K.; Machann, J.; Häring, H.U.; Andreas, F.; Hubert, P. Selective Insulin Resistance in Homeostatic and Cognitive Control Brain Areas in Overweight and Obese Adults. *Diabetes Care* **2015**, *38*, 1044–1050. [CrossRef]
137. Wingrove, J.; Swedrowska, M.; Scherließ, R.; Parry, M.; Ramjeeawon, M.; Taylor, D.; Gauthier, G.; Brown, L.; Amiel, S.; Zelaya, F.; et al. Characterisation of Nasal Devices for Delivery of Insulin to the Brain and Evaluation in Humans Using Functional Magnetic Resonance Imaging. *JCR* **2019**, *302*, 140–147. [CrossRef]
138. Mottolese, R.; Redouté, J.; Costes, N.; Le Bars, D.; Sirigu, A. Switching brain serotonin with oxytocin. *PNAS* **2014**, *111*, 8637–8642. [CrossRef] [PubMed]
139. Czerkinsky, C.; Holmgren, J. Topical Immunisation Strategies. *Mucosal Immunol* **2010**, *3*, 545–555. [CrossRef]
140. Hellings, P.; Jorissen, M.; Ceuppens, J.L. The Waldeyer's Ring. *Acta Otorhinolarngol. Belg.* **2000**, *54*, 237–241.
141. Pabst, R. Mucosal Vaccination by the Intranasal Route. Nose-Associated Lymphoid Tissue (NALT)—Structure, Function and Species Differences. *Vaccine* **2015**, *26*, 4406–4413.

142. Debertin, A.S.; Tschernig, T.; Tönjes, H.; Kleemann, W.J.; Tröger, H.D.; Pabst, R. Nasal-associated lymphoid tissue (NALT): Frequency and localization in young children. *Clin. Exp. Immunol.* **2003**, *134*, 503–507. [CrossRef]
143. Esposito, S.; Principi, N. Norovirus Vaccine: Priorities for Future Research and Development. *Front. Immunol.* **2020**, *11*, 1383. [CrossRef]
144. Moderna COVID-19 EUA Approval 2020. Available online: https://eua.modernatx.com/covid19vaccine-eua/fda-letter-eua.pdf (accessed on 11 March 2023).
145. Pfizer-BioNTech COVID-19 Vaccines 2021. Available online: https://www.fda.gov/emergency-preparedness-and-response/coronavirus-disease-2019-covid-19/pfizer-biontech-covid-19-vaccines (accessed on 11 March 2023).
146. Cohen, J. Chinese researchers reveal draft genome of virus implicated in Wuhan pneumonia outbreak. *Science* **2020**. [CrossRef]
147. Janssen COVID-19 Vaccine 2021. Available online: https://www.fda.gov/emergency-preparedness-and-response/coronavirus-disease-2019-covid-19/janssen-covid-19-vaccine (accessed on 11 March 2023).
148. Novavax COVID-19 Vaccine, Adjuvenated 2022. Available online: https://www.fda.gov/emergency-preparedness-and-response/coronavirus-disease-2019-covid-19/novavax-covid-19-vaccine-adjuvanted (accessed on 11 March 2023).
149. Waltz, E. China and India approve nasal COVID vaccines—Are they a game changer? *Nature* **2022**, *609*, 450. [CrossRef]
150. Sharifian-Dorche, M.; Bahmanyar, M.; Sharifian-Dorche, A.; Mohammadi, P.; Nomovi, M.; Mowla, A. Vaccine-induced immune thrombotic thrombocytopenia and cerebral venous sinus thrombosis post COVID-19 vaccination; a systematic review. *J. Neurol. Sci.* **2021**, *428*, 117607. [CrossRef]
151. Li, Y.-D.; Chi, W.-Y.; Su, J.-H.; Ferrall, L.; Hung, C.-F.; Wu, T.-C. Coronavirus vaccine development: From SARS and MERS to COVID-19. *J. Biomed. Sci.* **2020**, *27*, 104. [CrossRef]
152. Laffleur, F.; Bauer, B. Progress in nasal drug delivery systems. *Int. J. Pharm.* **2021**, *607*, 120994. [CrossRef]
153. Blakney, A.K.; McKay, P.F.; Hu, K.; Samnuan, K.; Jain, N.; Brown, A.; Thomas, A.; Rogers, P.; Polra, K.; Sallah, H.; et al. Polymeric and lipid nanoparticles for delivery of self-amplifying RNA vaccines. *J. Control. Release* **2021**, *338*, 201–210. [CrossRef] [PubMed]
154. Merkus, F.W.; van denBerg, M.P. Can Nasal Delivery Bypass the Blood-Brain Barrier?: Questionning the Direct Transport Theory. *Drugs* **2007**, *8*, 133–144. [CrossRef] [PubMed]
155. Alsarra, I.A.; Hamed, A.Y.; Alanazi, F.K.; El Maghraby, G.M. Vesicular Systems for Intranasal Drug Delivery. In *Drug Delivery to the Central Nervous System*; Jain, K.K., Ed.; Springer-Science: Berlin/Heidelberg, Germany, 2010; pp. 175–203.
156. Rowhani-Rahbar, A.; Fireman, B.; Lewis, N.; Ray, P.; Rasgon, B.; Klein, J.O.; Black, S.; Klein, N.P.; Baxter, R. Immunization and Bell's Palsy in Children: A Case-centered Analysis. *Am. J. Epidemiol.* **2012**, *175*, 878–885. [CrossRef]
157. Xu, H.; Alzhrani, R.F.; Warnken, Z.N.; Thakkar, S.G.; Zeng, M.; Smyth, H.D.; William, R.O., III; Cui, Z. Immunogenicity of Antigen Adjuvanted with AS04 and its Deposition in the Upper Respiratory Tract after Intranasal Administration. *Mol. Pharm.* **2020**, *17*, 3259–3269. [CrossRef] [PubMed]
158. Chaturvedi, M.; Kumar, M.; Pathak, K. A review on mucoadhesive polymer used in nasal drug delivery system. *J. Adv. Pharm. Technol. Res.* **2011**, *2*, 215–222. [CrossRef] [PubMed]
159. Mendoca, S.A.; Lorincz, R.; Boucher, P.; Curiel, D.T. Adenoviral vector platforms in the SARS-CoV-2 pandemic. *npj Vaccines* **2021**, *6*, 97. [CrossRef]

pharmaceutics

MDPI

Correction

Correction: Shrewsbury, S.B. The Upper Nasal Space: Option for Systemic Drug Delivery, Mucosal Vaccines and "Nose-to-Brain". *Pharmaceutics* 2023, *15*, 1720

Stephen B. Shrewsbury

Formerly of Impel Pharmaceuticals, 201 Elliott Ave West, Seattle, WA 98119, USA; steve.shrewsbury@me.com; Tel.: +1-(415)-250-1169

Error in Table

In the original publication [1], there was a mistake in Table 1 as published. The corrected Table 1 appears below. Specifically, the SipNose device is intended to deliver both liquid and powder formulations to the upper nasal space, although clinical data are yet to be generated to demonstrate that.

Table 1. Examples of Different Nasal Delivery Systems (in development or approved). The bottom four devices are basically syringes with different nozzles attached so that as a Healthcare Practitioner pushes the plunger of the syringe in, the liquid vaccine is forced out of the various tips creating a local mist or broad plume of particles 30–100 μm in diameter (in the case of the MAD).

Manufacturer	Device	Propellant	No. Doses	[Drug/Other Programs]	Pros	Cons	Reference/ Website
Aptar (Crystal Lake, IL, USA) (Device only) Multiple programs with drug companies	Unidose (UDS) Liquid Nasal Spray	None No spring. Finger squeeze pressure.	1 of up to 100 μL	Zomig® [zolmitriptan] Zavzpret® [zavegepant] Valtoco® [diazepam] Tosymra® [DHE] [+ several others + multiple partnered programs	One-handed operation. Low actuation force. No priming. No shaking. Multiple approved FDA/EMA products—for migraine (and other indications).	No distinction between UNS and LNS deposition. Diffuse "cloud" of droplets/particles.	[31]
	Bidose (BDS) Liquid Nasal Spray	None Spring	2 × 100 μL	Spravato® [esketamine]			[32]
	Unidose (UDS) Powder Nasal Spray	None No spring. Finger squeeze pressure	1	Baqsimi® [glucagon]	Ideal for low solubility molecules, minimizes excipient requirements, allows for larger dose administration, improves bioavailability and enhances drug diffusion/absorption. No shaking/priming.	No distinction between UNS and LNS deposition. Complex formulation and may increase irritability.	[33]
	Multi-Dose (preservative-free) VP3 Nasal Spray Systems	None	Multiple	Tyrvaya® [varenicline]	The "traditional" nasal spray for >40 years. Mechanical system. Reference pump for originator anti-allergy brands and their generic alternatives.	No distinction between UNS and LNS deposition.	[34]
Bausch Health (Laval, Canada) (Drug device combination product)	Traditional Nasal Spray	None	1	Migranal® [DHE]	Approved (>20 years) for delivery of 2.0 mg liquid DHE for acute treatment of migraines. Has a "traditional" pump spray.	Requires assembly and priming. No distinction between UNS and LNS deposition. Diffuse "cloud" of droplets/particles.	[35,36]

Table 1. *Cont.*

Manufacturer	Device	Propellant	No. Doses	[Drug/Other Programs]	Pros	Cons	Reference/ Website
Haleon (Weybridge, UK)	Sensimist (liquid)	None	60 doses	Flonase® [fluticasone] (generics and OTC focus)	Now OTC product. Designed to deliver a cloud of liquid fluticasone droplets to the LNS for allergic rhinitis. Systemic absorption is NOT desired.	Typical systemic corticosteroid effects are seen with long-term use and absorption.	[37]
Impel (Seattle, WA, USA) (Drug-device combination products)	Precision Olfactory Delivery (POD®) (Liquid)	HFA134a	1	Trudhesa® [DHE] INP102 [insulin]	Focus on UNS for N2B.Device adapted for each product. Approved for delivery of 1.45 mg liquid DHE formulation for acute treatment of migraine	First Generation device—requires assembly and priming.	[38]
	POD (Powder)	HFA134a	Multiple exchangeable tips	INP103 [levodopa] INP107 [car-bidopa/levodopa combination]	Several iterations of the device; research (which uses drug powder products in capsules) and single (no assembly) or multiple (changeable tip) dose design	Although delivering to UNS, there are no data on N2B delivery.Remains "in development."	[39]
	POD (Powder)	Nitrogen	1	INP105 [olanzapine]	Single-use, preloaded device (no priming or assembly)	Research and development halted Q1 2023 (for business reasons)	[40]
Kurve (Lynnwood, WA, USA) (Device only)	ViaNase™ (liquid)	None	1	N/A [insulin]	Focus on UNS for N2B. Device adapted for each product. Sixteen programs, fourteen in-clinic. Battery powered.	Unreliable performance in large NIH AD-insulin trial	[41,42]
OptiNose (Yardley, PA, USA) Drug-device combination products	Xhance® (OptiMist®) Bi-directional	None (breath powered)	120 sprays	Xhance® [fluticasone]	Approved for CRSwNP. Broader dispersion around the nasal cavity. The soft palate closes during use preventing the drug from entering the pharynx (or lungs).	Patient unfamiliarity with blowing into own nose. Initial priming is needed, and shaking before every dose. Focus on nasal disease—not systemic or N2B delivery.	[43]
	Bi-directional Exhalation Delivery System (EDS)—Onzetra® Xsail®		1	Onzetra®Xsail® [sumatriptan]	More of the drug reaches UNS. Approved for the delivery of sumatriptan powder (for migraine).	Patient unfamiliarity with blowing into own nose.	[44]

Table 1. *Cont.*

Manufacturer	Device	Propellant	No. Doses	[Drug/Other Programs]	Pros	Cons	Reference/ Website
Satsuma (Durham, NC, USA) (Drug-device combination product)	STS101—a manually squeezed plastic bottle	None	1	N/A [DHE]	Small, portable, and no assembly or priming, delivering 6.0 mg DHE powder	Two failed phase 3 studies, with device modifications in between to improve delivery. No distinction between UNS and LNS delivery	[45]
AeroPump (Hochheim am Main, Germany) (Device only)	AeroPump	None		N/A [insulin] (adaptable for use by OTC and generic drugs)	Requires priming. Simple. Easy to use.	Non-targeted, LNS delivery	[46]
PharmaSystems (Markham, ON, Canada) (Device only)	Metered Nasal Dispenser	None	Multiple	N/A [insulin] (Canadian pharmacy supplier)	Requires priming. Simple. Easy to use. Programs showed benefits in postoperative delirium and postoperative cognitive function	Non-targeted, LNS delivery	[47]
MeadWestvaco (Richmond, VA, USA)/Silgan (Richmond, VA, USA) (Device only)	Mistette MkII Pump	None	Single/Multiple?	N/A [insulin] (provide bottles/pumps for liquid formulation delivery)	Requires priming. Simple. Easy to use.	Non-targeted, LNS delivery.	[48]
Nemera (La Verpillière, France) (Device only)	SP270+	None	Single/Multiple	N/A [insulin]	Requires priming. Simple. Easy to use.	Program was discontinued due to variations in viscosity.	[49]
SipNose (Yokneam, Israel) (Drug-device combination products)	Sipnose	Compressed air	Single and Multiple dose	N/A [insulin] (seven programs; five in-clinic, three of their own, and two partnered)	Performed well in Patient-Centered Care Impact Analysis [50] compared to two invasive ROAs (intrathecal and intracerebroventricular injection. Liquid and powder formulations. Targeted for UNS delivery.	Clinical data awaited	[51]

Table 1. *Cont.*

Manufacturer	Device	Propellant	No. Doses	[Drug/Other Programs]	Pros	Cons	Reference/ Website
Teleflex (Wayne, PA, USA) (Device only)	Mucosal Atomisation Device (MAD)	None	1	N/A [vaccines] (Astra Zeneca: ChAdOx1nCoV-19 vaccine)	Fitted to the tip of a standard syringe in clinical trials of vaccines	Liquid (vaccines or drugs) administration by HCP	[52,53]
BD (Franklin Lakes, NJ, USA) (Device only)	Accuspray™	None	1	N/A [vaccines] 510(k) cleared	Fitted to the tip of a standard syringe in clinical trials of vaccines	Liquid (vaccines or drugs) administration by HCP	[54,55]
Aptar	BiVax	None	1 (either 200 μL or 500 μL—split across 2 nostrils)	N/A [vaccines]	The liquid vaccine can be transferred directly from vial to applicator.	Liquid (vaccines or drugs) administration by HCP	[56,57]
Aptar	LuerVax (nozzle only)	None	1	N/A [vaccines]	Fitted to the tip of a standard syringe in clinical trials of vaccines.	For HCP liquid administration	

AD = Alzheimer's disease; CRSwNP = chronic rhinosinusitis with nasal polyps; DHE = dihydroergotamine (for migraine); EMA = European Medicines Agency; FDA = Food and Drug Administration; HCP = healthcare practitioner; HFA = hydrofluoroalkane; LNS = lower nasal space; N/A = not applicable (no approved product); N2B = nose-to-brain delivery; NIH = National Institutes of Health; OTC = over the counter; POD = Precision Olfactory Delivery; UNS = upper nasal space.

Text Correction

There was an error in the original publication. The bioavailability ascribed in the original publication to nasal midazolam was from a program developed by another company with another product (and device), not Nayzilam (as developed and marketed by UCB). The bioavailability for the approved (Nayzilam) product is less than that claimed by the competitor product and that has now been corrected in the text of Section 3.1. Lower Nasal Space (LNS) Delivery.

Section 2.1. Local Nasal and Sinus Disease

Many local sino-nasal diseases, specifically allergic rhinitis and rhinosinusitis with or without nasal polyps, have responded to the development of numerous topical corticosteroid sprays, starting with triamcinolone in 1957 but followed by beclomethasone, budesonide, flunisolide, fluticasone, mometasone and ciclesonide. All were delivered with either a pressurized metered-dose inhaler (pMDI) that was originally chlorofluorocarbon (CFC)-propelled but later changed to hydrofluoroalkane (HFA) or an aqueous product delivered by a "traditional" pump-spray.

Although many cases of chronic rhinosinusitis, especially with the additional pathology of nasal polyposis, are perennial, many patients have seasonal allergy problems making year-round administration of potent corticosteroids unnecessary. The target of the respiratory epithelium on the turbinates (conchae) of the LNS has been effectively reached by the traditional nasal spray delivering a diffuse cloud of droplets. In addition, systemic absorption is not desired, allowing for simpler formulations and delivery systems. Most recently, fluticasone has been approved for delivery by the OptiNose bidirectional Exhalation Delivery System (EDS) specifically for the treatment of chronic rhinosinusitis with nasal polyps (CRSwNP) [29] and is able to deliver more of the potent steroid "higher and deeper" into the nasal cavity (compared to traditional sprays) where many polyps originate [30]. The OptiNose device generally distributes better throughout the nasal cavity (than traditional nasal sprays) with its bidirectional design and is propelled by the patient's own exhalation, which also elevates the vellum (soft palate), thus closing off the nose from the rest of the respiratory tract (Table 1). The nose piece directs the exhaled breath to push the drug product into one nostril, allowing it to reach the back of the nose, pass behind the septum and exit from the other nostril, hence creating the "bi-directional flow path" [16].

Section 3.1. Lower Nasal Space (LNS) Delivery

The delivery of drugs to the LNS can provide good bioavailability (BAV), i.e., access to the systemic circulation, with products such as Valtoco® (diazepam) through the Aptar Unit Dose System (UDS) reported at 97% [72], although this good bioavailability was obtained with the help of dodecyl maltoside (DDM) as an absorption/permeation enhancer and Vitamin E to increase solubility. Another product with good nasal bioavailability is Nayzilam® (midazolam), also delivered by Aptar's UDS. Section 12.3 of the Prescribing Information states the absolute bioavailability to be approximately 44%. However, other intranasal midazolam formulations have been independently investigated [73], delivered by a different unit dose device obtained from Ing. Erich Pfeiffer GmbH, demonstrating better bioavailability ranging from 76 to 92%. These different formulations contained different concentrations of randomly methylated-β5-cyclodextrin (0, 2, 4, or 12%); different concentrations of saline and with or without 0.5% chitosan added as an absorption enhancer. In contrast, a very recent approval of Zavzpret™ (vazegepant), also given by the Aptar UDS device [74], only reported ~5% bioavailability. The liquid formulation has the additional inactive ingredients: dextrose, hydrochloric acid, sodium hydroxide, succinic acid and water. In these examples, the same basic Aptar UDS delivery was used, presumably delivering to the same part of the nose (the LNS) with a diffuse nasal spray, showing that the addition of absorption enhancers was required to increase bioavailability. That, in turn, increases the complexity of the development program but does illustrate the extremes of the level of bioavailability that can be achieved through LNS delivery.

Section 3.2. Upper Nasal Space (UNS) Delivery

There is now a greater appreciation that drugs delivered to the upper nasal space (UNS) may experience faster and more extensive absorption than when delivered to the LNS. Data were initially generated with the OptiNose® bi-directional system and then, more recently, by several clinical programs using the Precision Olfactory Delivery (or POD®) system (Table 1), which specifically targets the upper nasal space (UNS). These programs have served as important steps as they highlighted the complex nasal architecture (Figure 1a) and showed one of the potential benefits of delivering drugs to the olfactory epithelium lining in the UNS. As can be appreciated, a cloud or broad plume of droplets delivered into the nose by a mechanical pump will coat the surfaces of the septum, inferior turbinate and lateral wall, with some penetrating to the middle turbinate but little to the superior turbinate and even less to the upper nasal space lying mostly above the superior turbinate. The nose is designed to convey volatile molecules to the olfactory epithelium in the UNS carried by inhaled air but not to allow a broad plume of droplets/particles to reach it. The olfactory epithelium has distinct differences from the respiratory epithelium of the nose's humidification and filtering system covering the three turbinates (or conchae), mostly located in the lower nasal space (Figure 1b). These differences lead to very different absorption profiles for drugs landing on different mucosae [75]. Few data have historically been generated looking at where nasal devices deliver their payloads, with options being to investigate in cadavers, nasal cavity replicas, nasal casts or by using in vivo gamma camera imaging [76].

Investigating the novel breath-actuated, bi-directional system, Djupesland and colleagues compared the systemic levels of midazolam with those obtained after traditional nasal spray delivery and IV delivery [77]. The 100 μL of bespoke formulation, including cyclodextrin, HPMC, EDTA and benzalkonium chloride, to 12 healthy adult subjects showed similar serum concentration curves for the two nasal devices, both with rapid T_{max} of 15 min and a geometric mean ratio (OptiMist/Traditional spray) of 97.6%, suggesting no difference in systemic delivery between the two devices. However, this group went on to deliver ^{99m}Technetium-labelled aerosol [78] to nine healthy subjects and showed increased delivery to the UNS, of 32%, versus 11% with a traditional spray. Subsequent work with the OptiNose® system reported 53.6% of the formulation reaching the UNS (upper and middle posterior regions) versus only 15.7% with the traditional liquid spray [79] with no lung deposition.

Hoekman and colleagues generated data supporting the differential delivery systems to the UNS with Precision Olfactory Delivery (POD®) using MAG-3 (^{99m}Technetium-labelled peptide) as determined by SPECT imaging in seven healthy subjects [80]. For this assessment, the nasal cavity was divided into four sections (Figure 1c): (1) vestibule, (2) lower nasal space, (3) UNS and (4) nasopharynx, determined from MRI imaging [81]. The UNS is where the olfactory epithelium is confined, which will be further discussed in the context of N2B delivery below—although there is also an approximately equal area of respiratory epithelium in the UNS, as it covers the superior turbinate. POD delivered substantially more (approaching 50%) to the UNS and less to the vestibule than the traditional spray (Figure 1d). The olfactory epithelium covers ~5 cm^2, representing ~3% of the total surface area of the nasal cavity [82]. The enhanced delivery of radioisotopes to the UNS then led to several clinical programs being launched with the POD system. The STOP 101 [83] clinical study specifically looked at the delivery of the same liquid formulation through an approved, traditional spray to the lower nasal space and compared it with POD (using the same device that was subsequently used in the phase 3 study [84] and thereafter approved and commercialized) delivering it to the UNS and showed a four-fold increase in (C_{max}), an almost four-fold increase in absolute bioavailability (59% vs. 15%) and an almost three-fold increase in $AUC_{0\text{-}inf}$ (Figure 2a). To accomplish this, the POD system has a novel design for the nozzle (dosing tip), which focuses the plume of emitted liquid droplets into a narrow plume [85], which is pictured in the publication. The differences in plume and aerosol characteristics between the two systems, with the same formulation of dihydroergotamine (DHE) mesylate, were further explained in a technical manuscript [86] as well as the Anderson Cascade Impactor data and using Spraytec technology, with a particle size distribution of Dv10 ranging from ~290 μm, Dv50 ranging from 402–472 μm across 10 samples from two lots and Dv90 ranging from 561–734 μm—all well above the respirable range. In addition, the novel nozzle of the POD device allows patients to position the device in the correct orientation if they follow the Instructions for Use and insert the device up to the "shoulder" of the actuator arm, which was confirmed to be easy to achieve in human factor testing.

To complete the clinical development for this INP104 program, the FDA required safety assessments of the UNS over 24 weeks with repeat dosing [84], which seemingly no other nasal delivery program had been asked to perform. This required the development of specific tools to assess the mucosal integrity of the olfactory epithelium and olfactory function, which detected no significant adverse effects over 24 and even 52 weeks [87].

A subsequent program, INP105, with a spray-dried powder formulation of olanzapine [88], showed in phase 1 a similar C_{max} and AUC as the same dose administered by intramuscular injection but with a faster T_{max}; however with no approved IV formulation of olanzapine to compare against, absolute bioavailability could not be determined in this study (Figure 2b). The POD powder programs (both INP105 and INP103/107 with levodopa/carbidopa) [89] benefited from the previous development of both rodent and primate versions of the POD which expedited formulation development and pharmacokinetic characterization before, or even during, human trials [90], with the structure and function of the non-human primate nose being most similar to that of humans [91].

References Correction

Additional references were included:

31. Unidose (UDS) Liquid Nasal Spray System. Available online: https://aptar.com/products/pharmaceutical/uds-unidose-liquid-nasal-spray-system/ (accessed on 9 June 2023).
32. Bidose (BDS) Liquid Nasal Spray System. Available online: https://aptar.com/products/pharmaceutical/bds-bidose-nasal-spray-system-manufacturer/ (accessed on 9 June 2023).
33. Unidose (UDS) Powder Nasal Spray System. Available online: https://aptar.com/products/pharmaceutical/unidose-nasal-powder-system-manufacturer/#:~:text=Aptar%20Pharma%E2%80%99s%20Unidose%20(UDS)%20Nasal,precise%20dose%20quickly%20and%20easily (accessed on 9 June 2023).
34. VP3 Multi-Dose Spray Pump. Available online: https://aptar.com/products/pharmaceutical/vp3-technology-platform/ (accessed on 9 June 2023).
35. Dihydroergotamine Mesylate. Available online: https://pi.bauschhealth.com/globalassets/BHC/PI/Migranal-PI.pdf (accessed on 9 June 2023).
36. Migranal. Available online: https://www.pdr.net/drug-summary/?drugLabelId=Migranal-dihydroergota-mine-mesylate-771 (accessed on 9 June 2023).
37. Flonase Allergy Relief Nasal Spray. Available online: https://www.flonase.com/products/flonase-allergy-relief/?gclid=CjwKCAi-Att2tBhBDEiwALZuhAEB-kI6eRoGWy2L-7zrmgp5zkSAX4ZcmpbvWvYIPwoRMvP0lijEufshoCvo8QAvD_BwE&gclsrc=aw.ds (accessed on 9 June 2023).
38. Trudhesa®. Available online: https://www.trudhesa.com/ (accessed on 9 June 2023).
39. Impel Pharmaceuticals. Available online: https://impelpharma.com/our-science/ (accessed on 9 June 2023).
40. INP105 Proof-of-concept Study for the Acute Treatment of Agitation in Adolescents and Young Adults With ASD (CALM 201). Available online: https://clinicaltrials.gov/study/NCT05163717?cond=Autism&term=NCT05163717&rank=1 (accessed on 9 June 2023).
41. The Future of Systemic and Central Nervous System (CNS) Therapies. Available online: https://kurvetx.com/ (accessed on 9 June 2023).

43. XHANCE® (Fluticasone Propionate). Available online: https://www.optinose.com/products/xhance-fluticasone-propionate/ (accessed on 9 June 2023).
44. ONZETRA Xsail. Available online: https://www.onzetra.com/ (accessed on 9 June 2023).
45. STS101 (DHE Nasal Powder). Available online: https://www.satsumarx.com/our-research/sts101/ (accessed on 9 June 2023).
46. Aero Pump. Available online: https://www.aeropump.de/en/products/nasal (accessed on 9 June 2023).
47. Metered Pump Nasal Spray Bottles, 1 oz. Available online: https://pharmasystems.com/metered-pump-nasal-spray-bottles-1-oz-10271 (accessed on 9 June 2023).
48. Healthcare Mark II™. Available online: https://silgandispensing.com/products/mark-ii (accessed on 9 June 2023).
49. Nemera Ear, Nose, Throat. Available online: https://www.nemera.net/wp-content/uploads/2021/11/Nemera-ENT-brochure-digital.pdf (accessed on 9 June 2023).
51. SipNose Nasal Delivery System. Available online: https://sipnose.com/products/ (accessed on 9 June 2023).
52. MAD Nasal™ Intranasal Mucosal Atomization Device. Available online: https://www.teleflex.com/usa/en/product-areas/anesthesia/atomization/mad-nasal-device/ (accessed on 9 June 2023).
53. Teleflex Intranasal Drug Delivery. 2023. Available online: https://teleflex.com/usa/en/product-areas/emergency-medicine/intranasal-drug-delivery/mad-nasal-intranasal-device/index.html (accessed on 24 March 2023).
54. BD Accuspray™ Nasal Spray System. Available online: https://www.bd.com/en-us/products-and-solutions/products/product-families/accuspray-nasal-spray-system (accessed on 9 June 2023).
55. Becton Dickinson. BD AccusprayTM Nasal Spray System. 2023. Available online: https://drugdeliverysystems.bd.com/products/prefillable-syringe-systems/vaccine-syringes/accuspray-nasal-spray-system (accessed on 24 March 2023).
56. The Potential and the Challenges of Nasal Vaccination. Available online: https://www.ondrugdelivery.com/the-potential-and-the-challenges-of-nasal-vaccination/ (accessed on 9 June 2023).
57. Suman, J. Intranasal Vaccination: Rationale, Progress and Challenges. RDD Online 2023. In Proceedings of the RDD 2023, Antibes (Nice), France, 2–5 May 2023.

With this correction, the order of some references has been adjusted accordingly. The authors state that the scientific conclusions are unaffected. This correction was approved by the Academic Editor. The original publication has also been updated.

Reference

1. Shrewsbury, S.B. The Upper Nasal Space: Option for Systemic Drug Delivery, Mucosal Vaccines and "Nose-to-Brain". *Pharmaceutics* **2023**, *15*, 1720. [CrossRef] [PubMed]

pharmaceutics

Article

Innovative Aqueous Nanoemulsion Prepared by Phase Inversion Emulsification with Exceptional Homogeneity

Patrícia C. Pires [1,2,3,†], Mariana Fernandes [1,4,†], Francisca Nina [1,4,†], Francisco Gama [1,4,†], Maria F. Gomes [1,4], Lina E. Rodrigues [1,4], Sara Meirinho [1,4], Samuel Silvestre [1,5], Gilberto Alves [1,4] and Adriana O. Santos [1,4,*]

1 CICS-UBI—Health Sciences Research Centre, University of Beira Interior, Av. Infante D. Henrique, 6200-506 Covilhã, Portugal; patriciapires93@gmail.com (P.C.P.); mariana-96@live.com.pt (M.F.); francisca.nina7@gmail.com (F.N.); franciscogama98@gmail.com (F.G.); mfsfgomes@hotmail.com (M.F.G.); linaisabelestevesrodrigues@gmail.com (L.E.R.); sara.alexandra92@gmail.com (S.M.); samuel@fcsaude.ubi.pt (S.S.); gilberto@fcsaude.ubi.pt (G.A.)

2 Department of Pharmaceutical Technology, Faculty of Pharmacy, University of Coimbra, 3000-548 Coimbra, Portugal

3 Associated Laboratory for Green Chemistry (LAQV) of the Network of Chemistry and Technology (REQUIMTE), Faculty of Pharmacy, University of Coimbra, 3000-548 Coimbra, Portugal

4 Faculty of Health Sciences, University of Beira Interior, Av. Infante D. Henrique, 6200-506 Covilhã, Portugal

5 Faculty of Sciences, University of Beira Interior, Rua Marquês d'Ávila e Bolama, 6201-001 Covilhã, Portugal

* Correspondence: asantos@fcsaude.ubi.pt

† These authors contributed equally to this work.

Abstract: Formulating low-solubility or low-permeability drugs is a challenge, particularly with the low administration volumes required in intranasal drug delivery. Nanoemulsions (NE) can solve both issues, but their production and physical stability can be challenging, particularly when a high proportion of lipids is necessary. Hence, the aim of the present work was to develop a NE with good solubilization capacity for lipophilic drugs like simvastatin and able to promote the absorption of drugs with low permeability like fosphenytoin. Compositions with high proportion of two lipids were screened and characterized. Surprisingly, one of the compositions did not require high energy methods for high droplet size homogeneity. To better understand formulation factors important for this feature, several related compositions were evaluated, and their relative cytotoxicity was screened. Optimized compositions contained a high proportion of propylene glycol monocaprylate NF, formed very homogenous NE using a low-energy phase inversion method, solubilized simvastatin at high drug strength, and promoted a faster intranasal absorption of the hydrophilic prodrug fosphenytoin. Hence, a new highly homogeneous NE obtained by a simple low-energy method was successfully developed, which is a potential alternative for industrial application for the solubilization and protection of lipophilic actives, as well as (co-)administration of hydrophilic molecules.

Keywords: nanoemulsion; intranasal; low energy; homogenous; phase inversion; propylene glycol monocaprylate type II

1. Introduction

Most drug candidates are highly lipophilic in nature, making their high strength solubilization in liquid dosage forms a challenge. Additionally, most drugs are easily susceptible to chemical and/or enzymatic degradation, which reduces their bioavailability at the action site. To tackle these issues, several strategies have been developed, with the encapsulation of molecules in nanosystems being one of the most successful [1,2].

Nanosystems are typically classified as colloidal structures with a size of less than 500 nm, inside which drugs are incorporated. This will allow not only to increase the preparation's drug strength, but also to protect the molecules from degradation, increase their permeability through biological membranes, promote bioavailability, reduce plasma protein binding, and allow a controlled drug release, with the possibility of targeting certain organs. There are many types of nanosystems, polymeric and lipid nanosystems being the most frequently used. There is a great variety of lipid nanosystems: liposomes and derived structures (transfersomes, niosomes, cubosomes, ethosomes, etc.), solid lipid nanoparticles, nanostructured lipid carriers, and nanometric emulsions [3,4]. Nevertheless, many of these nanocarriers have important disadvantages, such as being complex, time-consuming and having polluting preparation methods, low physical stability, low encapsulation efficiency, and lack of biocompatibility. However, these disadvantages are reduced or simply do not apply to nanometric emulsions, particularly those with the right formulas, which have good stability, solubilization capacity, and simple preparation methods.

Nanometric emulsions include nanoemulsions (NE) and microemulsions. Microemulsions, named as such since 1959 [5], are thermodynamically stable and spontaneously form liquid dispersions of lipids and water, generally implying high amounts of surfactants and co-solvents/co-surfactants [6,7]. The droplet size is usually inferior to 100 nm, often not much larger than simple surfactant micelles, in which case they may appear completely transparent. The nature of their composition makes them related to classic emulsions, which are, however, biphasic thermodynamically unstable systems.

In turn, NE are colloidal liquid-in-liquid dispersions, usually presenting a size below 200 nm and a higher kinetic stability than macroemulsions. Compared with microemulsions, NE are usually composed of a lower content of hydrophilic surfactants and co-solvents, and usually require high energy methods for shearing and homogenizing the lipid droplets. Nevertheless, specific NE compositions can also be prepared by low energy methods, but with some compromise in the amounts of surfactant and co-solvents that are used (which tends to be high, although not as much as in microemulsions), and in the degree of homogeneity, which is tendentially low [8].

Oil-in-water NE are a good strategy to deliver solubilized lipophilic drugs at high drug strengths. This is of high importance, especially for some delivery routes, such as in intranasal administration to the systemic circulation or to the brain, given the relatively short residence time and small volume of administration [9–12].

Hence, the purpose of this work was to develop a NE using low amounts of surfactants and/or cosolvents, thus with high lipid content and good solubilization of lipophilic drugs like simvastatin, while able to promote the absorption of drugs with low permeability like fosphenytoin. At the same time, it was aimed at a homogenous size under 200 nm and, preferably, a low energy preparation method. We screened NE compositions with a high proportion of relatively polar lipids aiming to achieve a good solubilization of drugs such as simvastatin and then characterized their droplet size. A composition with low proportion of hydrophilic surfactant to oils and no co-solvent originated a NE about 100 nm in droplet size using a simple low energy phase inversion method. Surprisingly, these NE spontaneously became highly homogenous upon refrigeration, with a polydispersity index (PDI) < 0.1, which is not usually found in NE without homogenization. Therefore, we secondarily aimed to establish which formulation factors were required for this attribute. The extremely low PDI was lost when changing excipients to similar ones or by changes in their proportion outside a narrow range. We also describe alternative compositions of the aqueous phase in which the NE display PDI < 0.1 already at room temperature. Given the high lipid content of such NEs, a high drug strength of lipophilic substances was obtained. Furthermore, the intranasal administration of the NE of a hydrophilic prodrug (fosphenytoin) to mice demonstrated a faster absorption than an aqueous solution of the drug.

2. Materials and Methods

2.1. Materials and Reagents

The hydrophilic surfactants Kolliphor® RH 40 (Macrogolglycerol hydroxy stearate), Kolliphor® EL (Macrogolglycerol ricinoleate), Kolliphor® P124 (Poloxamer 124), Kolliphor® HS 15 (Polyethylene glycol 660 12-hydoxystearate), and the oil Kollicream® IPM (Isopropyl Myristate) were kindly offered by BASF (Ludwigshafen, Germany); Transcutol®

HP (Diethylene glycol monoethyl ether), a cosolvent, Labrasol® ALF (Caprylocaproyl polyoxyl-8 glycerides), a hydrophilic surfactant, and the oils Capryol® 90 (Propylene Glycol Monocaprylate (type II) NF), Capryol® PGMC (Propylene glycol monocaprilate, Type I), LabrafacTM PG (Propylene glycol dicaprylocaprate), Maisine® CC (Glycerol monolinoleate), and PeceolTM (Glycerol mono-oleate) were kindly offered by Gattefossé (Saint-Priest, France); the oils Imwitor® 948 (Glyceryl mono-oleate), Imwitor® 988 (Glycerol monocaprilate, Type I), and Softisan® 645 (Bis-diglyceryl polyacyladipate-2) were kindly offered by IOI Oleo GmbH (Hamburg, Germany); Capmul® MCM (Glycerol monocaprilocaprate), Capmul® 808G EP/NF (Glycerol monocaprylate Type II), Capmul® PG-8 (Propylene glycol monocaprylate), and Capmul® PG-8-70 NF (Propylene glycol monocaprylate Type II) were kindly offered by Abitec; Miglyol® 812 (medium-chain triglycerides; Caprylic/Capric Triglyceride), Soybean oil, Span® 80 (Sorbitane mono-oleate), Vitamin E Acetate, Cetiol V (Decyl oleate), the hydrophilic surfactants Tween® 20 (Polysorbate 20) and Tween® 80 (polysorbate 80), and the polymers Polyethylene glycol (PEG) 4000, (Hydroxypropyl)methyl cellulose (HPMC, corresponding to Hypromellose Viscosity 4000 mPa·s), and Polyvinylpyrrolidone (PVP, corresponding to Povidone K30) were acquired from Acofarma® (Madrid, Spain); the surfactant Tyloxapol was from Acros Organics (Thermo Fisher ScientificGeel, Belgium); Malic acid was acquired from Applichem (Darmstadt, Germany). Ultra-pure water was obtained from a Mili-Q® purification system from Millipore (Billerica, MA, USA). Simvastatin (98.03% purity) was purchased from Bld Pharmatech GmbH. (Kaiserslautern, Germany.) and kept at 4 °C under a nitrogen atmosphere during utilization. The bovine serum albumin (BSA) was acquired from Sigma-Aldrich, Inc (St. Louis, MO, USA). Acetonitrile and methanol were high-performance liquid chromatography (HPLC) gradient grade. The symbols TM and® will be omitted from now on for simplification.

2.2. Nanoemulsions Preparation

The oil phase (preconcentrate) was prepared by weighing the lipids and surfactants and mixing them from a few seconds to a few minutes until a homogenous solution was obtained. Depending on the NE, the aqueous phase either consisted in water, a 30 mM pH 5 malate buffer, or a 20 mM pH 7 phosphate buffer, to which NaCl, BSA, PEG 4000, HPMC, or PVP were added at the indicated concentrations (presented with the respective data in the results section). To prepare the NE, a phase inversion method was used, in which about a quarter of the final aqueous phase mass was first added and mixed with e preconcentrate, followed by the addition and mixture of the remaining aqueous phase mass.

2.3. Nanoemulsion's Droplet Size and Zeta Potential

Both hydrodynamic diameter (droplet size) and PDI were measured by dynamic light scattering (DLS) technique associated with cumulants analysis. For that, a Zetasizer Nano ZS (Malvern®, United Kingdom) combined with the Zetasizer software (version 7.10) was used. Before each measurement, samples were diluted, about 500-fold, in ultra-pure water. For each tested formulation, two independent discardable cuvettes were prepared and three different measurements of each were automatically performed by the equipment set either at 20 or 25 °C. Measurements were typically performed within 30 min after dilution. As measurement parameters set in Zetasizer software, water was considered as the dispersant (Refractive Index = 1.330 and Viscosity = 0.8872 cP) and the material was set to a Refractive Index = 1.450, representing "lipid"). When assessing the role of refrigeration in mean droplet size and PDI, formulations were placed at 4 °C overnight (at least 12 h), and then measurements were performed exactly as stated before, after diluting the samples immediately upon removing them from the refrigerator.

Zeta potential was measured with Malvern's Dip Cell Kit in the same equipment, using the same preparation steps. Measurements were taken at 20 or 25 °C and water was selected as the dispersant (Dielectric Constant = 78.5) and "lipid" as the material.

2.4. Osmolality

Osmolality was measured using Osmomat® 3000 freezing point osmometer from Gonotec® GmbH (Berlin, Germany). Osmolality measurement was performed in independent triplicates. The device was previously calibrated using ultra-pure water and two standard solutions of 300 mOsmol/Kg and 850 mOsmol/Kg.

2.5. Viscosity

Viscosity measurements were performed at different rotational velocities in a Brookfield DV3T™ RV Cone Plate (DVTRVCP) Rheometer (Toronto, ON, Canada), using the CPA-40z cone spindle (viscosity range of 1.7–32,700 cP) and the Rheocalc T® software (version 1.1.13). Measurements were performed at controlled temperature using a thermostatic water bath (MultiTemp III Thermostatic Circulator, Thermo Fisher Scientific, Waltham, MA, USA). Before viscosity measurements, equipment calibration was verified using Ametek Brookfield Fluid 500 Viscosity Standard (Middleborough, MA, USA) with a standardized viscosity of 489 cP at 25 °C. At each velocity, viscosity was registered after the spindle had enough time to perform five complete rotations. For fluids with Newtonian rheological behavior, viscosity was determined at the shear rate corresponding to the highest torque value (just below 100%), due to the equipment's higher resolution and precision resulting in a lower measurement error. For non-Newtonian fluids, zero shear viscosity was estimated by the Y-intercept of the non-linear regressions based on the measurements performed at different shear rates at a constant temperature.

2.6. In Vitro Release of Model Drug

In vitro drug release studies, performed in horizontal Ussing Chambers (Harvard Apparatus, NaviCyte, Hugstetten, Germany), used phenytoin as a model drug. The methodology was adapted from Pires et al. [13]. Synthetic membranes were used, with a pore size of 0.2 µm (hydrophilic polyethersulfone Supor® membrane disc filters, Pall Life Sciences, MI, USA). The receiving chamber was filled with 1.8 mL of phosphate buffer (pH 7, 20 mM), plus albumin at 1% *w*/*w*, and 100 µL of this same solution was placed on the donor side of the membrane. The temperature was kept at 32 °C, the approximate temperature of the nasal cavity at the region of the middle turbinate [14], with a heating water bath (Grant Instruments, Cambridge, England), and receiving chamber homogenization was achieved through magnetic steering (Micro Stirring Bars, 2 mm, VWR, United Kingdom). When the intended temperature was reached, the buffer on the donor chamber was replaced with 100 µL of the test formulations. Afterwards, samples of 100 µL were taken from the receiving chamber and replaced by the same volume of buffer plus albumin solution at 10, 20, 40, 60, 90, 120, 180, and 240 min.

For phenytoin quantification, samples were diluted 5-fold in a water-Transcutol mixture (3:1), followed by addition of perchloric acid at 10% (*v*/*v*). Formulation's initial drug concentration was also quantified in a similar way, but the dilution was 500-fold. A previously developed and validated HPLC method [15] was used, comprising specific apparatus and conditions: LC-2010A HT Liquid Chromatography system, coupled with a SPD-M20A diode-array detector, controlled by LabSolutions (version 5.52) software (Shimadzu, Kyoto, Japan); analyte separation was performed in a reversed-phase column (3 µm particle size, 55 × 4 mm) protected by a guard column (5 µm particle size, 4 × 4 mm, C18, LiChroCART® Purospher® STAR, Merck, Darmstadt, Germany), with isocratic elution at 1 mL/min at 30 °C. Mobile phase was a mixture of 36% (*v*/*v*) methanol and 64% (*v*/*v*) sodium phosphate buffer (10 mM, pH 3, with 0.25% triethylamine), filtered (Nylaflo membrane, 0.2 µm pore size, Pall, NY, USA) and degassed in a ultrasound bath. Sample injection volume was 20 µL, and phenytoin was detected at 215 nm, with a retention time of 10–11 min, within 20 min runs.

2.7. Cell Culture and Cytotoxicity Evaluation

Normal Human Dermal Fibroblasts (NHDF, adult donor cells, Ref. C-12302 from PromoCell) were cultured in RPMI 1640 medium supplemented with inactivated fetal bovine serum at 10%, 2 mM *L*-glutamine, 10 mM 4-(2-hydroxyethyl)-1-piperazineethanesulfonic acid, 1 mM sodium pyruvate, and 1% antibiotic (10,000 U/mL penicillin G, 100 mg/mL streptomycin) at 37 °C in a cell incubator with a humidified atmosphere of 5% carbon dioxide. The culture media was renewed every two or three days, and cells were subcultured as required.

To evaluate formulations' cytotoxicity, 15,000 cells were seeded in 100 µL per well of 96-well culture plates the day preceding the experiment. Immediately before the experiment, the medium was replaced by 50 µL of complete fresh medium plus 50 µL of NE preconcentrates diluted in fresh medium at twice the concentration selected for treating the cells. Cells were then incubated for 30 min, after which the treatment medium was replaced by 200 µL of 10% (*w*/*v*) solution of resazurin prepared in Krebs Ringer Buffer ($NaH_2PO_4.H_2O$ 1.5 mM; Na_2HPO_4 0.83 mM, KCl 4.86 mM; NaCl 119.78 mM; $MgCl_2.6H_2O$ 1.67 mM; $NaHCO_3$ 15 mM; anhydrous *D*-Glucose 10 mM; $CaCl_2.2H_2O$ 1,2 mM) and plates incubated at 37 °C for the required time (until negative control wells had approximately a reference fluorescence level—10,000 RFU in our plate reader, as previously optimized). The fluorescence intensity of plate wells was measured using an excitation wavelength of 570 nm and emission wavelength of 590 nm in a microplate fluorophotometer (Spectramax GeminiTM EM, Molecular Devices, LLC, San Jose, CA, USA). After subtracting background fluorescence (wells with blank resazurin solution), cell viability data were expressed as a percentage of the negative control of non-treated cells. Each experiment was carried out in quadruplicate wells.

2.8. In Vivo Pharmacokinetic Study of Model Drugs through Intranasal or Subcutaneous Administration

Healthy adult CD-1 mice (8 to 11 weeks old, 39 to 42 g), originated from Faculty of Health Sciences' certified animal facility were housed with controlled environmental conditions (12 h light/dark cycle, 20 ± 2 °C, 50 ± 5% relative humidity). Mice had free access to acidified tap water and standard rodent diet. All experimental procedures were carried out in conformity with the regulations of the European Directive 2010/63/EU and approved both by the Local Animal Ethics Committee and the competent national authority [Portuguese National Authority for Animal Health, Phytosanitation and Food Safety (Direção Geral de Alimentação e Veterinária)].

Mice were randomly divided into 2 groups, receiving either intranasal or subcutaneous administration (12 animals, 3 time points, 2 mice per time point). All animals were anesthetized with an intraperitoneal dose of pentobarbital (60 mg/kg) prior to formulation administration. All administrations were carried out with the mouse's body lying on top of a heating pad (plus a DC Temperature Controller 40-90-8D, FHC, Bowdoin, ME, USA). The established administration volume was of 5 µL and 50 µL per 30 g of body weight, for intranasal and subcutaneous administrations, respectively. Afterwards the mice were left to recover in a supine position, in a temperature-controlled environment.

Euthanasia was conducted at specific time points (30, 240 and 720 min), after which mice blood and brain were collected. The blood was collected into K3 EDTA tubes (FL Medical, Italy), after which 300 µL were mixed with orthophosphoric acid 85% (*v*/*v*) in a 1:1 (*v*/*v*) blood/acid ratio. The brains were homogenized (Ika Ultra-Turrax® T25 Basic, Staufen, Germany) in a water-orthophosphoric acid [1:1 (*v*/*v*)] mixture (1 g of tissue per 4 mL of mixture), centrifuged (14,000 rpm, 4 °C, for 10 min, MIKRO 200R microcentrifuge, Hettich, Tuttlingen, Germany), and the supernatants were collected. Both acidified blood and brain homogenates were kept on ice and then stored at −20 °C.

Sample processing consisted of the addition of 20 µL of ketoprofen spiking solution (internal standard) to the sample (100 µL of acidified brain homogenate supernatant or 200 µL of acidified blood), followed by liquid–liquid extraction [addition of 1000 µL of diethyl ether, followed by vortexing for 30 s, and then by centrifugation for 5 min at 13,500 rpm at room temperature in a tabletop microcentrifuge (Gyrozen, Daejeon, Republic of Korea)]. Next the organic phase was transferred to a glass tube, and the aqueous phase was reextracted two more times, under the same conditions. The combined organic phases were then evaporated to dryness (gas stream, 45 °C) and reconstituted with 100 μL of mobile phase. The mobile phase was made of 36% (v/v) methanol and 64% (v/v) sodium acetate buffer (10 mM, pH 5, with 0.25% triethylamine). In each sample, phenytoin quantification was performed by HPLC, using a previously developed and validated method [15], and aside from a change in mobile phase composition most chromatographic apparatus and analyte separation conditions were the same as described in Section 2.6. for the drug release study. The only other parameter that was modified was the analytes' detection wavelength, which remained 215 nm for phenytoin and fosphenytoin, but was changed to 280 nm for the internal standard.

2.9. Statistical Analysis

Data are represented by means of replicate measurements or of independent formulations ± standard deviation. Cell viability data were fitted by a nonlinear regression model [log(inhibitor) vs. normalized response—Variable slope] using GraphPad Prism version 9.5.1 to determine half-inhibitory concentrations (IC_{50}).

3. Results

3.1. A Spontaneously Formed Nanometric Emulsion with Exceding Homogeneity

The purpose of this study was to develop NE with good solubilization capacity for several drugs with low water solubility, such as simvastatin and phenytoin. For that, we selected two relatively polar lipids (monoesters of propylene glycol or glycerol), Kolliphor RH 40 as surfactant and Transcutol as co-surfactant, further testing several compositions and proportions (Figure S1). NE were prepared by adding water in two steps to the mixture of organic excipients followed by homogenization by premix membrane emulsification. However, one of the tested formulas originated an emulsion already quite homogenous, prior to any homogenization (PDI close to 0.2, Figure S1), with a mean size lower than 200 nm, which was surprising given that it had a high lipid proportion and no co-surfactant. Furthermore, after refrigeration, that formulation became noticeably less opaque, suggesting a reduction in droplet size, a characteristic that reverted upon thawing back to room temperature.

To further understand this phenomenon, the effect of temperature on droplet size was thoroughly studied. It was found that upon 500-fold dilution for characterization by DLS, the temperature of the water and the temperature used during measurements was irrelevant (not shown). In fact, the factor with real impact on NE droplet size was the temperature of the concentrated emulsion at the time of its dilution into room temperature water, and whenever a temperature is mentioned (e.g., Figure 1A,B,E), it is the temperature of the concentrated emulsion before dilution into water at room temperature. At room temperature, membrane pre-emulsification had no relevant effect on the size of emulsions with 50% water content, only promoting a slight reduction in PDI from over 0.2 to slightly under 0.2 (Figure 1A). However, upon refrigeration, the exact same NE suffered a significant reduction in droplet mean size to around 100 nm, and in PDI to under 0.1, with homogenization being irrelevant (Figure 1A). This effect was not solely related to time since emulsions left overnight at room temperature did not become more homogeneous and thawing them back to room temperature after refrigeration reverted the droplet size (not shown). The authors are not aware of a similar phenomenon being previously described in the literature.

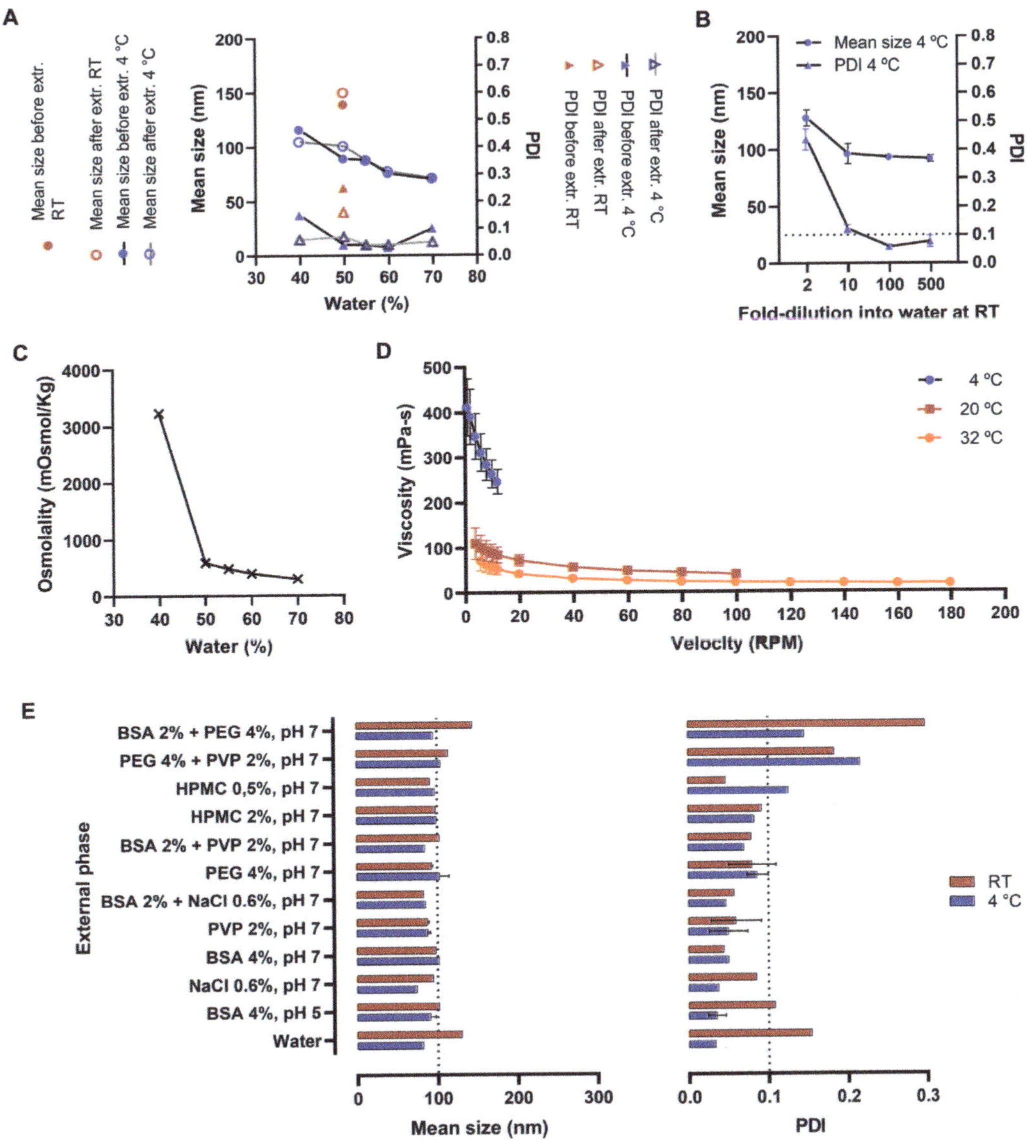

Figure 1. Characterization of the emulsions prepared from the selected preconcentrate with different aqueous phase proportions and composition. (**A**) Water proportion and temperature effect on the mean droplet size and polydispersity index (PDI) of the emulsions; (**B**) Water proportion effect on emulsion's osmolality; (**C**) Dilution effect of refrigerated concentrated emulsions (50% water) at room temperature (RT) water before measurement of the mean droplet size and PDI of the emulsions; (**D**) Viscosity of the nanoemulsion prepared with 50% aqueous malate buffer pH 5, at different temperatures; (**E**) Effect of the addition of different hydrophilic polymers and salt on the mean droplet size and PDI of the emulsions. Data corresponds to mean of replicate measurements/cuvettes (**A**,**C**,**E**) or mean ± standard deviation of four independent dilutions (**B**) or three independent formulation baches (**D**). Some of the data shown in (**E**) is mean ± standard deviation of two independent formulation baches.

In refrigerated NE, an increase in water content from 40% to 70% seemed to reduce droplet size. In NE containing between 50% and 60% water content, PDI was under 0.1 without membrane homogenization (Figure 1A). At least a 10-fold dilution appears to be required for refrigerated emulsions to maintain their low size and PDI (Figure 1B).

Formulations were slightly hypertonic but within a safe osmolality interval in the water range of 50–70% (Figure 1C), moderately viscous (up to around 100 mPa·s) at room temperate, and significantly more viscous after refrigeration (up to about 400 mPa·s, Figure 1D).

Next, we evaluated the effect of adding different hydrophilic polymers to the aqueous phase and found that several of them induced NE to have a droplet size under 100 nm and PDI under 0.1 without refrigeration (Figure 1E). This was the case with PVP, BSA (at pH 7 but less so at pH 5), HPMC at 0.5%, and PEG 4000.

3.2. The Very High Homogeneity in Nanoemulsion's Is Easily Lost by Small Changes in Preconcentrate Composition

To better understand which excipients of the present formula were related to the favorable size characteristics of the NE, several other formulas were screened by replacing each of the excipients with others of the same class. Concerning the minoritarian oil, glycerol mono-oleate (Imwitor 948), it was found that it could be replaced by another brand of glycerol mono-oleate (Peceol) or by glycerol monocaprylocaprate (Capmul MCM), but not by the closely related monolinoleate (Maisene CC) or any of the other tested lipids (Figure 2A).

It was found that Capryol, 90, the oil present in NE at higher proportion, could only be replaced by another brand of the exact same variety of propylene glycol monocaprylate type II—Capmul PG-8-70 NF—but not by other propylene glycol monocaprylates (type I or a variety not following pharmacopeia's specification), neither by glyceryl monocaprylates (Figure 2B).

The relative cytotoxicity of NE with different compositions was screened by exposing human fibroblasts (NHDF) cells to different preconcentrate concentrations (0.0016–0.16% or 0.16–45 or 50%) for 30 min. The obtained IC_{50} of the preconcentrate of the reference NE (without any drug) was about 0.04%. In fact, both Capryol 90 and Imwitor 948 are approved for cutaneous and oral administration, but not for parental use. Changing Imwitor 948 for other lipids did not significantly reduce formulation's cytotoxicity (all IC_{50} were $\leq$0.06%) (Table 1).

Table 1. Composition and half-inhibitory concentration (IC_{50}) of different nanoemulsions obtained by varying the secondary oil (16.7% *w*/*w*). All the NE also contained Carpyol 90 (25%) and Kolliphor RH 40 (8.3%). IC_{50} is expressed as % (*w*/*v*) of preconcentrate.

Secondary Oil		**Aqueous Phase**		**IC50 (%)**
Compendial Name	**Brand Name**	**BSA 4% * (%)**	**PEG 4% (%)**	
Glycerol mono-oleate	Imwitor 948	50		0.037
Glycerol mono-oleate	Peceol	50	-	0.027
Isopropyl myristate	Kollicream IPM	50	-	0.051
Glycerol mono-oleate	Imwitor 948	-	50	0.041
Glycerol monocaprilocaprate	Capmul MCM	-	50	0.021
Soybean oil	-	-	50	0.060
Glycerol monolinoleate	Maisine CC	-	50	0.026
Vitamin E acetate	-	-	50	0.037

* Malate buffer pH 5; BSA, bovine serum albumin; PEG, poly ethylene glycol 4000.

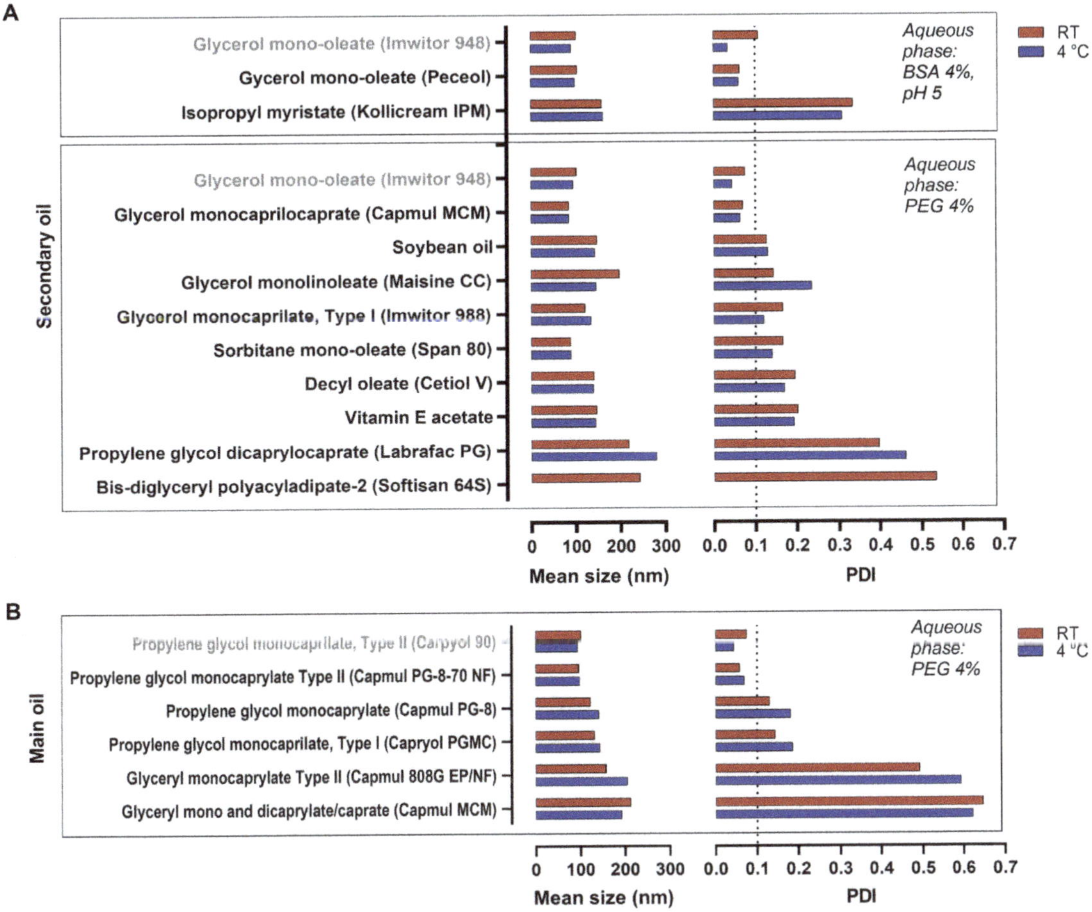

Figure 2. Mean droplet size characterization of emulsions obtained by changing one of the hydrophobic excipients in the selected preconcentrate. (**A**) Secondary oil and temperature effect on the mean droplet size and polydispersity index (PDI) of emulsions; (**B**) Main oil and temperature effect on the mean droplet size and PDI of emulsions. Data correspond to the mean of at least two independent dilutions of the same nanoemulsion.

To better rank the tested lipids according to their cytotoxicity, they were solubilized by mixing with Kolliphor RH 40:Transcutol:water (1:4:4:1), forming a self-microemulsifying preconcentrate, followed by cytotoxicity evaluation using the same method (Table 2). This allowed to rank several lipids from the less toxic to the more toxic: Vitamin E Acetate; Miglyol 812; Softisan 64S < Labrafac PG; Kollicream IPM; Maisine CC < Imwitor 948; Peceol < Capmul MCM; Capryol 90. Based on this, Capryol 90, which is the most toxic when compared to the other components, might account for the majority of the cytotoxicity of the NE.

Table 2. Lipidic composition and half-inhibitory concentration (IC_{50}) of different microemulsions prepared with different oils. Formulations are ranked from the least toxic to the most toxic. Other excipient's concentration (Kolliphor RH 40:Transcutol HP: and Water) was 40%:40%:10% (*w*/*w*). IC_{50} is expressed as % (*w*/*v*) of the preconcentrate without accounting for water.

Lipid (10%)		IC_{50}
Compendial Name	**Brand Name**	
No lipid (extra 10% water)		32.6
Vitamin E acetate		12.0
Medium chain triglycerides	Miglyol 812	10.6
Bis-diglyceryl polyacyladipate-2	Softisan 64S	10.5
Soybean oil		10.2
Propylene glycol dicaprylocaprate	Labrafac PG	7.34
Isopropyl myristate	Kollicream IPM	7.04
Glycerol monolinoleate	Maisine CC	6.71
Glycerol mono-oleate	Imwitor 948	1.67
Glycerol mono-oleate	Peceol	0.52
Glycerol monocaprilocaprate	Capmul MCM	<0.16 (0.08)
Propylene glycol monocaprylate Type II	Capryol 90	<0.16 (0.08)

Changing Capryol 90 for other propylene glycol monocaprylates or glycerol monocaprilocaprate did not change the outcome. However, the NE with glyceryl monocaprylate Type II was slightly less toxic (IC_{50} = 0.48%) (Table 3). Nonetheless, Figure 2 demonstrates that this NE lost its small and homogenous droplet size when replacing Capryol 90 with this lipid. Given that the most similar lipids could not replace Capryol 90, other lipids were not tested.

Table 3. Composition and half-inhibitory concentration (IC_{50}) of different NE obtained by varying the main oil (25%). The rest of the composition was Imwitor 948 (16.7%), Kolliphor RH 40 (8.3%) and as aqueous phase a solution of PEG 4000 at 4% (50%). IC_{50} is expressed as % (*w*/*v*) of the preconcentrate without accounting for the aqueous phase.

Main Oil		IC50 (%)
Compendial Name	**Brand Name**	
Propylene glycol monocaprylate NF (Type II)	Capryol 90	0.041
Propylene glycol monocaprylate NF (Type II)	Capmul PG-8-70 NF	<0.16
Propylene glycol monocaprylate	Capmul PG-8	<0.16
Propylene glycol monocaprylate Type I	Capryol PGMC	<0.16
Glyceryl monocaprylate Type II	Capmul 808G EP/NF	0.48
Glycerol monocaprilocaprate	Capmul MCM	0.08

We also tested many other hydrophilic surfactants for the replacement of Kolliphor RH 40. Still, at least at the proportion being used, neither of them gave comparable results (PDI were over 0.4 and sizes over 200 nm, Figure 3).

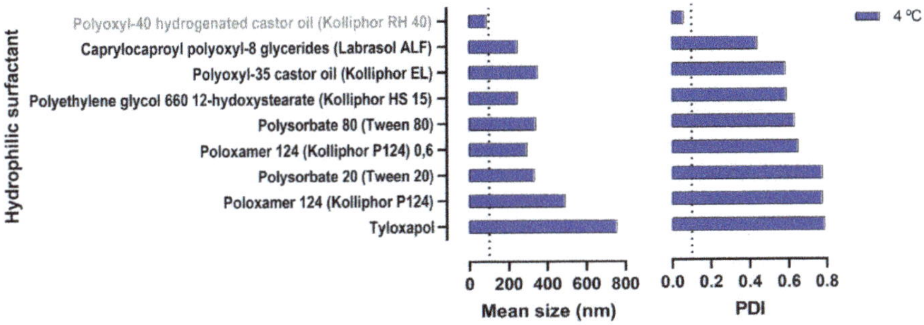

Figure 3. Droplet size characterization of emulsions obtained by changing the hydrophilic surfactant in the selected pre-concentrate. Mean droplet size and polydispersity index (PDI) were measured upon dilution of the refrigerated (4 °C) emulsions. Data correspond to the mean of independent dilutions of a same nanoemulsion.

The proportion of excipients in the formula was also varied. In these experiments, PEG 4000 at 4% was used as the aqueous phase, since it gave the NE a small homogenous droplet size already at room temperature. We started by changing the ratio between Capryol 90:Imwitor 948, originally set at 1.5:1. By doing that, a very small reduction or increase in Capryol 90 in the proportion of the two lipids produced a small but clear increase in both size and PDI, (Figure 4A). However, using refrigeration, the emulsions tolerated better the increase in Capryol 90 in the proportion of lipids, since PDI was still <0.1 with a Capryol 90/Imwitor 948 ratio of 2.333.

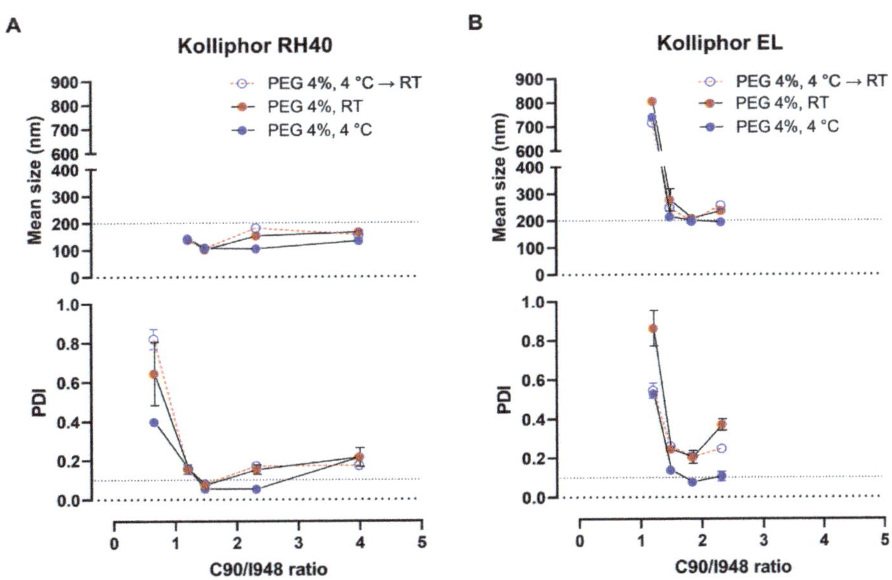

Figure 4. Droplet size characterization of emulsions after varying Capryol 90/Imwitor 948 (C90/I948) ratio. (**A**) Mean droplet size and PDI of nanoemulsions with a fixed amount of Kolliphor RH 40; (**B**) Mean droplet size and PDI of nanoemulsions with a fixed amount of Kolliphor EL. Measurements were made after the emulsions were kept at room temperature (RT), under refrigeration (4 °C), or at room temperature after being kept under refrigeration (4 °C → RT). PEG 4%, polyethylene glycol 4000 aqueous solution at 4% as external phase Data correspond to at least two independent dilutions of the same nanoemulsion.

Still insisting on the optimization of the compositions containing Kolliphor EL, the variation of the lipids' ratio was also tested. Slightly better results were obtained after a small increase in Capryol 90 proportion. However, droplet sizes remained higher (about 200 nm), and the emulsion remained dependent on refrigeration to achieve PDI under 0.1 (Figure 4B), even in the presence of PEG in the aqueous phase (Figure 4B).

The effect of varying the proportion between the oils and the hydrophilic surfactant (originally at a proportion of 5:1) was also tested. In formulations containing Kolliphor RH 40, the increase in the ratio of oils/surfactant from five to seven or higher led to the increase in droplets' mean size. However, in the presence of PEG, PDI values remained low until the ratio was 10 (Figure 5A). On the other sense, the ratio should not be less than four for optimal PDI values.

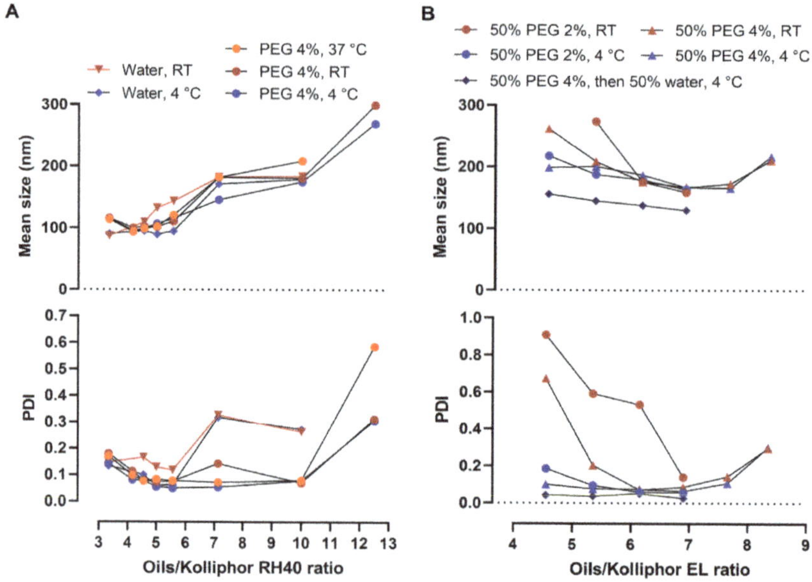

Figure 5. Mean droplet size characterization of emulsions having a varying oils/Kolliphor ratio. (**A**) Data with Kolliphor RH 40; (**B**) Data with Kolliphor EL. Measurements were made after the emulsions were kept at room temperature (RT), under refrigeration (4 °C), or at 37 °C. Data correspond to at least two independent dilutions of the same nanoemulsion.

When using Kolliphor EL as surfactant, the behavior was somewhat different. While the optimum ratio range of oils/surfactant was similar (4.5 to ~7), and refrigeration and PEG were both required, droplet sizes tended to decrease with the increase in oils' proportion (Figure 5B). Also, the lower mean droplet size and PDI were obtained when preparing the emulsion using a 4% PEG solution and then diluting it again two-fold with water (Figure 5B).

3.3. *The Nanoemulsion Allows the Incorporation of Both Hydrophilic and Lipophilic Molecules at High Strength*

It was possible to solubilize simvastatin, a lipophilic drug (XLogP3 of 4.7 according to Pubchem), at about 5.2% (*w*/*w*) of the final NE (with 50% aqueous phase). An acidic malate buffer (pH 5) in the aqueous phase was used to maximize the chemical stability of simvastatin [16]. Despite refrigeration of the NE, simvastatin increased the mean droplet size and PDI of the NE, which was significantly reduced back by addition of albumin to the aqueous phase (Figure 6).

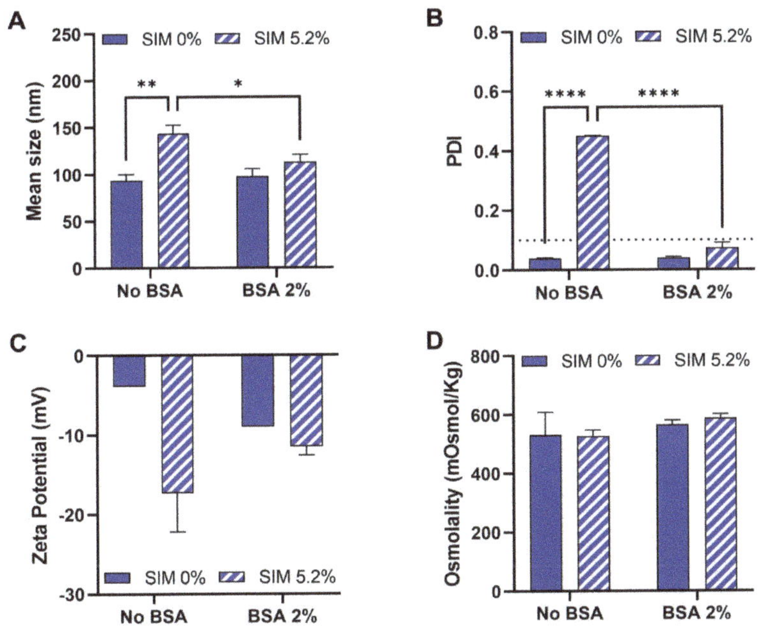

Figure 6. Simvastatin (SIM) and bovine serum albumin (BSA) effect in nanoemulsions' attributes. Droplet's mean size (**A**), polydispersity index (PDI, **B**), zeta potential (**C**), and preparation osmolality (**D**) are shown. Measurements were made upon dilution of the refrigerated (4 °C) emulsions. Data correspond to mean ± standard deviation of three independent preparation baches, each measured in two independent dilutions (**A–C**) or at least in three replicate measurements (**D**). Statistical significance of differences was tested by two-way ANOVA with Tukey's multiple comparisons test and given by asterisks: * $p < 0.05$; ** $p < 0.01$; **** $p < 0.0001$.

Other substances were also solubilized in the NE vehicle at relatively high final strengths (Table 4), mainly very lipophilic ones (cholesterol). Hydrophilic molecules like the prodrug fosphenytoyin sodium can also be added to the aqueous phase at relatively high drug strengths (here the intention was to keep the preparation in a safe osmolality range, but a higher concentration would be possible to obtain).

Next, we also tested if it was possible to remove refrigeration or use other polymers (PEG 4000 and PVP) in simvastatin nanoemulsions while also testing the presence of NaCl in the aqueous phase. While at 4 °C, all tested compositions led to extremely low PDI (≤0.053), at room temperature size and PDI tended to increase and were lower when PEG 4000 was used in the aqueous phase (Table 5).

The effects of temperature, simvastatin concentration, and albumin concentration were evaluated in more detail. We hypothesized that increasing BSA in the aqueous phase would improve simvastatin solubilization. BSA is able to bind poorly soluble drugs, such as simvastatin, and enhance their solubility. BSA seems to bind to simvastatin in a 1:1 mol ratio due to very strong hydrophobic and hydrogen bond interactions [17]. First, the impact of different BSA concentrations (2–8%) in the water phase on the physical attributes of NE was evaluated (Figure 7A). At room temperature, the NE mean droplet size was very similar among all formulations. On the other hand, larger differences in the PDI values were observed. BSA at 2% originated a lower PDI compared to the NE without BSA. However, PDI remained over 0.1, likely because of pH 5, close to BSAs isoelectric point. At higher BSA concentrations, PDI values increased but were still within the homogenous range (PDI < 0.2). After refrigeration, mean droplet size and PDI decreased in all the formulations, becoming extremely homogenous (PDI < 0.1). The effect of refrigeration on PDI was still visible even if the NE remained for 30 min at room temperature before dilution, although it was sufficient to observe a slight increase in the mean droplet size.

Table 4. Composition and mean droplet size characterization of nanoemulsions solubilizing chemicals with different lipophilia. Preconcentrate to external phase proportion of 1:1, with the preconcentrate composition in excipients being Capryol 90: Imwitor 948: Kolliphor RH 40 in a 3:2:1 ratio (weight), and the external phase a BSA aqueous dispersion (at 2 or 4% in 20 mM phosphate buffer, pH 7). In the case of fosphenytoin sodium solubilization, it was dissolved in the aqueous phase and the pH titrated to neutrality.

External Phase's BSA Concentration	Solubilized Molecule	XLogP3 *	%	RT		4 °C	
				Mean Size (nm)	PDI	Mean Size (nm)	PDI
2%	Cholesterol	8.7	5	110	0.064	n.d.	n.d.
2%	Cholesterol	8.7	7.5	138	0.097	111	0.075
4%	Segesterone Acetate	2.9	1.12	100	0.074	80	0.092
2%	Phenytoin	2.5	0.35	94	0.042	90	0.029
4%	Phenytoin	2.5	0.35	124	0.144	89	0.021
4%	Fosphenytoin sodium	0.6 **	4.25	85	0.177	61	0.082

BSA—bovine serum albumin; CHOL—cholesterol; FOS—fosphenytoin; n.d.—not determined; PDI—polydispersity index; PHT—phenytoin; RT—room temperature; * LogP valued are according to Pubcehm; ** this is not the maximum concentration, just the one required for an isotonic preparation.

Table 5. Composition and mean droplet size characterization of additional simvastatin emulsions having a preconcentrate to external phase proportion of 1:1. The preconcentrate was made of Capryol 90: Imwitor 948: Kolliphor RH 40 in a 3:2:1 ratio (weight), and the external phase was made of saline malate buffer (pH 5, containing 0.4% malic acid and 0.8% sodium chloride) with either bovine serum albumin (BSA), poly ethylene glycol 4000 (PEG) or polyvinylpyrrolidone (PVP) at 4%.

Simvastatin (%)	Polymer in the aq. Phase	RT		4 °C	
		Mean Size (nm)	PDI	Mean Size (nm)	PDI
5.20	BSA 4%	160.4	0.104	102.8	0.041
4.56	PEG 4%	106.2	0.060	101.4	0.042
4.46	PVP 4%	110.1	0.192	101.8	0.053
5.66	PVP 4%	-	-	115.1	0.046

BSA—bovine serum albumin; PEG—poly ethylene glycol 4000; PDI—polydispersity index; PVP—polyvinylpyrrolidone; RT—room temperature.

A series of simvastatin increments were then performed to determine the maximum amount of simvastatin capable of being loaded without precipitation when using a BSA 6% solution as the aqueous phase (Figure 7B). Simvastatin increments produced an overall increase in the mean droplet size. At room temperature, all the simvastatin concentrations resulted in PDI values higher than 0.1 but can still be considered homogenous (PDI < 0.2). Once again, refrigeration of the NE produced a decrease in both mean droplet size and PDI, an effect extended for at least 30 min when NE were placed at room temperature again regarding PDI. A final concentration of 9.09% of simvastatin was reached. At higher concentrations of 9.50% simvastatin started to precipitate after the dilution needed for mean droplet size and PDI measurements. Also, at 4 °C, formulations with concentrations higher than 7.41% precipitated in 1–2 days.

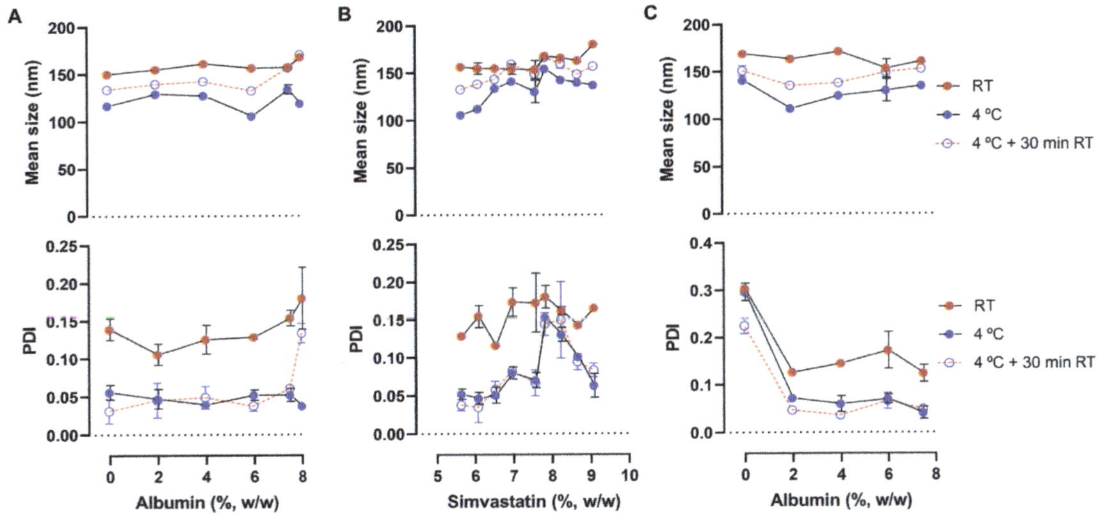

Figure 7. Influence of bovine serum albumin (BSA) and simvastatin (SIM) concentration on nanoemulsions' mean droplet size. Mean diameter and polydispersity index (PDI) of formulations containing simvastatin at 5.66% (**A**), albumin in the aqueous phase at 6% (**B**) or simvastatin at 7.41% (**C**). Measurements were performed at room temperature (RT), after refrigeration (4 °C), and 30 min at RT after being refrigerated. Data correspond to the mean ± standard deviation of two independent dilutions of one formulation.

In order to further improve the characteristics of NE, BSA was once again tested at different concentrations but, this time, only with 7.41% of simvastatin (Figure 7C). This time it was no longer possible to have a homogenous emulsion without using BSA, even after refrigeration. Even at the lowest concentration (2%) of BSA in the aqueous phase, PDI values decreased from 0.3 to under 0.1 at 4 °C, demonstrating the importance of BSAs presence.

We further evaluated the role of BSA on the physical stability of the refrigerated NE containing simvastatin at 5.66% or 7.41%. Formulations were observed daily until precipitation occurred. To prove the role of temperature in the loss of physical stability, this test was conducted at room temperature and 4 °C (Table 6). With 5.66% simvastatin concentration, both formulations had physical stability (absence of drug precipitation) for at least for 30 days at room temperature and 4 °C. It means that at lower simvastatin concentrations, BSA does not play a major role in increasing physical stability. At 7.41%, the role of temperature in speeding up simvastatin's precipitation is visible because all formulations achieved better stability at room temperature than at 4 °C. Using BSA at a concentration of 2% did not seem to affect its physical stability because it had exactly the same precipitation day as the NE without BSA (nine days at room temperature and one day at 4 °C). However, with BSA concentrations of 4% and 7.5%, physical stability at room temperature increased to 24 days and over 30 days when at room temperature and 2 days and 6 days at 4 °C, respectively. Despite six days being a short amount of time, the experiment was carried out in microtubes where some solvent evaporation is possible, and the use of BSA at 7.5% could delay precipitation for five more days than when no BSA was used, proving the role of BSA in simvastatin solubilization/stabilization.

Table 6. Time at which precipitation was observed at room temperature and 4 °C in different nanoemulsions containing albumin (BSA) at different concentrations (0%, 2%, 4%, and 7.5%) and simvastatin at 5.66% or 7.41%. Preconcentrate to external phase proportion of 1:1. The preconcentrate was made of Capryol 90: Imwitor 948: Kolliphor RH 40 in a 3:2:1 ratio (weight), and the external phase was made of malate buffer (pH 5) with BSA.

Nanoemulsions		Time for Precipitation (Days)	
Simvastatin	**BSA**	**Room Temperature**	**4 °C**
5.66%	0%	>30	>30
	2%	-	>30
	4%	-	>30
	7.5%	>30	>30
7.41%	0%	9	1
	2%	9	1
	4%	24	2
	6%	-	3
	7.5%	>30	6

3.4. Sustained In Vitro Drug Release and In Vivo Performance after Intranasal or Subcutaneous Administration

In vitro drug release from the selected nanoemulsion containing phenytoin as a model drug and albumin at 2% in the aqueous phase was studied ($NE^{PHT + BSA\ 2\%}$, Figure 8). The formulation showed sustained phenytoin release, when compared to a drug solution (0.2 mg/g, in 30% Transcutol), releasing only 30% of phenytoin after 4 h (as opposed to the drug solution, which released over 80%). A sustained drug release capacity could be a means to provide a prolonged therapeutic effect.

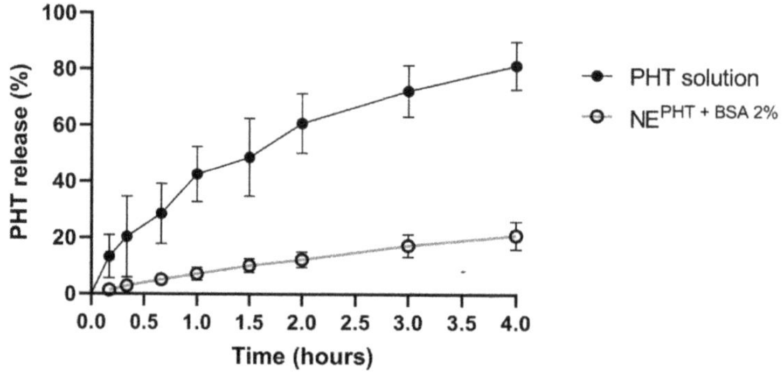

Figure 8. In vitro drug release profile of the developed optimized nanoemulsion, containing bovine serum albumin (BSA) at 2% in the aqueous phase, and phenytoin (PHT) at 3.5 mg/g ($NE^{PHT + BSA\ 2\%}$) in comparison to a solution (in water with 30% Transcutol). Preconcentrate to external phase proportion of 1:1. The preconcentrate was made of Capryol 90: Imwitor 948: Kolliphor RH 40 in a 3:2:1 ratio (weight), and the external phase was 20 mM pH 7 phosphate buffer with BSA.

Additionally, in order to demonstrate the relevance of using the NE for hydrophilic drugs and not only lipophilic ones, the fosfenytoin NE was administered intranasally to a small number of mice at comparable conditions to previously published work [15]. The brains and plasma were collected at three time points, and phenytoin (the active form) was quantified and plotted together with previously obtained data for comparison purposes. As demonstrated in Figure 9, phenytoin attained a higher concentration at 30 min after the intranasal administration of the NE than after the intranasal administration of a solution of the same drug. Since the drug strength was not high enough for intranasal administration, a NE containing phenytoin was also subcutaneously administered at a similar dose, demonstrating, however, that subcutaneous administration is less favorable (lower concentrations were achieved at 30 min and 4 h) than intranasal administration.

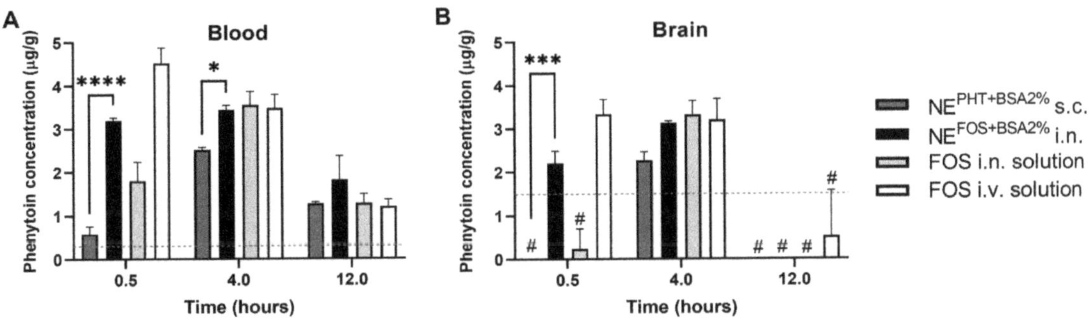

Figure 9. Comparison of phenytoin concentrations in blood and brain after administration of nanoemulsions and solutions of phenytoin and fosphenytoin to mice through different routes. (**A**) Blood phenytoin concentration. (**B**) Brain phenytoin concentration. Administered formulations were either nanoemulsion with bovine serum albumin (BSA) at 2% and phenytoin (PHT) ($NE^{PHT+BSA2\%}$), subcutaneously (s.c.) or a nanoemulsion with BSA at 2% and fosphenytoin ($NE^{FOS+BSA2\%}$) intranasally (i.n.). Data with a fosphenytoin (FOS) solution [intranasally and intravenously (i.v.)] from previously published results is shown for comparison purposes [15]. The data correspond to mean ± standard deviation. The statistical significance of differences between means was tested by two-way ANOVA with Tukey's multiple comparisons test and indicated by asterisks only in the comparison of the 2 novel experimental groups: * $p < 0.05$; *** $p < 0.001$; **** $p < 0.0001$. The dashed line represents the limit of quantification (LOQ). # In all samples, phenytoin was detected, but below the LOQ it was considered as equal to zero.

4. Discussion

Several related low energy methods of NE production have been described [18]. The most closely related to the process we used here with this novel NE is the reverse phase emulsification method, also named phase inversion emulsification [19]. We claim this because we observed smaller and more homogenous droplet size by adding the aqueous phase in two steps (a very low amount first to force the formation of a water-in-oil emulsion, and then the rest to inverted it to oil-in-water) than in a single step. Since long ago, this strategy has been used in the traditional continental method of oral emulsion preparation to obtain finer droplet dispersions [20]. This is also one of the reasons why we describe our system as a NE and not a microemulsion, since for microemulsions formation the order of excipients addition is not supposed have an effect.

Temperature is known to induce phase inversion of some emulsions with neutral surfactants (phase inversion temperature or PIT method [21]), and refrigeration is known to increase emulsions' physical stability. However, a particular composition that spontaneously forms smaller and more homogeneous droplets upon refrigeration without phase inversion has, as far as we know, not been previously described. The fact that after dilution (at least 10-fold) the small and homogeneous size is maintained at room temperature is likely due to the slower rearrangement of droplets at a greater distance.

It was also very surprising that the optimum mass proportion of oils to hydrophilic surfactant was between four and six to one. In fact, it is important to emphasize that the optimized preconcentrate has a composition of 83% of lipids or, more precisely, water-insoluble surfactants, and only 17% of a hydrophilic surfactant, which has no correspondence in the classification of lipid based formulations by Colin Pouton [22]. The explanation of why the aqueous dispersion of this particular composition has this behavior and how refrigeration or the composition of the aqueous phase can modulate a droplet's size and PDI is beyond the scope of our work. What has been shown, however, is how narrow the optimum design space seems to be.

Regarding the potential utility of the NE or of its preconcentrate, much remains to be explored in future works. One of the drugs that was demonstrated to solubilize at high strength in this vehicle was simvastatin, a lipophilic statin with low oral availability. This is a drug with pleiotropic effects and many potential applications beyond the control of dyslipidemia, like anti-cancer [23], anti-fibrotic [24], neuroprotective [25,26], and bone regeneration [27] applications, among others. Some of these applications could benefit from an alternative liquid formulation for, for example, intranasal administration, which has the potential to enhance brain delivery [28]. However, a limiting factor should be the relative cytotoxicity of the NE lipids Capryol 90 and Imwitor 948 compared to other lipids, as shown here. In fact, both Capryol 90 and Imwitor 948 are approved for cutaneous and oral administration and not for parental use. Therefore, the cutaneous and oral use of this NE, or of the preconcentrate as a self-nanoemulsifying drug delivery system, should not pose safety concerns since all excipients are well established and approved for these routes. Therefore, many possible applications could be envisioned in cosmetic or oral medicinal products. However, their safety for intranasal, ophthalmic, vaginal or parenteral delivery must still be established. For these routes, it is likely that there are limitations to the concentration/dose of the vehicle itself that can be safely used. Nevertheless, given the high content in Capryol 90:Imwitor 948, the studied NE might have the potential to provide a means to obtain a high concentration of lipophilic substances with a good solubility profile in this oil mixture. When compared to other oils, Capryol 90, in higher proportion in our formula, has shown to be the better solubilizer (among those tested) for very lipophilic drugs such as simvastatin (105 mg/mL [29]), clofazimine (18 mg/mL, [30]), luliconazole [~75 mg/mL [31]), terconazole (116 mg/mL [32]), tolvaptan (11 mg/g [33]), and even novel drug candidates such as JIN-001 (41 mg/mL [34]) and AC1497 (45 to 50 mg/mL [35]), to mention just a few examples. Precipitation upon dilution is not expected to occur since no water-miscible co-solvents account for the initial drug solubilization, and droplet size does not reduce upon dilution and is shown to provide a slow release of phenytoin used as the model drug. Furthermore, the small size and optimal homogeneity are in favor of long-term physical stability for these compositions. As we have demonstrated, it can also promote the mucosal absorption of hydrophilic substances. This effect was similar to what was previously observed by us with a microemulsion of fosphenytoin [36].

5. Conclusions

A novel composition with a high lipid/surfactant ratio was described for the first time, comprising Capryol 90 and preferentially Imwitor 948 and Kolliphor RH 40 in the optimum proportion of 3:2:1. This composition (preconcentrate) surprisingly formed an extremely homogeneous NE (PDI < 0.1) upon addition of the aqueous phase at about 50% using only mild manual agitation, not allowing much variation of excipients and their proportions for optimal physical attributes. This novel NE could be most suitable for the dissolution of lipophilic drugs such as simvastatin or for increasing the absorption of hydrophilic ones like fosphenytoin. Its low PDI, along with small droplet size, is expected to contribute favorably to the formulation's physical stability during storage. Using plain water, refrigeration was necessary to obtain the lowest PDI values, but several hydrophilic polymers could be used in the aqueous phase to promote the greatest homogeneity at room temperature or even higher temperatures. Future work will explore the usefulness of this novel formulation in the delivery of simvastatin and other drugs.

6. Patents

WO2022259205A1—WIPO (PCT). Self-emulsifying composition, production methods and uses thereof. Inventors: Adriana Oliveira dos Santos, Mariana Carvalho Fernandes, Patrícia Sofia Cabral Pires, Gilberto Lourenço Alves, Ana Carolina Maricoto Fazendeiro, Francisca Matos Silva Pereira Nina, Maria De Fátima Da Silva Ferreira Gomes, Lina Isabel

Esteves Rodrigues. Publication date: 15 December 2022. International Application Number: PCT/IB2022/055385. International filling date 9 June 2022; Applicant: University of Beira Interior. Status: pending.

Supplementary Materials: The following supporting information can be downloaded at: https://www.mdpi.com/article/10.3390/pharmaceutics15071878/s1, Figure S1: Droplet size characterization of the initial screen emulsion formulas before and after extrusion.

Author Contributions: Conceptualization, A.O.S., L.E.R., M.F., P.C.P. and S.S.; methodology, A.O.S., G.A. and P.C.P.; formal analysis, A.O.S. and P.C.P.; investigation, M.F., P.C.P., F.N., M.F.G., F.G., S.M. and L.E.R.; visualization, P.C.P., F.G., F.N. and M.F. writing—original draft preparation, A.O.S., M.F., F.N., F.G., L.E.R. and P.C.P.; writing—review and editing, P.C.P., A.O.S., G.A., S.M. and S.S; supervision, A.O.S., P.C.P., G.A., S.M. and S.S., funding acquisition and resources G.A. and A.O.S., project administration A.O.S. All authors have read and agreed to the published version of the manuscript.

Funding: This research was funded by Fundação para a Ciência e a Tecnologia (FCT), through funds from the Portuguese State Budget (grant numbers UIDB/00709/2020, UIDP/00709/2020), and by the European Regional Development Fund, under the Portugal 2020 Program, through the Regional Operational Program of the Center (Centro2020), (CENTRO-01-0145-FEDER-000013 and CENTRO-01-0145-FEDER-181231). SM was funded by FCT (PhD fellowship number SFRH/BD/136028/2018). FG was funded by FCT (BII fellowship from the program "Verão com Ciência", MERCI project).

Institutional Review Board Statement: The animal experimental protocols were reviewed and approved by the Portuguese National Authority for Animal Health, Phytosanitation, and Food Safety (DGAV—Direção Geral de Alimentação e Veterinária) in agreement with the regulations of the European Directive 2010/63/EU (protocol code 0421/000/000/2016, 14 November 2016).

Informed Consent Statement: Not applicable.

Data Availability Statement: Data is contained within the article or Supplementary Material in the summarized form (graphs and tables). The corresponding raw data are available on request from the corresponding author.

Acknowledgments: Ana C. Fazendeiro (CICS-UBI) had a small contribution to this work. Several excipients used in this work were kindly donated by BASF (Ludwigshafen, Germany), Gattefossé (Saint-Priest, France); IOI Oleo GmbH (Hamburg, Germany), and Abitec Corporation (Columbus, OH, USA).

Conflicts of Interest: The authors declare no conflict of interest. The funders had no role in the design of the study; in the collection, analyses, or interpretation of data; in the writing of the manuscript; or in the decision to publish the results.

References

1. Elhassan, E.; Devnarain, N.; Mohammed, M.; Govender, T.; Omolo, C.A. Engineering Hybrid Nanosystems for Efficient and Targeted Delivery against Bacterial Infections. *J. Control. Release* **2022**, *351*, 598–622. [CrossRef]
2. Li, C.; Wang, Z.; Lei, H.; Zhang, D. Recent Progress in Nanotechnology-Based Drug Carriers for Resveratrol Delivery. *Drug Delivery* **2023**, *30*, 2174206. [CrossRef] [PubMed]
3. Pires, P.C.; Santos, A.O. Nanosystems in Nose-to-Brain Drug Delivery: A Review of Non-Clinical Brain Targeting Studies. *J. Control. Release* **2018**, *270*, 89–100. [CrossRef] [PubMed]
4. Md, S.; Mustafa, G.; Baboota, S.; Ali, J. Nanoneurotherapeutics Approach Intended for Direct Nose to Brain Delivery. *Drug Dev. Ind. Pharm.* **2015**, *41*, 1922–1934. [CrossRef]
5. Schulman, J.H.; Stoeckenius, W.; Prince, L.M. Mechanism of Formation and Structure of Micro Emulsions by Electron Microscopy. *J. Phys. Chem.* **1959**, *63*, 1677–1680. [CrossRef]
6. Ruckenstein, E.; Chi, J.C. Stability of Microemulsions. *J. Chem. Soc. Faraday Trans.* **1975**, *71*, 1690. [CrossRef]
7. Schulman, J.H.; Montagne, J.B. FORMATION OF MICROEMULSIONS BY AMINO ALKYL ALCOHOLS. *Ann. N. Y. Acad. Sci.* **1961**, *92*, 366–371. [CrossRef] [PubMed]
8. Singh, Y.; Meher, J.G.; Raval, K.; Khan, F.A.; Chaurasia, M.; Jain, N.K.; Chourasia, M.K. Nanoemulsion: Concepts, Development and Applications in Drug Delivery. *J. Control. Release* **2017**, *252*, 28–49. [CrossRef]

9. Chatterjee, B.; Gorain, B.; Mohananaidu, K.; Sengupta, P.; Mandal, U.K.; Choudhury, H. Targeted Drug Delivery to the Brain via Intranasal Nanoemulsion: Available Proof of Concept and Existing Challenges. *Int. J. Pharm.* **2019**, *565*, 258–268. [CrossRef]
10. Kashyap, K.; Shukla, R. Drug Delivery and Targeting to the Brain Through Nasal Route: Mechanisms, Applications and Challenges. *Curr. Drug Deliv.* **2019**, *16*, 887–901. [CrossRef]
11. Bonferoni, M.; Rossi, S.; Sandri, G.; Ferrari, F.; Gavini, E.; Rassu, G.; Giunchedi, P. Nanoemulsions for "Nose-to-Brain" Drug Delivery. *Pharmaceutics* **2019**, *11*, 84. [CrossRef]
12. Costa, C.P.; Moreira, J.N.; Sousa Lobo, J.M.; Silva, A.C. Intranasal Delivery of Nanostructured Lipid Carriers, Solid Lipid Nanoparticles and Nanoemulsions: A Current Overview of in Vivo Studies. *Acta Pharm. Sin. B* **2021**, *11*, 925–940. [CrossRef]
13. Pires, P.C.; Peixoto, D.; Teixeira, I.; Rodrigues, M.; Alves, G.; Santos, A.O. Nanoemulsions and Thermosensitive Nanoemulgels of Phenytoin and Fosphenytoin for Intranasal Administration: Formulation Development and in Vitro Characterization. *Eur. J. Pharm. Sci.* **2020**, *141*, 105099. [CrossRef]
14. Lindemann, J.; Keck, T.; Wiesmiller, K.; Sander, B.; Brambs, H.-J.; Rettinger, G.; Pless, D. A Numerical Simulation of Intranasal Air Temperature During Inspiration. *Laryngoscope* **2004**, *114*, 1037–1041. [CrossRef] [PubMed]
15. Pires, P.C.; Santos, L.T.; Rodrigues, M.; Alves, G.; Santos, A.O. Intranasal Fosphenytoin: The Promise of Phosphate Esters in Nose-to-Brain Delivery of Poorly Soluble Drugs. *Int. J. Pharm.* **2021**, *592*, 120040. [CrossRef]
16. Jemal, M.; Ouyang, Z.; Powell, M.L. Direct-Injection LC–MS–MS Method for High-Throughput Simultaneous Quantitation of Simvastatin and Simvastatin Acid in Human Plasma. *J. Pharm. Biomed. Anal.* **2000**, *23*, 323–340. [CrossRef]
17. Shi, J.-H.; Wang, Q.; Pan, D.-Q.; Liu, T.-T.; Jiang, M. Characterization of Interactions of Simvastatin, Pravastatin, Fluvastatin, and Pitavastatin with Bovine Serum Albumin: Multiple Spectroscopic and Molecular Docking. *J. Biomol. Struct. Dyn.* **2017**, *35*, 1529–1546. [CrossRef] [PubMed]
18. Anton, N.; Vandamme, T.F. The Universality of Low-Energy Nano-Emulsification. *Int. J. Pharm.* **2009**, *377*, 142–147. [CrossRef]
19. Kumar, A.; Li, S.; Cheng, C.-M.; Lee, D. Recent Developments in Phase Inversion Emulsification. *Ind. Eng. Chem. Res.* **2015**, *54*, 8375–8396. [CrossRef]
20. Nogueira Prista, L.; Correia Alves, A.; Ramos Morgado, R.; Sousa Lobo, J. *Tecnologia Farmacêutica*, 8th ed.; Fundação Calouste Gulbenkian: Lisboa, Portugal, 2011; Volume I.
21. Perazzo, A.; Preziosi, V.; Guido, S. Phase Inversion Emulsification: Current Understanding and Applications. *Adv. Colloid Interface Sci.* **2015**, *222*, 581–599. [CrossRef]
22. Pouton, C.W. Formulation of Poorly Water-Soluble Drugs for Oral Administration: Physicochemical and Physiological Issues and the Lipid Formulation Classification System. *Eur. J. Pharm. Sci.* **2006**, *29*, 278–287. [CrossRef]
23. Fuentes-Fayos, A.C.; G-García, M.E.; Pérez-Gómez, J.M.; Montero-Hidalgo, A.J.; Martín-Colom, J.; Doval-Rosa, C.; Blanco-Acevedo, C.; Torres, E.; Toledano-Delgado, Á.; Sánchez-Sánchez, R.; et al. Metformin and Simvastatin Exert Additive Antitumour Effects in Glioblastoma via Senescence-State: Clinical and Translational Evidence. *eBioMedicine* **2023**, *90*, 104484. [CrossRef]
24. Dolivo, D.M.; Reed, C.R.; Gargiulo, K.A.; Rodrigues, A.E.; Galiano, R.D.; Mustoe, T.A.; Hong, S.J. Anti-Fibrotic Effects of Statin Drugs: A Review of Evidence and Mechanisms. *Biochem. Pharmacol.* **2023**, *214*, 115644. [CrossRef]
25. Hanin, A.; Roussel, D.; Lecas, S.; Baudin, P.; Navarro, V. Repurposing of Cholesterol-Lowering Agents in Status Epilepticus: A Neuroprotective Effect of Simvastatin. *Epilepsy Behav.* **2023**, *141*, 109133. [CrossRef]
26. Susanto, M.; Pangihutan Siahaan, A.M.; Wirjomartani, B.A.; Setiawan, H.; Aryanti, C. Michael The Neuroprotective Effect of Statin in Traumatic Brain Injury: A Systematic Review. *World Neurosurg. X* **2023**, *19*, 100211. [CrossRef] [PubMed]
27. Jin, H.; Ji, Y.; Cui, Y.; Xu, L.; Liu, H.; Wang, J. Simvastatin-Incorporated Drug Delivery Systems for Bone Regeneration. *ACS Biomater. Sci. Eng.* **2021**, *7*, 2177–2191. [CrossRef] [PubMed]
28. Pires, P.C.; Rodrigues, M.; Alves, G.; Santos, A.O. Strategies to Improve Drug Strength in Nasal Preparations for Brain Delivery of Low Aqueous Solubility Drugs. *Pharmaceutics* **2022**, *14*, 588. [CrossRef]
29. Karim, F.T.; Kalam, A.; Anwar, R.; Miah, M.M.; Rahman, M.S.; Islam, S.M.A. Preparation and Evaluation of SEDDS of Simvastatin by *in Vivo, in Vitro* and *Ex Vivo* Technique. *Drug Dev. Ind. Pharm.* **2015**, *41*, 1338–1342. [CrossRef]
30. Yamanouchi, K.; Ishimaru, T.; Kakuno, T.; Takemoto, Y.; Kawatsu, S.; Kondo, K.; Maruyama, M.; Higaki, K. Improvement and Characterization of Oral Absorption Behavior of Clofazimine by SNEDDS: Quantitative Evaluation of Extensive Lymphatic Transport. *Eur. J. Pharm. Biopharm.* **2023**, *187*, 141–155. [CrossRef] [PubMed]
31. Yang, J.; Liang, Z.; Lu, P.; Song, F.; Zhang, Z.; Zhou, T.; Li, J.; Zhang, J. Development of a Luliconazole Nanoemulsion as a Prospective Ophthalmic Delivery System for the Treatment of Fungal Keratitis: In Vitro and In Vivo Evaluation. *Pharmaceutics* **2022**, *14*, 2052. [CrossRef]
32. Yousry, C.; Zikry, P.M.; Basalious, E.B.; El-Gazayerly, O.N. Self-Nanoemulsifying System Optimization for Higher Terconazole Solubilization and Non-Irritant Ocular Administration. *Adv. Pharm. Bull.* **2020**, *10*, 389–398. [CrossRef] [PubMed]
33. Lee, J.-H.; Lee, G.-W. Formulation Approaches for Improving the Dissolution Behavior and Bioavailability of Tolvaptan Using SMEDDS. *Pharmaceutics* **2022**, *14*, 415. [CrossRef] [PubMed]
34. Kim, H.-S.; Kim, C.-M.; Jo, A.-N.; Kim, J.-E. Studies on Preformulation and Formulation of JIN-001 Liquisolid Tablet with Enhanced Solubility. *Pharmaceuticals* **2022**, *15*, 412. [CrossRef]

35. Baral, K.C.; Song, J.-G.; Lee, S.H.; Bajracharya, R.; Sreenivasulu, G.; Kim, M.; Lee, K.; Han, H.-K. Enhanced Bioavailability of AC1497, a Novel Anticancer Drug Candidate, via a Self-Nanoemulsifying Drug Delivery System. *Pharmaceutics* **2021**, *13*, 1142. [CrossRef]
36. Pires, P.C.; Fazendeiro, A.C.; Rodrigues, M.; Alves, G.; Santos, A.O. Nose-to-Brain Delivery of Phenytoin and Its Hydrophilic Prodrug Fosphenytoin Combined in a Microemulsion—Formulation Development and in Vivo Pharmacokinetics. *Eur. J. Pharm. Sci.* **2021**, *164*, 105918. [CrossRef] [PubMed]

pharmaceutics

MDPI

Review

Optimizing Absorption for Intranasal Delivery of Drugs Targeting the Central Nervous System Using Alkylsaccharide Permeation Enhancers

Stuart Madden [1,*], Enrique Carrazana [1,2] and Adrian L. Rabinowicz [1]

1 Neurelis, Inc., San Diego, CA 92121, USA; ecarrazana@neurelis.com (E.C.); arabinowicz@neurelis.com (A.L.R.)
2 John A. Burns School of Medicine, University of Hawaii, Honolulu, HI 96813, USA
* Correspondence: smadden@neurelis.com; Tel.: +1-858-251-2100

Abstract: Intranasal delivery of drugs offers several potential benefits related to ease of delivery, rapid onset, and patient experience, which may be of particular relevance to patients with central nervous system (CNS) conditions who experience acute events. Intranasal formulations must be adapted to address anatomical and physiological characteristics of the nasal cavity, including restricted dose volume, limited surface area, and barriers to mucosal absorption, in addition to constraints on the absorption window due to mucociliary clearance. Development of an effective formulation may utilize strategies including the addition of excipients to address the physicochemical properties of the drug within the constraints of nasal delivery. Dodecyl maltoside (DDM) and tetradecyl maltoside are alkylsaccharide permeation enhancers with well-established safety profiles, and studies have demonstrated transiently improved absorption and favorable bioavailability of several compounds in preclinical and clinical trials. Dodecyl maltoside is a component of three US Food and Drug Administration (FDA)–approved intranasal medications: diazepam for the treatment of seizure cluster in epilepsy, nalmefene for the treatment of acute opioid overdose, and sumatriptan for the treatment of migraine. Another drug product with DDM as an excipient is currently under FDA review, and numerous investigational drugs are in early-stage development. Here, we review factors related to the delivery of intranasal drugs and the role of alkylsaccharide permeation enhancers in the context of approved and future intranasal formulations of drugs for CNS conditions.

Keywords: absorption; central nervous system; dodecyl maltoside; intranasal; Intravail; nasal cavity; rescue therapy; route of administration; solubility; tetradecyl maltoside

1. Introduction

Intranasal drug delivery is a promising option for an increasing number of drugs for systemic absorption and, importantly, for targeting the central nervous system (CNS). Formulating treatments for intranasal delivery must take into account the unique features of nasal anatomy and physiology, which offer potential benefits and present specific challenges to be addressed by a successful formulation. The intranasal route is noninvasive, and prefilled devices can offer the benefits of quick administration for acute events and ease of use by nonmedical caregivers in the community, including the potential for self-administration [1]. Surveys report positive impressions and satisfaction with existing intranasal formulations among patients and caregivers and preference over other routes of delivery, such as rectal administration [2]. Intranasal formulations also offer potential benefits in terms of favorable pharmacokinetics, including potentially high bioavailability while bypassing variable gastrointestinal absorption and first-pass metabolism [3]. At the same time, intranasal delivery necessitates a specific formulation that is adapted to the unique characteristics of the nasal anatomy and physiology, including a surface area that limits dosing volume, permeability of nasal mucosa, mucociliary clearance, and issues of tolerability from either the drug substance or the formulation itself [3].

A growing number of intranasal drug formulations for the treatment of neurologic conditions have been developed in recent years. One treatment, esketamine nasal spray, is administered regularly under the supervision of a healthcare provider as an ongoing adjunct treatment for depression [4]. However, many are treatments for acute conditions, such as triptans dihydroergotamine and zavegepant for migraine, naloxone and nalmefene for opioid overdose, and diazepam and midazolam for seizure cluster in epilepsy [5–13]. In the first half of 2023 alone, the intranasal formulations of zavegepant (for migraine) and nalmefene (for opioid overdose) were approved by the US Food and Drug Administration (FDA), and naloxone nasal spray has been approved for nonprescription use in the US and is being made available directly to the public [10,13,14]. While intranasal formulations are becoming increasingly available, there remains a lack of awareness among researchers, clinicians, and patients of their unique characteristics for intranasal administration and drug delivery. Understanding intranasal delivery and strategies for the development of intranasal drug formulations will help clinicians assess and differentiate intranasal formulations and ultimately facilitate working with their patients to choose the most appropriate treatment option. In this review, we address aspects of nasal anatomy and physiology that are particularly relevant to intranasal delivery of CNS drugs. Within the broad context of strategies to facilitate intranasal absorption, which also include nanocarriers [15], gels [16], and devices [17], we focus on the development of alkylsaccharides as permeation-enhancing excipients and the data supporting their clinical use in a growing number of intranasal formulations that are increasingly available in different regions.

2. Challenges of Nasal Drug Delivery

2.1. Nasal Anatomy and Physiology

Structures of the nose heat and humidify air for respiration; clear foreign particles, including pathogens; and facilitate olfaction [3]. The two nasal cavities are irregularly shaped internal structures lying between the roof of the mouth and the skull bones encasing the bottom of the brain (Figure 1) [18]. They are separated by the septum, while the outer cavity walls are folded to form three turbinates on each side [18]. The nasal cavity contains four general areas: the vestibule, the respiratory mucosa, the olfactory mucosa, and the nasopharynx-associated lymphatic tissue [3].

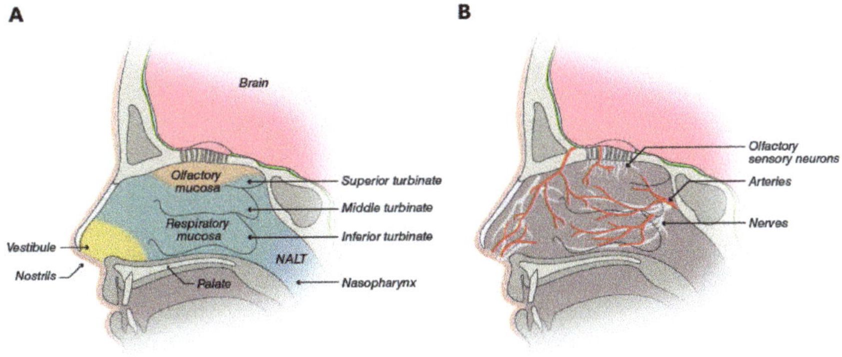

Figure 1. (**A**) The nasal cavity is partitioned into four areas: the vestibule is the area inside the nostrils; the respiratory mucosa and the olfactory mucosa cover the central portion, including the turbinates; and the nasopharynx-associated lymphatic tissue (NALT). (**B**) The respiratory mucosa is the most vascularized part of the nasal cavity, and it is innervated by the trigeminal, palantine, and maxillary nerves. The olfactory mucosa additionally contains olfactory sensory neurons [3].

The central portion of the nasal cavity is covered by the respiratory and olfactory mucosa and represents the area most relevant for drug absorption after intranasal administration. The respiratory mucosa overlays the inferior and middle turbinates, as well as the lower part of the septum [3]. It is the largest portion of the nasal cavity and is highly vascularized by a rich bed of blood vessels containing pores (fenestrations) in the vessel walls [3,18]. The characteristics of these vessels make them a prime potential site for drug absorption into general circulation. In addition, the presence of the turbinates increases the overall surface area of the nasal cavity to approximately 160 cm^2, which is available for drug absorption.

The olfactory mucosa constitutes $\leq$10% of the nasal cavity surface area and covers the upper portion of the cavity [3,18]. This region contains olfactory sensory neurons, which are the only neurons of the CNS on the surface of the body exposed to the external environment [18]. This exposure offers the potential for direct delivery of CNS drugs to the brain, although the location may present an obstacle to the efficient deposition of intranasal drugs. The trigeminal nerve, lying beneath the nasal mucosa, also innervates the nasal cavity and offers the potential for direct-to-brain delivery of drugs [3,18]. In this context, it is important to note the differences in nasal anatomy and physiology between humans and animal (e.g., rat) models used to study nasal delivery systems [19]. These differences, such as a proportionally larger olfactory region in rats, may limit the direct applicability of findings from animal models to humans but can be used to assess the rank order of nose-to-brain delivery of analogs, for example [20].

2.2. *Considerations for Nasal Drug Formulations*

2.2.1. Anatomic and Physiologic Constraints

Although the nasal cavity may effectively capture intranasally delivered medications, it also creates a finite volume for dose delivery. The optimal volume for a dose of intranasal drug is no more than 100 to 150 μL per nostril [1,18]. Larger volumes risk the partial loss of drug dose either anteriorly through the nostrils or posteriorly into the nasopharynx, which is then swallowed and absorbed as an oral drug, subject to variability in bioavailability based on fed state and first-pass metabolism [3]

Second, mucus coating the epithelium of the nasal cavity acts as a defense against pathogens and particulates. Beating cilia continuously move mucus into the nasopharynx, and it is estimated that the mucus layer in the nasal cavity renews every 10 to 20 min [21]. This may reduce residence time in the nasal cavity and affect drug absorption.

Third, the mucosal lining of the nose is sensitive to irritation by drugs or other compounds, which can lead to inflammation, secretions, itching, sneezing, and pain [17]. This may constrain the choice of drug for intranasal delivery or the addition of certain excipients [22]. Although there is concern that seasonal allergies or rhinitis may negatively affect intranasal drug delivery and absorption, several studies of different intranasal formulations have demonstrated a similar extent of absorption or bioavailability between patients with and without allergic rhinitis [23–25]. No clinical impact of rhinitis or seasonal allergies was observed in separate safety studies of zolmitriptan and diazepam nasal sprays [26,27]. Finally, for intranasal deposition, droplets of 10 to 120 μm in diameter may be ideal because smaller droplets may be inhaled and deposited in pulmonary tissue, while larger droplets may deposit predominantly in the anterior nasal cavity [28,29].

2.2.2. Formulation and Physiochemical Constraints

An optimal intranasal dose of no more than 100 to 150 μL translates into a requirement for adequate drug solubility in a fixed and relatively small dose volume. Physiochemical properties of a drug, such as its lipophilic-hydrophilic properties, and its molecular weight and size affect how it can be formulated for intranasal delivery and its absorption across nasal mucosa to ensure adequate and consistent bioavailability [30]. In general, small, lipophilic drugs are more easily absorbed across the nasal mucosa; however, they are less soluble in the aqueous delivery systems commonly used in nasal formulations [1,29,31].

Excipients may be used to modify drug solubility, membrane permeation capacity, mucosal tolerability, mucosal adhesion, or formulation stability [30]. These agents include buffers, cosolvents, absorption enhancers, mucoadhesives, and viscosity enhancers, which must balance the desired effect with the potential for toxicity and/or irritation in the formulation. For example, decreasing pH may increase the intranasal absorption of some drugs and decrease it for others, while sensitizing the nasal cavity as the formulation deviates from the natural pH of the nasal cavity (pH 5.5–6.5) [30,32,33], which carries a risk of local irritation [1].

2.2.3. Delivery Device Constraints

The intranasal delivery system must create reproducible parameters of dose delivered, droplet size distribution, and spray pattern and plume geometry to ensure consistent dosing to the intended target tissue [34]. Several delivery systems are available, from droppers and mucosal atomization devices (MADs) attached to syringes to prefilled unit-dose or unidose pumps, multidose pumps, and propellent-activated devices. With droppers and MADs, administration may be inconvenient, requiring awkward positioning of the patient, and precise dosing may be difficult [31]. Unidose pumps are single-use devices delivering a precise dose of the drug with simple actuation, whereas multidose pumps have the capability for repeat use during the course of treatment. A propellent-powered device is also being studied with a limited number of CNS drugs [35,36].

The delivery system must provide ease of use for patients who self-administer treatment or for care partners responsible for administration. The device should function reliably in any orientation; have proven biocompatibility so as not to cause irritation to the lining of the nostrils; and, for delivery to incapacitated patients, be able to be used without their active participation [1,31]. Unidose delivery systems are optimized for easy handling and intuitive use. Finally, the drug–device combination product should have an acceptable drug shelf life at controlled room temperature and be sufficiently robust to withstand shipping.

3. Focus on Absorption Optimization

To overcome the constraints imposed by nasal anatomy and physiology, including small volume, continual mucociliary clearance, and potential low drug permeability through the nasal mucosal membranes, intranasal formulations may use two broad strategies to optimize drug absorption and bioavailability: increase residence time in the nasal cavity or increase the rate of absorption across the mucosal membrane [30]. Both strategies employ specialized excipients and may be used together in a single formulation. Increasing drug permeation carries the advantages of increased bioavailability with lower drug load within the dose volume, which in turn may reduce the solubility burden on the formulation. Increased permeation may also be associated with less variability in the total dose delivered and has the potential to deliver higher-molecular-weight molecules that are typically poorly absorbed intranasally. An ideal permeation enhancer is compatible with the drug, soluble and stable in a range of solvent systems, and commercially available with appropriate labeling by a regulatory body (Figure 2).

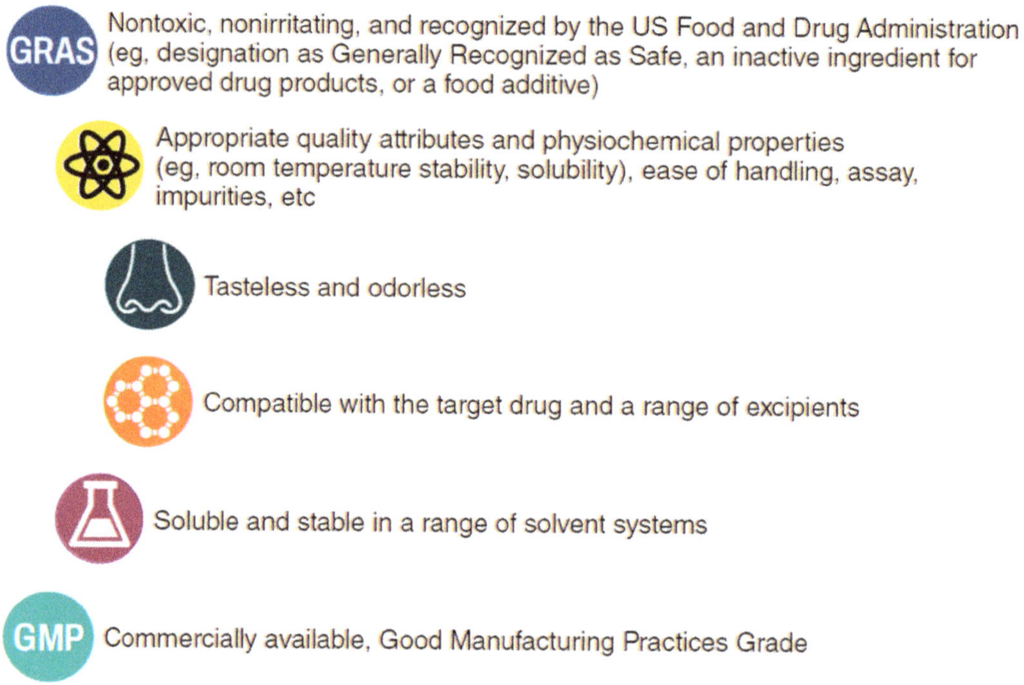

Figure 2. Ideal characteristics of a permeation enhancer for intranasal drug formulations.

3.1. Biochemistry of the Alkylsaccharides Dodecyl Maltoside and Tetradecyl Maltoside

Alkylsaccharides are a family of sugars characterized by covalent linkages to $\geq$1 alkyl chain (Figure 3) [37], several of which have been developed as transmucosal delivery enhancement agents. They are classed as nonionic surfactants and used in food and personal care products. In particular, dodecyl maltoside (DDM; 511 Da) and tetradecyl maltoside (TDM; 539 Da) are examples of Intravail® (Neurelis, Inc., San Diego, CA, USA) alkylsaccharide absorption enhancers [38]. These excipients are considered safe, nontoxic, nonmutagenic, tasteless, odorless, and nonsensitizing (up to 25% concentration in the Draize test); they are designated as Generally Recognized as Safe (GRAS) for oral consumption and meet all the requirements listed in Figure 2 [37]. Sucrose esters have a no-observed-effect level (NOEL) of 2000 mg/kg body weight and a World Health Organization oral allowable daily intake (ADI) of $\leq$40 mg/kg body weight, supporting their use as an excipient [39]. In the body, alkylsaccharides are metabolized to their constituent sugars and fatty acids, and ultimately to carbon dioxide and water [40]. DDM is soluble in oils and water, making it appropriate for formulations of hydrophilic and hydrophobic compounds [40]. DDM is compatible with routine liquid formulation and dispensing processes for ease of scale-up and production. Intravail is composed of synthetic pure chemical entities prepared under good manufacturing practices (GMP) in Europe and Asia to ensure uniform composition between lots and below-threshold levels of residual reactants or solvents [37].

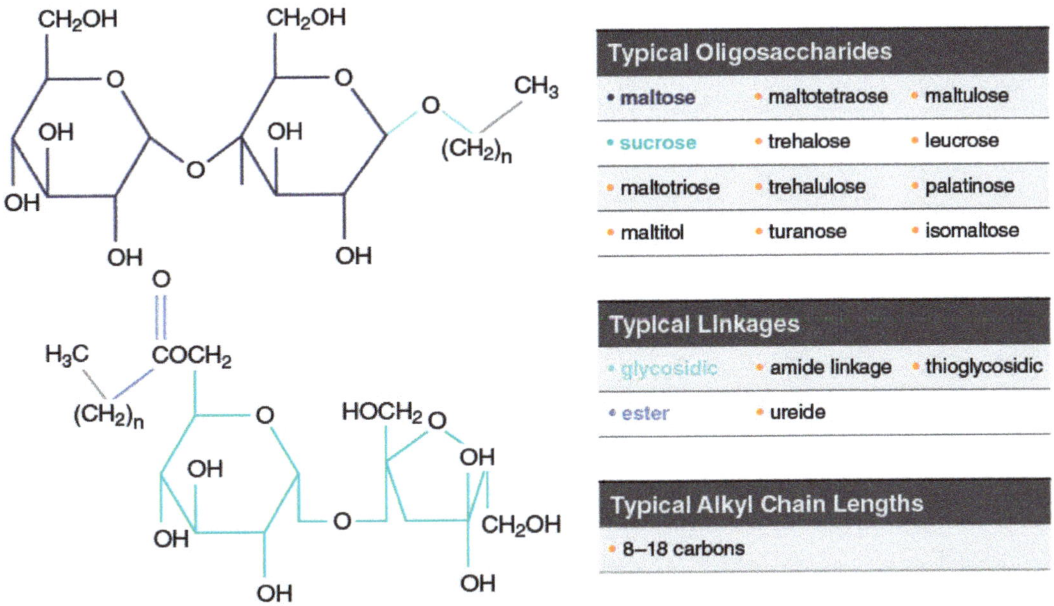

Figure 3. Examples of typical alkylsaccharide structures comprising Intravail® excipients. Used with permission from Maggio & Pillion, 2013 [37].

3.2. DDM and TDM Mechanism of Action

Two possible mechanisms of action have been proposed for Intravail excipients' effect of increased transmucosal transport. The first involves paracellular transport via transient loosening of tight junctions between epithelial cells by DDM to permit mucosal barrier permeation, which has been demonstrated in several human cell lines and epithelial tissue [38]. A study in the rat demonstrated a transient permeation effect on nasal epithelia after the application of TDM with successful transport of molecules up to 22 kDa (human growth hormone analog somatropin) [41]. The temporary opening and then closing of tight junctions was observed through the time-dependent exclusion of successively smaller molecules after treatment (Figure 4). When calcitonin (4 kDa) was administered 60 and 120 min after TDM, absorption was reduced but not halted, indicating that the tight junctions remained sufficiently open to allow passage of the small molecule. However, when somatropin (22 kDa) was administered 60 and 120 min after TDM, absorption was prevented, suggesting that the tight junctions had closed sufficiently to exclude the larger compound. The second mechanism of action involves transcellular transport across the mucosa via vesicle-mediated mechanisms, as observed in electron micrographs of the rat nasal septum tissue treated with TDM (Figure 5) [42]. DDM has also demonstrated vesicular transport effects in a tissue explant system [38].

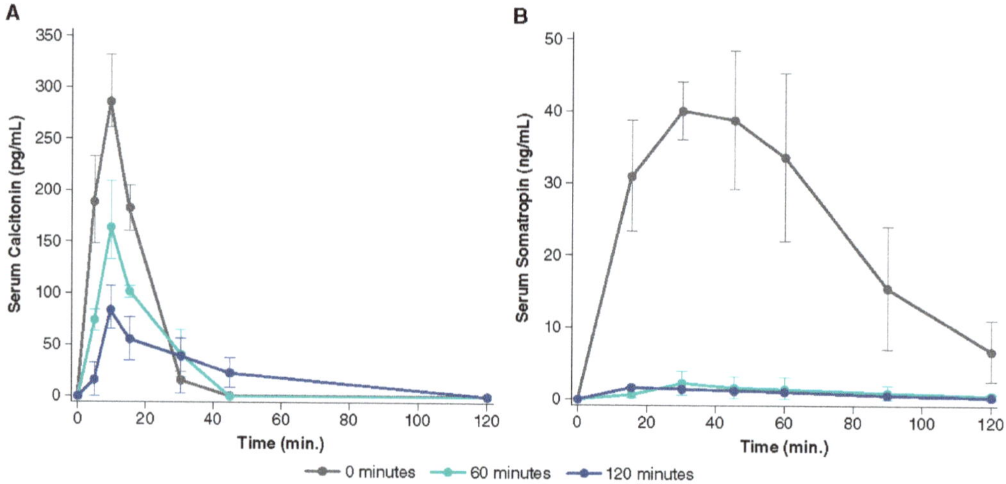

Figure 4. Serum concentration over time after administration of 0.125% tetradecyl maltoside (TDM) with (**A**) calcitonin (2.2 U) and (**B**) somatropin (100 µg) in rats. The uppermost line shows the simultaneous administration of TDM and drug, while the lower lines show administration of TDM alone followed by drug administration after 60 or 120 min. The permeation-enhancing effect of TDM is reversed within 2 h after nasal administration as evidenced by lower serum drug concentration with a longer delay after TDM administration. Used with permission from Arnold et al., 2010 [41].

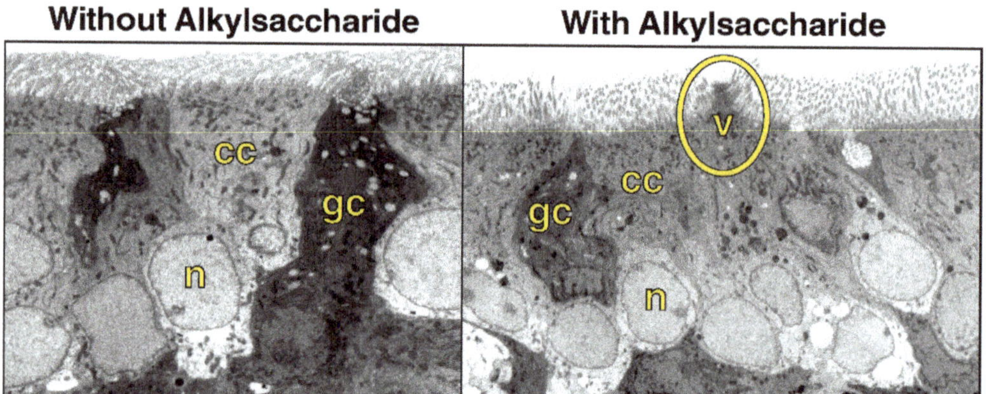

Figure 5. Electron microscopy (original magnification 3500×) of rat nasal mucosa without administration of the alkylsaccharide tetradecyl maltoside (0.125%) and 10 min after alkylsaccharide administration, showing vesicle formation. Note vesicular formation (circled) in right image and cilia at the top of both images. cc, ciliated cell; gc, goblet cell; n, nucleus, v, vesicle. Used with permission from Arnold et al., 2004 [42].

3.3. Preclinical Studies of DDM and TDM

In animal studies of intranasal absorption, the use of TDM was associated with increased absorption of calcitonin (3.5 kDa), enoxaparin (4.5 kDa), and dalteparin (5 kDa) [41,43,44]. The calcitonin study measured plasma levels in rats over time after nasal administration of formulations containing saline, a medium-chain-length alkylsaccharide, octylmaltoside, or TDM [43]. The lipophilic characteristics of an alkylsaccharide are related to alkyl chain length, and lipophilicity increased with increasing chain length. Saline and octylmaltoside (C_8 chain length) formulations resulted in little to no absorption of calcitonin, whereas

TDM (C_{14} chain length) formulations (0.125–0.25%) resulted in increased calcitonin plasma levels, peaking 7.5 to 10 min after administration [43]. Using low-molecular-weight heparin composed of enoxaparin and dalteparin, researchers tested the absorption-enhancing effect of TDM (0.25%) in rats. Intranasal administration of a formulation containing TDM resulted in a significant increase in peak plasma concentration and area under the curve for anti–factor Xa activity (a surrogate for heparin absorption) and higher bioavailability compared with saline alone, as well as reversibility [44]. Building on those findings, researchers then tested formulations of enoxaparin and four different alkylsaccharides, including DDM and TDM [45]. Intranasal administration with these alkylsaccharides resulted in dose-dependent and chain length–dependent increases in the absorption of enoxaparin, while all had a reversible effect [45]. Subsequent animal studies have assessed the bioavailability of several molecules ($\leq$30 kDa) delivered intranasally with different concentrations of TDM [37]. The studies demonstrated two notable qualities: (1) a dose-dependent relationship between TDM concentration and bioavailability of the drug and (2) an inverse relationship between molecular weight and drug bioavailability (Figure 6) [37]. For some molecules, bioavailability after intranasal delivery with DDM or TDM is comparable to intravenous delivery [37,46].

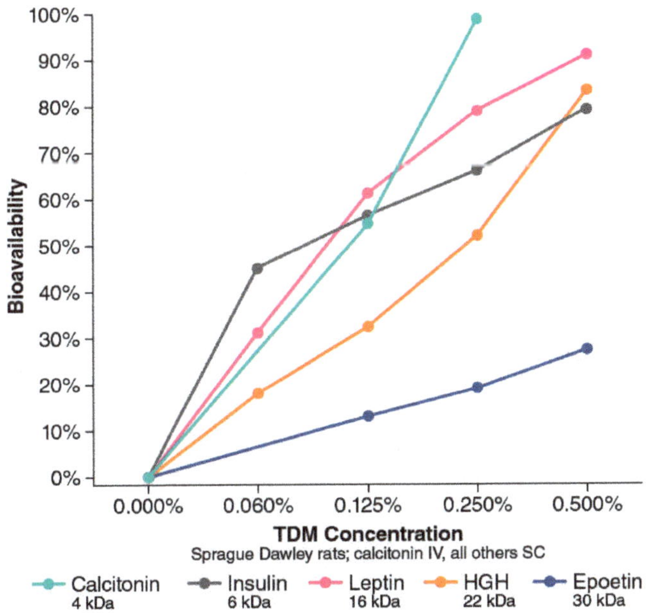

Figure 6. Bioavailability (compared with intravenous delivery) of various intranasally administered proteins ranging from 4 kDa to 30 kDa based on Intravail concentration. HGH, human growth hormone; IV, intravenous; SC, subcutaneous; TDM, tetradecyl maltoside. Adapted with permission from Maggio & Pillion, 2013 [37].

3.4. DDM: Currently Approved Treatments

To date, three intranasal medications containing DDM have been approved by the US Food and Drug Administration (FDA). They are treatments for migraine, seizure cluster in epilepsy, and opioid overdose. Clinical trials of these treatments support the favorable safety profile of DDM as an excipient. Currently, no intranasal treatments containing DDM are approved by the European Medicines Agency for use in Europe.

3.4.1. Sumatriptan Nasal Spray with Intravail (Tosymra®)

Sumatriptan nasal spray with DDM (Tosymra®, Upsher-Smith Laboratories, Maple Grove, MN, USA) is indicated for the treatment of acute migraine headaches with or without aura in adults [9]. A randomized crossover study compared intranasal sumatriptan 10 mg containing 0.20% DDM with the earlier commercially available intranasal sumatriptan 20 mg without DDM (n = 18 healthy volunteers) [47]. The earlier formulation is characterized by low bioavailability (17%) [8] and slow absorption, whereas the newer formulation with DDM has a bioavailability of 58% to 87% [9]. In the crossover study, the median time to maximum plasma concentration (C_{max}) for the DDM formulation was 10.2 min, while for sumatriptan 20 mg without DDM, the median time was 2 h. The concentration-time profile of the formulation without DDM registered two peaks. The researchers interpreted the early peak in plasma levels as an indication of nasally absorbed drug, while the second later peak was likely due to most of the dose being swallowed and absorbed through the gastrointestinal tract (Figure 7). In contrast, the DDM formulations demonstrated a single early peak of absorption, suggesting nasal absorption [47].

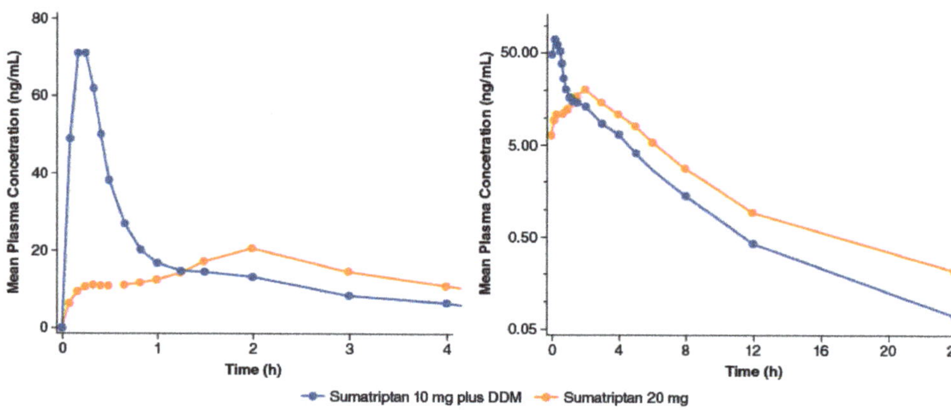

Figure 7. Intranasal sumatriptan 10 mg plus 0.2% dodecyl maltoside (DDM) vs. intranasal sumatriptan 20 mg: mean plasma sumatriptan concentration-time profiles. Panels differ by the span of the x-axis; in addition, the y-axis of the right panel is on a log scale. Adapted with permission from Munjal et al., 2016 [47].

The efficacy, safety, and tolerability of sumatriptan plus DDM were assessed in phase 2, a double-blind, 2-period, placebo-controlled study of sumatriptan 10 mg with 0.20% DDM [48]. The study, which enrolled 107 patients with migraine, met its primary endpoint: the proportion of patients free from headache pain at 2 h postdose was statistically significantly higher in the sumatriptan with DDM group than in the placebo group (last observation carried forward: 43.8% vs. 22.5%, $p = 0.044$; observed cases: 43.8% vs. 20.5%, $p = 0.025$). Treatment-emergent adverse events (TEAEs) were reported in 9/93 (9.7%) patients, and 7/93 (7.5%) reported a TEAE that was considered to be treatment-related. The most commonly reported TEAEs were dysgeusia (3 patients) and application site pain (2 patients) [48].

In the same report, researchers described a 3-way crossover study comparing pharmacokinetic parameters of intranasal sumatriptan plus DDM and 4 or 6 mg sumatriptan administered subcutaneously in 78 healthy volunteers. Intranasal sumatriptan with DDM provided significantly faster time to maximum concentration (t_{max}) than subcutaneous dosing (10 vs. 15 min; $p < 0.0001$), with similar overall exposure, measured as the mean area under the curve (AUC), between intranasal sumatriptan 10 mg with DDM and the 4- mg subcutaneous dose. TEAEs occurring in $\geq$10% of patients in the trial overall study were dysgeusia (19%, n = 15 [13 occurred with the intranasal formulation]), headache (18%, n = 14 [5 intranasal]), nausea (15%, n = 12 [2 intranasal]), paresthesia (15%, n = 12 [0 intranasal]), and dizziness (12%, n = 9 [2 intranasal]). In an open-label, long-term, repeat-dose safety study of the intranasal formulation of sumatriptan 10 mg with DDM, 51 of 167 (30.5%) patients reported application site pain (including nasal burning or stinging), usually of mild severity [49]. Incidences of application site reaction and irritation were 5.4% and 4.2%, respectively. It is important to note that these studies did not assess the safety of DDM alone compared with sumatriptan plus DDM, so the contribution of active drug vs. excipient to treatment safety and tolerability cannot be determined.

3.4.2. Diazepam Nasal Spray (Valtoco®)

Dodecyl maltoside is also a component of diazepam nasal spray (Valtoco®, Neurelis, Inc., San Diego, CA, USA), which is indicated for the acute treatment of intermittent, stereotypic episodes of frequent seizure activity (i.e., seizure clusters, acute repetitive seizures) that are distinct from a patient's usual seizure pattern in patients with epilepsy 6 years of age and older [5]. It includes vitamin E to increase diazepam solubility without the use of potentially irritating organic cosolvents that would be used in conventional aqueous systems [50]. An early crossover pharmacokinetic study compared two intranasal diazepam 10-mg formulations that contained DDM with commercially available intravenous diazepam in healthy volunteers (n = 24). Diazepam nasal spray solution had an absolute bioavailability of 97% relative to the intravenous formulation with similar variability in exposure, as measured by AUC [46].

A phase 1 open-label crossover study in healthy volunteers (n = 48) assessed the bioavailability of diazepam nasal spray compared with oral and rectal diazepam [51]. Intranasal delivery was associated with less interpatient variability in bioavailability (as measured by AUC) than rectal delivery, while overall bioavailability was slightly less. The pharmacokinetics of diazepam nasal spray was also studied in patients with epilepsy with seizure clusters [52]. There was little impact of the epileptic state (ictal/peri-ictal vs. interictal) on pharmacokinetics or safety [52]. The study also assessed levels of DDM in a subset of patients (n = 25) with epilepsy after treatment with diazepam nasal spray [53]. At any time point, ≤5 patients had detectable DDM plasma concentrations (>500 pg/mL; maximum concentration 741 pg/mL), with levels returning to undetectable by 1.75 h postdose, confirming that residual plasma concentrations of DDM are low and transient following use of diazepam nasal spray [53].

The safety of diazepam nasal spray was assessed in a long-term, open-label, repeat-dose phase 3 study of patients aged 6 to 65 years with epilepsy and seizure clusters (n = 163 safety population) [50]. Overall, the safety profile of diazepam nasal spray was comparable to that of rectal diazepam. Over the course of the 12-month study, 134 (82.2%) patients reported any TEAE. Treatment-related TEAEs were reported by 30 (18.4%) patients: events reported by ≥3 patients were nasal discomfort (n = 10 patients [6.1%]); headache (n = 4 [2.5%]); and dysgeusia, epistaxis, and somnolence (n = 3 each [1.8%]). There were no clinically significant toxicities of the nasal cavity. Nasal irritation was assessed by a trained observer. Most patients experienced no sign of irritation (764 of 781 tests), with the remaining cases of irritation being transient. No significant olfactory changes were observed by the NIH Toolbox Odor Identification Test. Finally, rates of TEAEs, serious TEAEs, and treatment-related TEAEs were similar between patients with and without seasonal allergies/rhinitis [50]. As with the studies of sumatriptan with DDM, this study did not assess the safety of DDM alone; thus, the relationship to DDM cannot be determined.

Finally, surveys of patients with seizure clusters and their caregivers who used intranasal diazepam rescue therapy delivered in unidose pumps reported favorable impressions of the treatment. Patients and caregivers found it comfortable to carry and use outside the home, and they preferred the convenience of the nasal spray over rectal diazepam [2]. Of note, a study of a prefilled intranasal spray pump (naloxone) found it to be easier to use than an assembled MAD or an intramuscular autoinjector [54]. The intranasal device was also associated with a shorter time to successful delivery (16 s) than either the MAD (113 s; $p = 0.012$) or the autoinjector (58 s; $p < 0.001$) [54].

3.4.3. Nalmefene Nasal Spray (Opvee®)

In May 2023, nalmefene nasal spray with DDM (Opvee®, Indivior Inc., Chesterfield, VA, USA) received FDA approval for healthcare and community use as an emergency treatment for known or suspected opioid overdose in adults and pediatric patients 12 years of age and older. In a preclinical study assessing three absorption enhancers including DDM in an animal model, absolute nalmefene bioavailability with 0.5% and 0.25% DDM was 76.5% and 71.0%, respectively, a significant increase ($p < 0.05$) over the bioavailability of nalmefene administered alone (47.7%) [55]. Nalmefene plus DDM reported good safety in nasal ciliotoxicity models [55]. A phase 1 pharmacokinetic study of nalmefene in healthy volunteers (n = 14) compared four formulations: intranasal nalmefene 1.5 mg, intranasal nalmefene 3 mg, intranasal nalmefene 3 mg plus 0.25% DDM, and intramuscular nalmefene 1.5 mg [56]. Median t_{max} of intranasal nalmefene 3 mg was 2 h. The addition of DDM reduced t_{max} to 15 min and more than doubled C_{max} (4.45 vs. 1.99 ng/mL for nalmefene 3 mg). DDM had no apparent effect on nalmefene half-life. The onset of action with nalmefene with DDM was comparable to the intramuscular injection, with a higher C_{max}. TEAEs were mild, with no apparent changes in olfaction [56].

Three clinical trials (2 pharmacokinetic trials and 1 pharmacodynamic study) support the safety of nalmefene nasal spray. The most common treatment-related TEAEs (>5%) associated with nalmefene 2.7 mg nasal spray in healthy volunteers (n = 150) were nasal discomfort (28.7%), headache (26.7%), nausea (16.7%), dizziness (9.3%), hot flush (8.0%), and vomiting (6.0%) [13]. These studies did not assess the safety of DDM alone; thus, the relationship to DDM cannot be determined.

3.5. DDM: Future Directions

3.5.1. Epinephrine Nasal Spray (Neffy™)

Intramuscular injection of epinephrine is the standard of care for the treatment of severe allergic reactions, including anaphylaxis. Epinephrine nasal spray (neffy™, ARS Pharmaceuticals, Inc., San Diego, CA, USA) is under development as a noninvasive alternative to injection for use in community settings [57]. Epinephrine nasal spray contains 0.275% DDM, which was chosen based on optimal epinephrine bioavailability in phase 1 studies [58]. A recent publication presented an integrated analysis of data from four phase 1 studies comparing the pharmacodynamic and pharmacokinetic properties of intramuscular epinephrine 0.3 mg injection either manually or with autoinjectors and epinephrine 1 mg nasal spray. Within the context of the emerging understanding that epinephrine pharmacokinetics can vary among different injection devices, epinephrine nasal spray with DDM demonstrated a mean C_{max} that was similar to manually injected epinephrine, with a shorter median t_{max}. Overall, the nasal spray produced similar or more pronounced pharmacodynamic changes compared with the injected formulations [57]. Epinephrine nasal spray is currently under review with the FDA.

3.5.2. Other Treatments

Naltrexone with DDM (Indivior, Chesterfield, VA, USA) is in development as a nasal spray for the treatment of patients with alcohol use disorder. Based on a pharmacokinetic study in healthy volunteers that showed a decrease in t_{max} from 30 to 10 min and a ~3-fold increase in C_{max} with the addition of DDM to intranasal naltrexone [59], a phase 2 study is underway. The randomized, double-blind, placebo-controlled trial will evaluate the effects of naltrexone nasal spray on alcohol use disorder, with preliminary results expected in 2023 [60,61]. Finally, other intranasal formulations containing DDM in the early stages of development include intranasal olanzapine plus DDM for the treatment of acute agitation in patients with schizophrenia or bipolar disorder [62].

4. Future Perspectives and Conclusions

Intranasal delivery is becoming an increasingly common route of administration for drugs that treat CNS conditions. As of mid-2023, the FDA has approved ten intranasal formulations of CNS drugs as treatments [4–7,9–13,63], with the three discussed above containing DDM as a permeation enhancer (Figure 8). Intranasal delivery offers several benefits related to ease of delivery, favorable pharmacokinetics, and patient experience. To optimize these benefits, intranasal formulations must address the specific anatomic and physiologic constraints of the nasal cavity, as well as the physicochemical constraints of the drug formulation.

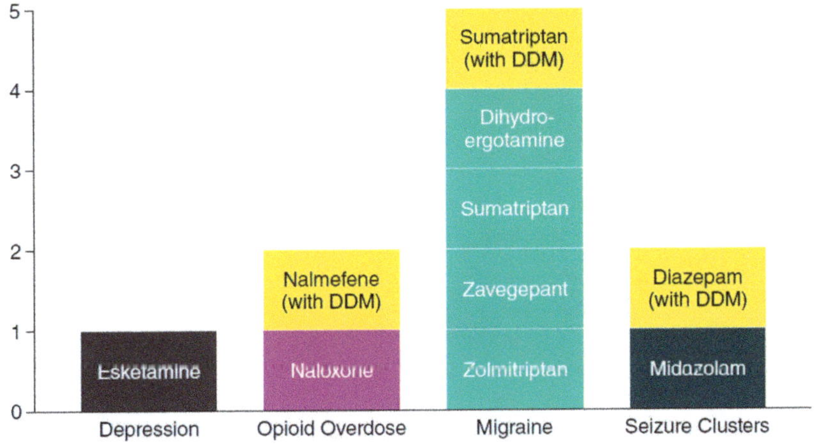

Figure 8. Central nervous system drugs approved by the US FDA as intranasal formulations by mid-2023. CNS, central nervous system; DDM, dodecyl maltoside [4–7,9–13,63].

Permeation enhancers such as DDM and TDM are valuable excipients in a growing number of FDA-approved intranasal treatments. They have been shown to enhance drug absorption and bioavailability. DDM has a proven record of preclinical and clinical safety as an excipient in intranasal formulations. Moreover, the physicochemical characteristics of alkylsaccharides offer the potential for the development of other intranasal drug therapies for non-CNS and nonemergency conditions, incorporating hydrophilic and hydrophobic formulations of small molecules, peptides, and proteins. In the CNS, in particular, direct nose-to-brain delivery of drugs with intranasal delivery is an important potential benefit for certain molecules. As real-world experience with these newer intranasal formulations grows, additional potential benefits to patients and healthcare utilization may become apparent. Finally, DDM may also have potential applications in buccal, dermal, oral, and other pharmaceutical agents. While approved intranasal formulations have made progress in providing effective and acceptable treatment for patients with some conditions, significant unmet needs remain for many other conditions that range from allergy to psychiatry. Ongoing research and development of intranasal formulations offers future novel and alternative therapies, thereby broadening the choice of treatment options and improving the experience and outcomes for patients living with a number of acute CNS conditions.

Author Contributions: Conceptualization, S.M., E.C. and A.L.R.; writing—original draft preparation, S.M.; writing—review and editing, S.M., E.C. and A.L.R. All authors have read and agreed to the published version of the manuscript.

Funding: This project was funded by Neurelis, Inc. (San Diego, CA, USA).

Institutional Review Board Statement: Not applicable.

Informed Consent Statement: Not applicable.

Data Availability Statement: Not applicable.

Acknowledgments: Editorial support was provided by David McLay, of The Curry Rockefeller Group, LLC (Tarrytown, NY, USA), and was funded by Neurelis, Inc. (San Diego, CA, USA).

Conflicts of Interest: S.M. and E.C. are employees of and have received stock and stock options from Neurelis, Inc. A.L.R. is an employee of and has received stock options from Neurelis, Inc.

Abbreviations

ADI	Allowable daily intake
AUC	Area under the curve
C_{max}	Maximum plasma concentration
CNS	Central nervous system
DDM	Dodecyl maltoside
FDA	US Food and Drug Administration
GMP	Good manufacturing practices
GRAS	Generally recognized as safe
MAD	Mucosal atomization device
NALT	Nasopharynx-associated lymphatic tissue
NOEL	No-observed-effect level
TDM	Tetradecyl maltoside
TEAE	Treatment-emergent adverse event
t_{max}	Time to maximum plasma concentration

References

1. Cloyd, J.; Haut, S.; Carrazana, E.; Rabinowicz, A.L. Overcoming the challenges of developing an intranasal diazepam rescue therapy for the treatment of seizure clusters. *Epilepsia* **2021**, *62*, 846–856. [CrossRef] [PubMed]
2. Penovich, P.; Wheless, J.W.; Hogan, R.E.; Guerra, C.; Cook, D.F.; Carrazana, E.; Rabinowicz, A.L. Examining the patient and caregiver experience with diazepam nasal spray for seizure clusters: Results from an exit survey of a phase 3, open-label, repeat-dose safety study. *Epilepsy Behav.* **2021**, *121*, 108013.
3. Chung, S.; Peters, J.M.; Detyniecki, K.; Tatum, W.; Rabinowicz, A.L.; Carrazana, E. The nose has it: Opportunities and challenges for intranasal drug administration for neurologic conditions including seizure clusters. *Epilepsy Behav. Rep.* **2023**, *21*, 100581. [PubMed]
4. Janssen Pharmaceuticals. *Spravato (Esketamine Nasal Spray, CII)*; Janssen Pharmaceutical Companies: Titusville, NJ, USA, 2020.
5. Neurelis, Inc. *VALTOCO®(Diazepam Nasal Spray)*; Neurelis, Inc.: San Diego, CA, USA, 2023.
6. UCB, Inc. *Nayzilam®(Midazolam Nasal Spray)*; UCB, Inc.: Smyrna, GA, USA, 2023.
7. Bausch Health US, LLC. *Migranal®(Dihydroergotamine Mesylate Nasal Spray)*; Bausch Health US, LLC: Bridgewater, NJ, USA, 2022.
8. GlaxoSmithKline. *Imitrex Nasal Spray (Sumatriptan)*; GlaxoSmithKline: Research Triangle Park, NC, USA, 2017.
9. Upsher-Smith Laboratories, LLC. *TOSYMRA®(Sumatriptan)*; Upsher-Smith Laboratories, LLC: Maple Grove, MN, USA, 2021.
10. Pfizer Inc. *Zavzpret (Zavegepant)*; Pfizer Inc.: New York, NY, USA, 2023.
11. Amneal Pharmaceuticals. *Zomig (Zolmitriptan Spray, Metered)*; Amneal Pharmaceuticals: Bridgewater, NJ, USA, 2019.
12. Adapt Pharma, Inc. *Narcan®Nasal Spray (Naloxone Hydrochloride)*; Adapt Pharma, Inc.: Plymouth Meeting, PA, USA, 2020.
13. Opiant Pharmaceuticals, Inc. *Opvee (Nalmefene Nasal Spray)*; Opiant Pharmaceuticals, Inc.: Santa Monica, CA, USA, 2023.
14. US Food & Drug Administration. FDA Approves First Over-the-Counter Naloxone Nasal Spray [Press Release]. Available online: https://www.fda.gov/news-events/press-announcements/fda-approves-first-over-counter-naloxone-nasal-spray (accessed on 14 July 2023).
15. Tripathi, S.; Gupta, U.; Ujjwal, R.R.; Yadav, A.K. Nano-lipidic formulation and therapeutic strategies for Alzheimer's disease via intranasal route. *J. Microencapsul.* **2021**, *38*, 572–593. [CrossRef]
16. Nair, A.B.; Chaudhary, S.; Shah, H.; Jacob, S.; Mewada, V.; Shinu, P.; Aldhubiab, B.; Sreeharsha, N.; Venugopala, K.N.; Attimarad, M.; et al. Intranasal Delivery of Darunavir-Loaded Mucoadhesive In Situ Gel: Experimental Design, In Vitro Evaluation, and Pharmacokinetic Studies. *Gels* **2022**, *8*, 342. [CrossRef] [PubMed]
17. Djupesland, P.G. Nasal drug delivery devices: Characteristics and performance in a clinical perspective-a review. *Drug Deliv. Transl. Res.* **2013**, *3*, 42–62. [CrossRef]
18. Gizurarson, S. Anatomical and histological factors affecting intranasal drug and vaccine delivery. *Curr. Drug Deliv.* **2012**, *9*, 566–582.
19. Erdo, F.; Bors, L.A.; Farkas, D.; Bajza, A.; Gizurarson, S. Evaluation of intranasal delivery route of drug administration for brain targeting. *Brain Res. Bull.* **2018**, *143*, 155–170.

20. Sharma, D.; Sharma, R.K.; Sharma, N.; Gabrani, R.; Sharma, S.K.; Ali, J.; Dang, S. Nose-to-brain delivery of PLGA-diazepam nanoparticles. *AAPS PharmSciTech* **2015**, *16*, 1108–1121. [CrossRef]
21. Edizer, D.T.; Yigit, O.; Rudenko, M. Mucociliary clearance and its importance. In *All Around the Nose*; Cingi, C., Bayar Muluk, N., Eds.; Springer International Publishing: Cham, Switzerland, 2020; pp. 65–70.
22. Maggio, E.T. Intravail: Highly effective intranasal delivery of peptide and protein drugs. *Expert. Opin. Drug Deliv.* **2006**, *3*, 529–539. [CrossRef]
23. Shyu, W.C.; Pittman, K.A.; Robinson, D.S.; Barbhaiya, R.H. The absolute bioavailability of transnasal butorphanol in patients experiencing rhinitis. *Eur. J. Clin. Pharmacol.* **1993**, *45*, 559–562. [CrossRef] [PubMed]
24. Davis, G.A.; Rudy, A.C.; Archer, S.M.; Wermeling, D.P.; McNamara, P.J. Bioavailability and pharmacokinetics of intranasal hydromorphone in patients experiencing vasomotor rhinitis. *Clin. Drug Investig.* **2004**, *24*, 633–639. [CrossRef] [PubMed]
25. Lunell, E.; Molander, L.; Andersson, M. Relative bioavailability of nicotine from a nasal spray in infectious rhinitis and after use of a topical decongestant. *Eur. J. Clin. Pharmacol.* **1995**, *48*, 71–75. [PubMed]
26. Dowson, A.J.; Charlesworth, B.R.; Green, J.; Färkkilä, M.; Diener, H.-C.; Hansen, S.B.; Gawel, M.; INDEX Study Group. Zolmitriptan nasal spray exhibits good long-term safety and tolerability in migraine: Results of the INDEX trial. *Headache* **2005**, *45*, 17–24.
27. Vazquez, B.; Wheless, J.; Desai, J.; Rabinowicz, A.L.; Carrazana, E. Lack of observed impact of history or concomitant treatment of seasonal allergies or rhinitis on repeated doses of diazepam nasal spray administered per seizure episode in a day, safety, and tolerability: Interim results from a phase 3, open-label, 12-month repeat-dose safety study. *Epilepsy Behav.* **2021**, *118*, 107898.
28. Trows, S.; Wuchner, K.; Spycher, R.; Steckel, H. Analytical challenges and regulatory requirements for nasal drug products in Europe and the U.S. *Pharmaceutics* **2014**, *6*, 195–219.
29. Keller, L.A.; Merkel, O.; Popp, A. Intranasal drug delivery: Opportunities and toxicologic challenges during drug development. *Drug Deliv. Transl. Res.* **2022**, *12*, 735–757.
30. Lofts, A.; Abu-Hijleh, F.; Rigg, N.; Mishra, R.K.; Hoare, T. Using the intranasal route to administer drugs to treat neurological and psychiatric illnesses: Rationale, successes, and future needs. *CNS Drugs* **2022**, *36*, 739–770.
31. Marx, D.; Williams, G.; Birkhoff, M. Intranasal drug administration—An attractive delivery route for some drugs. In *Drug Discovery and Development—From Molecules to Medicine*; Vallisuta, O., Olimat, S., Eds.; InTech Open: London, UK, 2015; pp. 299–320.
32. Ahmed, S.; Sileno, A.P.; de Meireles, J.C.; Dua, R.; Pimplaskar, H.K.; Xia, W.J.; Marinaro, J.; Langenback, E.; Matos, F.J.; Putcha, L.; et al. Effects of pH and dose on nasal absorption of scopolamine hydrobromide in human subjects. *Pharm. Res.* **2000**, *17*, 974–977. [CrossRef]
33. Tengamnuay, P.; Sahamethapat, A.; Sailasuta, A.; Mitra, A.K. Chitosans as nasal absorption enhancers of peptides: Comparison between free amine chitosans and soluble salts. *Int. J. Pharm.* **2000**, *197*, 53–67. [CrossRef]
34. US Department of Health and Human Services, US Food and Drug Administration, Center for Drug Evaluation and Research (CDER). *Guidance for Industry: Nasal Spray and Inhalation Solution, Suspension, and Spray Drug Products—Chemistry, Manufacturing, and Controls Documentation*; Center for Drug Evaluation and Research: Rockville, MD, USA, 2002.
35. Shrewsbury, S.; Davies, G.; McConnachie, L.; Hoekman, J. The pharmacokinetics of drug delivery to the upper nasal space: A review of INP105 development. *Med. Res. Arch.* **2022**, *10*. [CrossRef]
36. Cooper, W.; Ray, S.; Aurora, S.K.; Shrewsbury, S.B.; Fuller, C.; Davies, G.; Hoekman, J. Delivery of dihydroergotamine mesylate to the upper nasal space for the acute treatment of migraine: Technology in action. *J. Aerosol Med. Pulm. Drug Deliv.* **2022**, *35*, 321–332.
37. Maggio, E.T.; Pillion, D.J. High efficiency intranasal drug delivery using Intravail® alkylsaccharide absorption enhancers. *Drug Deliv. Transl. Res.* **2013**, *3*, 16–25.
38. Rabinowicz, A.L.; Carrazana, E.; Maggio, E.T. Improvement of intranasal drug delivery with Intravail® alkylsaccharide excipient as a mucosal absorption enhancer aiding in the treatment of conditions of the central nervous system. *Drugs RD* **2021**, *21*, 361–369.
39. World Health Organization. The forty-ninth meeting of the Joint FAO/WHO Expert Committee on Food Additives (JECFA). In *Sucrose Esters of Fatty Acids and Sucroglycerides (WHO Food Additives Series 40)*; World Health Organization: Geneva, Switzerland, 1998.
40. Maggio, E.T. Absorption enhancing excipients in systemic nasal drug delivery. *J. Excip. Food Chem.* **2014**, *5*, 100–112.
41. Arnold, J.J.; Fyrberg, M.D.; Meezan, E.; Pillion, D.J. Reestablishment of the nasal permeability barrier to several peptides following exposure to the absorption enhancer tetradecyl-beta-D-maltoside. *J. Pharm. Sci.* **2010**, *99*, 1912–1920. [PubMed]
42. Arnold, J.J.; Ahsan, F.; Meezan, E.; Pillion, D.J. Correlation of tetradecylmaltoside induced increases in nasal peptide drug delivery with morphological changes in nasal epithelial cells. *J. Pharm. Sci.* **2004**, *93*, 2205–2213. [PubMed]
43. Ahsan, F.; Arnold, J.; Meezan, E.; Pillion, D.J. Enhanced bioavailability of calcitonin formulated with alkylglycosides following nasal and ocular administration in rats. *Pharm. Res.* **2001**, *18*, 1742–1746.
44. Arnold, J.; Ahsan, F.; Meezan, E.; Pillion, D.J. Nasal administration of low molecular weight heparin. *J. Pharm. Sci.* **2002**, *91*, 1707–1714.
45. Mustafa, F.; Yang, T.; Khan, M.A.; Ahsan, F. Chain length-dependent effects of alkylmaltosides on nasal absorption of enoxaparin. *J. Pharm. Sci.* **2004**, *93*, 675–683.
46. Agarwal, S.K.; Kriel, R.L.; Brundage, R.C.; Ivaturi, V.D.; Cloyd, J.C. A pilot study assessing the bioavailability and pharmacokinetics of diazepam after intranasal and intravenous administration in healthy volunteers. *Epilepsy Res.* **2013**, *105*, 362–367.

47. Munjal, S.; Gautam, A.; Offman, E.; Brand-Schieber, E.; Allenby, K.; Fisher, D.M. A randomized trial comparing the pharmacokinetics, safety, and tolerability of DFN-02, an intranasal sumatriptan spray containing a permeation enhancer, with intranasal and subcutaneous sumatriptan in healthy adults. *Headache* **2016**, *56*, 1455–1465. [PubMed]
48. Lipton, R.B.; Munjal, S.; Brand-Schieber, E.; Rapoport, A.M. DFN-02 (sumatriptan 10 mg with a permeation enhancer) nasal spray vs placebo in the acute treatment of migraine: A double-blind, placebo-controlled study. *Headache* **2018**, *58*, 676–687. [PubMed]
49. Munjal, S.; Brand-Schieber, E.; Allenby, K.; Spierings, E.L.H.; Cady, R.K.; Rapoport, A.M. A multicenter, open-label, long-term safety and tolerability study of DFN-02, an intranasal spray of sumatriptan 10 mg plus permeation enhancer DDM, for the acute treatment of episodic migraine. *J. Headache Pain.* **2017**, *18*, 31.
50. Wheless, J.W.; Miller, I.; Hogan, R.E.; Dlugos, D.; Biton, V.; Cascino, G.D.; Sperling, M.R.; Liow, K.; Vazquez, B.; Segal, E.B.; et al. Final results from a phase 3, long-term, open-label, repeat-dose safety study of diazepam nasal spray for seizure clusters in patients with epilepsy. *Epilepsia* **2021**, *62*, 2485–2495. [PubMed]
51. Hogan, R.E.; Gidal, B.E.; Koplowitz, B.; Koplowitz, L.P.; Lowenthal, R.E.; Carrazana, E. Bioavailability and safety of diazepam intranasal solution compared to oral and rectal diazepam in healthy volunteers. *Epilepsia* **2020**, *61*, 455–464. [PubMed]
52. Hogan, R.E.; Tarquinio, D.; Sperling, M.R.; Klein, P.; Miller, I.; Segal, E.B.; Rabinowicz, A.L.; Carrazana, E. Pharmacokinetics and safety of VALTOCO (NRL-1; diazepam nasal spray) in patients with epilepsy during seizure (ictal/peri-ictal) and nonseizure (interictal) conditions: A phase 1, open-label study. *Epilepsia* **2020**, *61*, 935–943.
53. Klein, P.; Sperling, M.R.; Hogan, R.E.; Tarquinio, D.; Miller, I.; Segal, E.B.; Rabinowicz, A.L.; Carrazana, E. Pharmacokinetics of Intravail® A3 (n-dodecyl-beta-D-maltoside), a mucosal absorption enabler, after intranasal administration of NRL-1 in patients with epilepsy. *Neurology* **2020**, *94*, 1918.
54. Eggleston, W.; Calleo, V.; Kim, M.; Wojcik, S. Naloxone administration by untrained community members. *Pharmacotherapy* **2020**, *40*, 84–88.
55. Zhang, T.; Li, M.; Han, X.; Nie, G.; Zheng, A. Effect of different absorption enhancers on the nasal absorption of nalmefene hydrochloride. *AAPS PharmSciTech* **2022**, *23*, 143.
56. Krieter, P.; Gyaw, S.; Crystal, R.; Skolnick, P. Fighting fire with fire: Development of intranasal nalmefene to treat synthetic opioid overdose. *J. Pharmacol. Exp. Ther.* **2019**, *371*, 409–415. [CrossRef] [PubMed]
57. Tanimoto, S.; Kaliner, M.; Lockey, R.F.; Ebisawa, M.; Koplowitz, L.P.; Koplowitz, B.; Lowenthal, R. Pharmacokinetic and pharmacodynamic comparison of epinephrine, administered intranasally and intramuscularly: An integrated analysis. *Ann. Allergy Asthma Immunol.* **2023**, *130*, 508–514.e501. [CrossRef] [PubMed]
58. ARS Pharamceuticals, Inc. *neffyTM (Epinephrine Nasal Spray) for the Treatment of Type I Allergic Reactions, Including Anaphylaxis: FDA Advisory Board Briefing Document*; US Food and Drug Administration: Silver Spring, MD, USA, 2023.
59. Krieter, P.; Gyaw, S.; Chiang, C.N.; Crystal, R.; Skolnick, P. Enhanced intranasal absorption of naltrexone by dodecyl maltopyranoside: Implications for the treatment of opioid overdose. *J. Clin. Pharmacol.* **2019**, *59*, 947–957. [CrossRef] [PubMed]
60. Opiant Pharmaceuticals, Inc. Opiant Pharmaceuticals Announces Completion of Enrollment in Phase 2 Clinical Trial of OPNT002, Nasal Naltrexone, in Patients with Alcohol Use Disorder. Available online: https://www.globenewswire.com/en/news-release/2022/10/06/2529493/0/en/Opiant-Pharmaceuticals-Announces-Completion-of-Enrollment-in-Phase-2-Clinical-Trial-of-OPNT002-Nasal-Naltrexone-in-Patients-with-Alcohol-Use-Disorder.html (accessed on 5 June 2023).
61. EudraCT Number: 2019-002859-42. Available online: https://www.clinicaltrialsregister.eu/ctr-search/search?query=2019-002859-42 (accessed on 5 June 2023).
62. Neurelis, Inc. Neurelis Completes Pre-IND Meeting with FDA to Establish Clinical Development Program for NRL-4 in the Treatment of Acute Agitation Associated with Schizophrenia and Bipolar 1 Mania in Adults. Available online: https://www.neurelis.com/neurelis-news/neurelis-completes-pre-ind-meeting (accessed on 5 June 2023).
63. GSK group of companies. Imitrex Nasal Spray. Available online: https://www.drugs.com/pro/imitrex-nasal-spray.html (accessed on 26 January 2022).

pharmaceutics

MDPI

Article

Utility of a Novel Micro-Spraying Device for Intranasal Administration of Drug Solutions to Mice

Naoto Suzuki [1,*], Hiroaki Tanigawa [1], Taiki Nagatomo [1], Hiroko Miyagishi [2], Takanori Kanazawa [3], Toyofumi Suzuki [1] and Yasuhiro Kosuge [2,*]

1 Laboratory of Pharmaceutics, School of Pharmacy, Nihon University, 7-7-1 Narashinodai, Funabashi 274-8555, Chiba, Japan; phhi20001@g.nihon-u.ac.jp (H.T.); nagatomo.taiki@nihon-u.ac.jp (T.N.); suzuki.toyofumi@nihon-u.ac.jp (T.S.)
2 Laboratory of Pharmacology, School of Pharmacy, Nihon University, 7-7-1 Narashinodai, Funabashi 274-8555, Chiba, Japan; miyagishi.hiroko@nihon-u.ac.jp
3 Department of Clinical Pharmacology, Graduate School of Biomedical Sciences, Tokushima University, 1-78-1 Shoumachi, Tokushima 770-8505, Tokushima, Japan; kanazawa@tokushima-u.ac.jp
* Correspondence: suzuki.naoto65@nihon-u.ac.jp (N.S.); kosuge.yasuhiro@nihon-u.ac.jp (Y.K.); Tel.: +81-47-465-6699 (N.S.); +81-47-465-4027 (Y.K.)

Abstract: Intranasal administration has attracted attention as a means of delivering drugs because it bypasses the blood–brain barrier. However, conventional intranasal administration of drug solutions to mice using the micropipette method (MP method) is complicated and time-consuming because it requires small doses to be administered under inhalation anesthesia. This study evaluated the effectiveness of a novel intranasal administration method using Micro FPS™, a novel micro-spraying device (the MSD method). The MSD method allowed more reliable administration of the solution to the nasal mucosa than the MP method did. The transfer of inulin, a model water-soluble macromolecule compound, to the olfactory bulb and brain (cerebrum, cerebellum, brainstem, and striatum) was similar with the two methods. It also allowed the drug to be administered in a shorter time. These results suggest that the MSD method is simpler and more rapid than the MP method for intranasal administration of drugs to mice and achieves comparable delivery of inulin to the olfactory bulb and brain. Therefore, the Micro FPS™ device is a potentially useful tool for intranasal drug administration to rodents and could facilitate the development of intranasal formulations, contributing to drug development for central nervous system diseases.

Keywords: intranasal administration; micro-spraying device; nose-to-brain; mice; inulin

1. Introduction

1.1. Background

Intranasal administration of drugs through the nostrils to the nasal mucosa enables drug delivery to the systemic circulation via capillaries distributed locally in the nasal cavity and mucosa [1]. The nasal surface to which the drug adheres is covered with a thin mucosal layer with fewer proteolytic enzymes than the oral mucosa [2]. In addition, intranasal administration avoids hepatic first-pass effects. One of the most notable features of intranasal administration is the direct nose-to-brain (N2B) pathway, which enables efficient brain delivery of drugs with a significantly limited blood-to-brain transfer, bypassing the blood–brain barrier [3–6]. These features enable the delivery of novel modalities, such as peptides and nucleic acid drugs, to the central nervous system [7,8] and suppress systemic side effects of drugs that occur when administered via conventional administration methods [6,9]. Therefore, intranasal administration presents the potential for further development of formulations targeting the central nervous system, local nasal cavity, and systemic circulation.

In drug development, pharmacological evaluation of new drugs is generally conducted in rodent species such as mice and rats. However, standardized administration conditions (e.g., volume, time, and administration rate) for intranasal administration to rodents have not yet been established, and administration methods differ among researchers [10]. The lack of standardized administration methods is a cause for concern because differences in administration methods among researchers may have a considerable effect on drug retention in the nasal mucosa and drug delivery to the brain due to the complexity of the nasal cavity [11]. The most common method of intranasal administration to rodents is the micropipette (MP) method. In this method, 10–20 μL of drug solution is administered into the nasal cavity of mice, which has a volume of approximately 30 μL, under inhalation anesthesia with isoflurane [12] using a micropipette 10–20 times into alternating nostrils, and the drug is absorbed into the nasal mucosa without an excess amount of solution being excreted into the pharynx.

1.2. Rationale

Previously, we developed an openable inhalation mask that allows intranasal administration even under inhalation anesthesia. This method enabled the administration of drug solutions in the same position to rodents under inhalation anesthesia. Moreover, this minimized the leakage of drug solutions from the nasal cavity to the pharynx and variability due to the technique [10,13]. Fukuda et al. [14] evaluated the brain translocation of inulin, which is a model water-soluble macromolecule, using these MP-technology-based dosing methods. Kurano et al. [15,16] demonstrated the migration of liposomes with different surface charges intranasally administered via the MP method to the brain and spinal cord and the therapeutic effect of intranasal administration of N-acetyl-L-cysteine, an antioxidant loaded on a polymeric nanocarrier, in a mouse model of amyotrophic sclerosis. The MP method is widely used to evaluate the kinetics or therapeutic effects of intranasally administered formulations based on their physical properties. However, these MP methods are complicated because the maximum volume that can be administered per dose is minimal (1–2 μL) and is administered into the right and left nostrils at 1 min intervals, implying that 10–20 min are required to administer the entire solution. Moreover, as there is always a time lag between the start and end of administration, the amount of drug distributed on the nasal surface and its residence time may differ from those of actual intranasal administration, which may affect pharmacokinetics and drug effects. To resolve these issues, Ullah et al. [17] investigated intranasal administration under awake conditions. Intranasal administration under awake conditions can be performed in a shorter time because it eliminates the need for anesthesia and other time-consuming procedures [17,18]. However, the results depend on the specific equipment used and the technical proficiency of the operator. Therefore, this method cannot be universally applied. Additionally, mice require time to acclimatize before intranasal administration under awake conditions. Notably, the distribution of the administered drug is highly variable; therefore, awake administration is not a satisfactory method.

1.3. Objectives

Micro FPS™, a new micro-spraying device (MSD; Figure 1) for intranasal administration of drugs to mice [19], is capable of spraying drug solutions in the range of 1–5 μL in 1 μL increments. This is otherwise difficult to achieve with the fine particle sprayers used for transpulmonary administration to rodents. This new MSD is expected to reduce differences in intranasal administration techniques among experimenters and simplify intranasal administration. Therefore, to clarify the usefulness of Micro FPS™ as a new intranasal administration device, we compared the time required for intranasal administration, nature of the distribution of the drug solution in the nasal cavity of mice, and transfer of inulin, a model water-soluble macromolecule compound, into the olfactory bulb or brain (cerebrum, cerebellum, brainstem, and striatum) to those of the MP method.

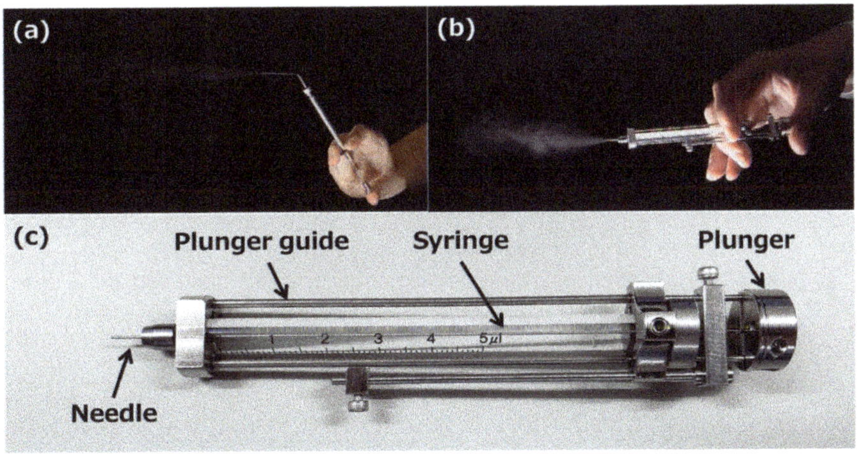

Figure 1. Spraying demonstration of (**a**) fine particle sprayer and (**b**) Micro FPS™. (**c**) Structure of Micro FPS™.

In this study, we investigated the intranasal distribution of drug solution in the nasal cavity of mice and brain migration of inulin, a model water-soluble middle molecule, administered intranasally using Micro FPS™ MSD to evaluate the usefulness of this MSD for intranasal delivery of drug solutions to mice.

2. Materials and Methods

2.1. Reagents and Materials

A solution of 0.4% trypan blue and radiolabeled inulin ([Carboxyl-14C]-inulin, molecular weight approximately 5000, 2 mCi/g; purity > 99%, Muromachi Kikai Co. Ltd., Tokyo, Japan) added to the drug solution was purchased from Thermo Fisher Scientific Corporation (Tokyo, Japan) and American Radiolabeled Chemicals (St Louis, MO, USA), respectively. The Micro FPS™ (MFPS-01-A1, MSD) microdose atomizer (Toray Precision, Inc., Shiga, Japan) was used for intranasal administration of the solution to mice. Table 1 lists the spray characteristics of Micro FPS™.

Table 1. Specifications (spray characteristics, needle size, and device weight) of the novel microspraying device Micro FPS™ [19].

Spray Characteristics	
Minimum spray volume	1 µL
Maximum spray volume	5 µL
Average spray angle	43.8°
Average atomizing particle size	12.97 µm
Needle size and device weight	
Sprayable viscosity at 20 °C	1.000 mPa·s
Needle outer diameter	0.52 mm
Needle length	7.0 mm
Device weight	45.5 g

2.2. Animals

All animal experiments were conducted under the guidelines approved by the Nihon University Animal Care and Use Committee (Tokyo, Japan, experiment number #AP22PHA013-1). Seven-week-old male mice (Deutschland, Denken, and Yoken strains) were obtained from Japan SLC, Inc. (Shizuoka, Japan). Mice were housed under a light–dark cycle of 25 ± 1 °C, 55 ± 10% humidity, and 12 h of illumination (8:00–20:00), with ad libitum access to feed and water. Male mice weighing 35–45 g were used in the subsequent studies.

2.3. Intranasal Distribution of Trypan Blue Solution

In the MSD method, the needle of the MSD was inserted into the right nostril of a mouse immobilized in the supine position under inhalation anesthesia with isoflurane using an openable inhalation mask (SN-487-70-09, Shinano Seisakusyo, Tokyo, Japan) [10] and 4 μL of 0.4% trypan blue, an azo dye similar to that used for nasal staining in the previous report [20], and the solution was sprayed into the nasal cavity of the mouse (Figure 2a). Mice were removed from the anesthesia mask during administration. In the MP method as a reference method, droplets of 0.4% trypan blue solution were formed at the tip of a micropipette and aspirated by spontaneous breathing of the anesthetized mice [10] (Figure 2b). After opening the silicon cap of the mask, 1 μL of 0.4% trypan blue solution was administered into the right nostril of the mouse at 1-min intervals from the opening of the inhalation mask to make a total volume of 4 μL. After the administration of each method, the head was cut in a sagittal plane, and the distribution of trypan blue adhering to the inside of the nasal cavity was captured. This image was analyzed using ImageJ software downloaded from the NIH website [21], and the adhesion rate of the trypan blue solution to the entire nasal cavity was calculated using Equation (1):

$$\text{Adhesion ratio of trypan blue solution in the mice nasal cavity } (\%) = \frac{\text{Trypan blue adhered area}}{\text{Nasal cavity area}} \quad (1)$$

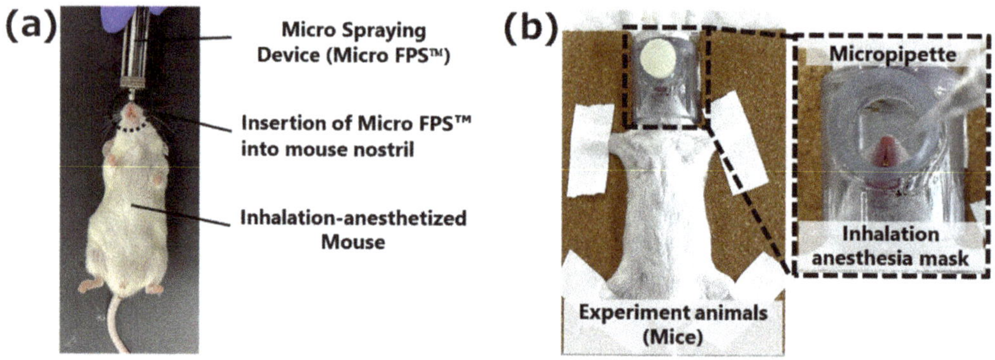

Figure 2. Comparison of intranasal administration methodologies and dosing schedule of each method. (**a**) Micro-spraying device (MSD) method: 1–5 μL administered into each nostril at a time using Micro FPS^{TM}. (**b**) Micropipette (MP) method: 1–2 μL administered into each nostril at 1-min intervals via micropipette.

2.4. Measurement of the Amount of [14C]-Inulin to the Brain and Olfactory Bulb after Intranasal Administration

A total of 10 μL of phosphate-buffered saline solution containing 5 μCi/mL (400 μM) of [14C]-inulin was administered intranasally to the mice using the MP or MSD method. In the MSD method, Micro FPS™ was filled with 5 μL of the drug solution and administered intranasally into the right and left nasal cavities once each. In the MP method, 1.25 μL of drug solution was administered eight times into the right and left nasal cavities at 1-min intervals, based on the methods used in previous studies [10,14]. Thirty minutes after each administration, isolated brain tissue was divided into two parts: the olfactory bulb and the rest of the brain, including the cerebrum, cerebellum, brainstem, and striatum. Each sample was dissolved in Solusol™ (National Diagnostics, GA, USA), a tissue solubilizer, at 55 °C for 2 h. Then, 10 mL of Hionic-flour™ (Waltham, MA, USA) known as the liquid scintillation cocktail was added to the samples. The drug solution equivalent to the dosage was dissolved in 3 mL of Pico-flour™ 40 (Waltham, MA, USA). To determine the [14C]-inulin radioactivity in the olfactory bulb and brain, a liquid scintillation counter was used (Tri-Carb 4810TR, PerkinElmer, Shelton, CT, USA). All experiments using isotopes were conducted in accordance with the Isotope Center Use Plan, which was reviewed and approved by the Isotope Center of Nihon University, School of Pharmacy (experiment #23-01, 02).

2.5. Statistical Analysis

JMP Version 14 (SAS Institute Inc., Cary, NC, USA) was used for statistical analysis. The significance of the difference among three groups (untreated or treated using the MP or MSD method) in the adhesion ratio of trypan blue solution in the nasal cavity of the mice was determined using analysis of variance with Tukey's test for multiple comparisons. p values < 0.05 were considered statistically significant. Additionally, the t-test for independent samples was used to evaluate the significance of the difference between the MP and MSD methods in the transfer of [14C]-inulin to the olfactory bulb and brain.

3. Results

3.1. Adhesion of 0.4% Trypan Blue Solution to the Nasal Cavity of Mice

In this experiment, the 0.4% trypan blue solution was administered intranasally to stain the nasal cavity, as reported by Kumar et al. [20], and the adhesion of the trypan blue solution to the nasal cavity was calculated. We confirmed that 0.4% trypan blue solution can be sprayed using Micro FPS™. Unlike that in the mice with no administered trypan blue solution (Figure 3a), the administered trypan blue was distributed between the nostrils and nasal cavity and in the anterior part of the nasal cavity using the MP method (Figure 3b). In contrast, the MSD method showed no distribution of trypan blue between the nostrils and nasal cavity, and most of the sprayed trypan blue solution reached deep within the nasal cavity, physically close to the brain tissue (Figure 3c). Compared with that using the MP method, the adhesion rate of trypan blue in the nasal cavity using the MSD method increased significantly by approximately 1.5 times (Figure 3d).

3.2. Transfer of Inulin from the Nasal Cavity to the Brain of Mice

Subsequently, we compared the brain transfer of inulin. This water-soluble macromolecule model compound has previously been shown to be transferred to the brain via the N2B route using the MP method of intranasal administration [14]. Micro FPS™ is also capable of spraying an inulin-containing drug solution. The results showed no significant difference between the MP and MSD methods in the amount of inulin transferred to the olfactory bulb and brain 30 min after intranasal administration, indicating that the method of administration did not affect the transfer of inulin to the brain (Figure 4).

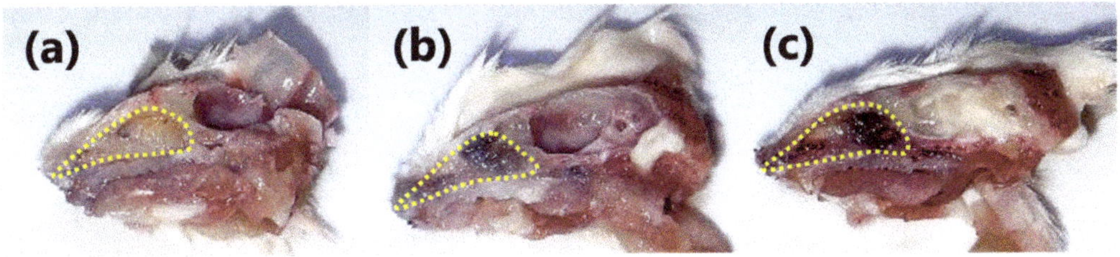

Figure 3. *Cont.*

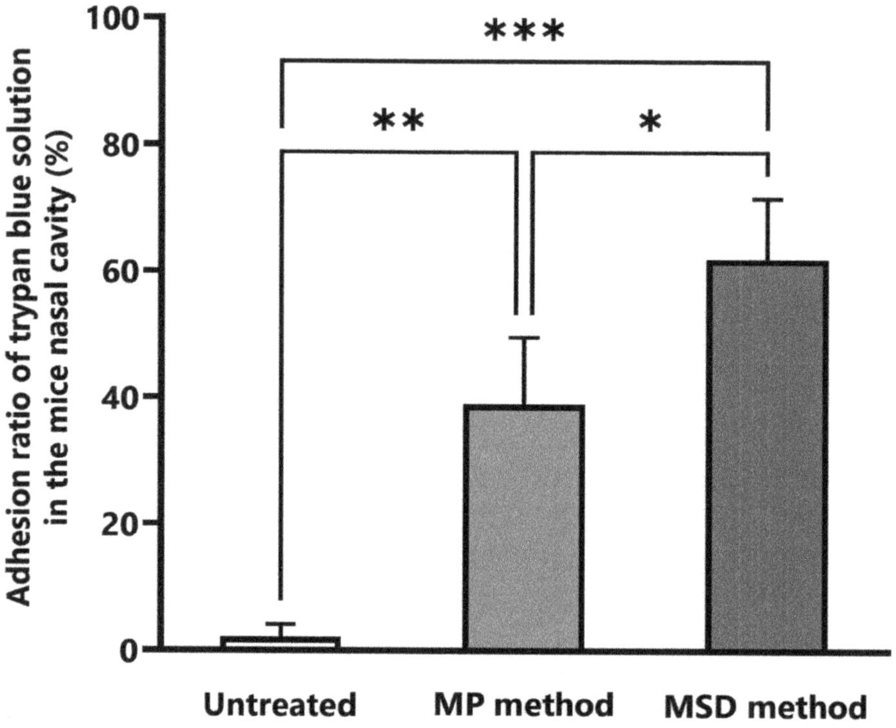

(d)

Figure 3. Distribution of the dosing solution in the nasal cavity of mice according to the intranasal administration methods. (**a**) Untreated; (**b**) MP method; (**c**) MSD method. (**d**) Adhesion ratio according to the intranasal administration methods. The distribution of trypan blue in the nasal cavity was confirmed from a sagittal section of the head of mice administered 0.4% trypan blue intranasally. In (**a**–**c**), the yellow dotted line indicates the nasal cavity of mice. The significance of the differences in the mean values of the three groups was estimated using analysis of variance with Tukey's test. * $p < 0.05$, ** $p < 0.01$, *** $p < 0.001$. Each bar represents mean ± standard error of three treated mice. MP, micropipette; MSD, micro-spraying device.

Compared with that of the MP method, the MSD method significantly reduced the time required for administration (Table 2). In this experiment, the time required for intranasal administration of 10 μL of drug solution was approximately 60 s for the MSD method and approximately 190 s for the MP method.

Table 2. Time for intranasal administration of drug solution by each method. S.E.M., standard error of the mean.

Time for Administration (s)	*n*								Mean	S.E.M.
	1	2	3	4	5	6	7	8		
MSD method	57	55	51	57	63	57	...	...	56.67	3.54
MP method	197	191	194	191	190	192	193	194	192.75	2.11

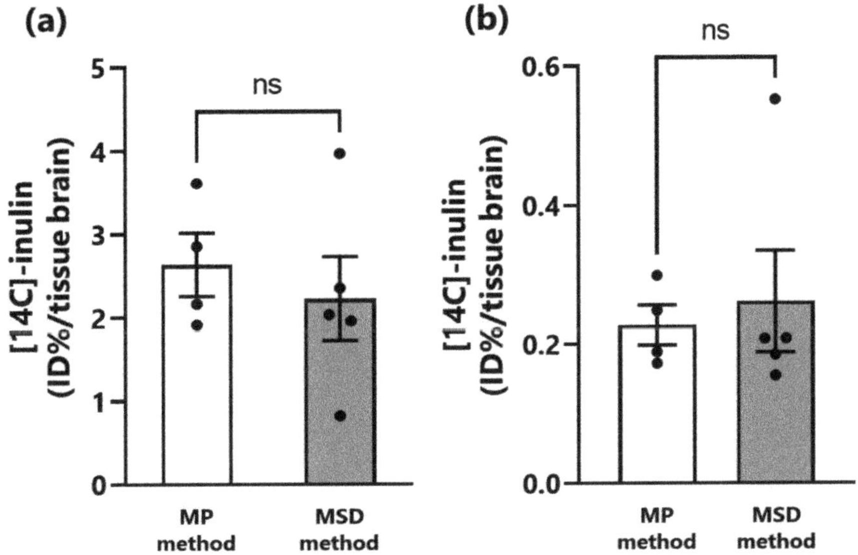

Figure 4. Comparison of the transfer of inulin to the olfactory bulb and brain of mice using the MP and MSD methods of intranasal administration. (**a**) The olfactory bulb; (**b**) the brain. The ratio of [14C]-inulin distributed to the olfactory bulb and brain relative to the total amount of [14C]-inulin administered by each method was divided by the tissue weight and expressed as %ID/g. Each bar represents the mean ± standard error of four mice treated using the micropipette (MP) method or five mice treated using the micro-spraying device (MSD) method. ns; not significant ($p > 0.05$).

4. Discussion

Recently, intranasal administration has been attracting attention as an administration method that can deliver drugs directly to the central nervous system [22]. Notably, the blood–brain barrier, comprising brain capillary endothelial cells, pericytes, and astrocytes [23–25], restricts the delivery of drugs to the brain using conventional methods. The therapeutic effects of these drugs administered intranasally to rodents using the micropipette (MP) method and their translocation into the brain and blood have been reported [11,14,26–28]. The MP method is more widely used than other intranasal administration methods because it is simple and relatively easy. However, the time required for administration through the MP method and differences in the proficiency of the administration technique among the experimenters are barriers to research. Our research group has reported the development of masks for inhalation anesthesia and a reverse canulation method to shorten the administration time and minimize the influence of inter-experimenter skills [10]. However, these investigations only solve some of the problems associated with intranasal administration. In this study, we focused on Micro FPS™, a new micro-atomizer developed by Toray Precision Inc. We examined its applicability for intranasal administration of drugs to mice, which are commonly used as experimental animals.

First, we observed the intranasal distribution of the drug solution administered using each intranasal administration method. Similar to Evans blue, trypan blue, which is also an azo dye, could clearly stain the nasal cavity. The MSD method showed no distribution of trypan blue between the nostrils and nasal cavity, and most of the drug solution reached deep within the nasal cavity adjacent to the brain tissue. This is because the length of the Micro FPS™ needle is approximately 7 mm, which corresponds to the length between the nostrils and nasal cavity of a mouse, allowing the needle tip to be inserted into the nasal cavity and spray the drug solution. In contrast, with the MP method, the trypan blue was administered intranasally as the mice spontaneously breathed, and trypan blue remained in the nostril and the anterior part of the nasal cavity. Therefore, the adhesion rate of trypan blue solution in the nasal cavity of mice was significantly higher using the MSD method than using the MP method. The MSD method was able to administer drugs intensively deep into the nasal cavity, to the area where the olfactory nerve endings are distributed. The olfactory nerve pathway via the olfactory nerve from the olfactory region located in the deepest part of the nasal cavity and the trigeminal pathway via the trigeminal nerve distributed in the submucosa of the nasal cavity are important pathways in N2B drug transfer [11,29,30]. Additionally, differences in the volume of the rodent's nasal cavity may affect drug delivery to the olfactory bulb [31]. The MSD method using Micro FPS™, which allows intensive spray of drug solution into the olfactory region, facilitates N2B transfer, without the distribution of drug solution between the nostril and nasal cavity, suggesting that drug solution can be efficiently administered to the olfactory area regardless of the nasal cavity volume. Flamm et al. [32] developed a catheter-based application that can deliver drugs precisely to the olfactory region. This device is beneficial from a pharmacokinetic or formulation perspective because it allows direct administration of drug solutions with various physical properties. However, drugs are administered to the nasal cavity as droplets using atomizers in most practical applications. It has been reported that the size of the sprayed droplet affects drug deposition in the nasal cavity [33,34]. Therefore, intranasal administration using Micro FPS™, which can atomize the drug solution as fine droplets, is a beneficial method for designing intranasal formulations. Additionally, when the drug is sprayed as droplets using Micro FPS™, fine particles may reach respiratory organs such as the airways, lungs and gastrointestinal tract when the mice inhale. Since A sprays droplets measuring several tens of micrometers, the risk of reaching the pharyngeal side or respiratory tract is considered low. However, along with the nasal cavity, the respiratory and gastrointestinal tracts also need to be evaluated in further studies for the possibility of secondary side effects owing to inhalation or swallowing of the drug.

The brain transfer of inulin to the olfactory bulb and brain after intranasal administration was compared between the two methods. Our group has previously reported that intranasal administration of 25 μL of inulin solution using the MP or reverse canulation method resulted in the transfer of 1.5–3.5% ID/g tissue to the olfactory bulb and 0.1–2.7% ID/g tissue to the brain and that the rate of inulin transfer to each tissue increased with decreasing volume of administration using the reverse canulation method [14]. In the current study, the degree of inulin brain transfer using the MP method was similar to that reported previously. The level of inulin transfer to the olfactory bulb and brain was similar using the MP and MSD methods. These results indicate that the MSD method is as effective as the MP method for the delivery of drug solution into the nasal cavity of mice. Despite differences in the nasal distribution of the drug solution due to the administration method, the brain transfer of inulin did not differ regardless of the method used. Intranasal administration is a useful method of administration to improve brain delivery of water-soluble low-molecular-weight drugs with low mucosal permeability [35]. However, the nasal mucosal permeability of drugs generally tends to decrease with increasing molecular weight [36–38]. In addition, we confirmed that the amount of intranasally administered inulin transferred to the olfactory bulb and brain was constant regardless of the dose of inulin. The inulin used in this study as a model drug is water-soluble and has a molecular weight of 5000 Da, because of which the efficiency of intranasal delivery to the brain was limited, and the difference in the distribution of the administered solution in the nasal cavity due to the intranasal administration method did not affect the transfer of inulin to the olfactory bulb or brain. Therefore, despite the differences in the distribution of the drug in the nasal cavity, no difference in the amount of inulin transferred from the nose to the olfactory bulb or brain was observed. Further research is required to examine the effects of the method of intranasal administration and nasal distribution of the drug solution on the transfer of low-molecular-weight or lipophilic compounds with a high contribution to brain delivery via the N2B route to the blood and various tissues, especially into various regions of the central brain [39,40]. Micro FPS™ has not yet been evaluated in rats. Rats have a larger nasal cavity volume than that of mice. Micro FPS™ can also be used in rats for intranasal administration of candidate compounds for new drugs. However, the needle length of Micro FPS™ may need to be changed because the length from the nostrils to the nasal cavity is longer in rats than in mice.

In addition, we compared the time required for intranasal administration of 10 μL of drug solution to mice. The MSD method reduced the time required for intranasal administration by 2 min, from 3 min to 1 min, compared with that of the MP method, in which 1.25 μL of the drug was administered into the right and left nasal cavities alternately, followed by a 1-min interval between administrations. This is because the maximum volume of Micro FPS™ is 5 μL per spray and only one spray in each nostril was needed to administer the total drug dose. Therefore, intranasal administration to rats, which have a larger nasal cavity volume than that of mice, using the MSD method is likely to shorten the administration time further. Micro FPS™ also allowed for one-handed syringe filling and spraying from the device. Ullah et al. [17] reported a novel method in which mice are immobilized in a particular device that maintains them in a condition suitable for brain delivery [41] of siRNA by intranasal administration. This administration method is efficient, allowing the substance to be administered intranasally to 4–8 mice at the same time. However, it requires a special device to immobilize the mice and a micropipette for intranasal administration; therefore, it requires approximately the same amount of time as the MP method. In contrast, Micro FPS™ allows 1–5 μL of drug solution to be sprayed intranasally at a time, thus reducing the administration time (Table 2). These advantages of increased speed and reduced costs are extremely important in terms of practical application. While the nasal retention property is essential for brain-targeted formulations by adding high-molecular-weight thickener or gelling agents, spraying viscous solutions with MSD has been difficult, so further improvement of the device is expected in the future. The development of an MSD that can spray a viscous solution is expected to accelerate the design of intranasal formulations for N2B administration. This could contribute to the development of drugs to treat central nervous system diseases in humans.

5. Conclusions

In this study, we investigated the usefulness of an intranasal administration method using Micro FPS™, a novel micro-atomizer, as an alternative to the MP method for intranasal administration of drug solutions to rodents, in this case using mice. Intranasal administration of drug solutions was more rapid and simpler using the MSD method than that using the MP method. Using the MSD method, all of the administered drug solution could be sprayed into the nasal cavity, and most of it was deposited in the olfactory area, which is involved in N2B transfer. Furthermore, there was no difference in the amount of inulin transferred to the brain after intranasal administration by each method, suggesting that Micro FPS™ can be used for intranasal administration of drug solutions to rodents in the same way as the conventional MP method. In conclusion, intranasal administration of drugs to mice using Micro FPS™ is a useful method to investigate drug delivery to the central nervous system via the N2B pathway. Further studies using water-soluble middle-molecule model compounds and drugs with various characteristics are expected to provide a useful tool for developing nasal formulations based on tests using rodents.

Author Contributions: Conceptualization, N.S. and Y.K.; methodology, N.S. and Y.K.; validation, N.S., H.T. and T.N.; formal analysis, N.S., H.T. and T.N.; investigation, N.S., H.T. and T.N.; resources, N.S., H.M. and Y.K.; data curation, N.S., H.T. and T.N.; writing—original draft preparation, N.S.; writing—review and editing, H.T., T.N., H.M., T.K., T.S. and Y.K.; visualization, N.S., H.T. and T.N.; supervision, N.S., T.S. and Y.K.; project administration, N.S. and Y.K.; funding acquisition, N.S., T.K., T.S. and Y.K. All authors have read and agreed to the published version of the manuscript.

Funding: This research was supported in part by a Nihon University Multidisciplinary Research Grant for 2019–2020 (to N.S. and T.S.) and 2022–2023 (to Y.K. and H.M.), by JSPS KAKENHI, a

Grant-in-Aid for Early-Career Scientists, Grant Number 20K16059 and 23K14395 (to N.S.), and by OTC Self-Medication Promotion Foundation (to N.S. and Y.K.).

Institutional Review Board Statement: The animal study protocol was approved by the Nihon University Animal Care and Use Committee (Tokyo, Japan, experiment number #AP22PHA013-1).

Informed Consent Statement: Not applicable.

Data Availability Statement: Not applicable.

Acknowledgments: We thank Toray Precision Co., Ltd., for lending us the Micro FPS™ device (MFPS-01-A1) used in this study.

Conflicts of Interest: Yasuhiro Kosuge and Naoto Suzuki received Micro FPS™ from Toray Precision, Inc.

Abbreviations

MP	micropipette
MSD	micro-spraying device
N2B	nose-to-brain

References

1. Bitter, C.; Suter-Zimmermann, K.; Surber, C. Nasal drug delivery in humans. *Curr. Probl. Dermatol.* **2011**, *40*, 20–35. [CrossRef] [PubMed]
2. Joukhadar, C.; Schenk, B.; Kaehler, S.T.; Kollenz, C.J.; Bauer, P.; Muller, M.; Eichler, H.G. A replicate study design for testing bioequivalence: A case study on two desmopressin nasal spray preparations. *Eur. J. Clin. Pharmacol.* **2003**, *59*, 631–636. [CrossRef] [PubMed]
3. Illum, L. Transport of drugs from the nasal cavity to the central nervous system. *Eur. J. Pharm. Sci.* **2000**, *11*, 1–18. [CrossRef] [PubMed]
4. Hanson, L.R.; Frey, W.H., 2nd. Intranasal delivery bypasses the blood-brain barrier to target therapeutic agents to the central nervous system and treat neurodegenerative disease. *BMC Neurosci.* **2008**, *9* (Suppl. S3), S5. [CrossRef]
5. Chapman, C.D.; Frey, W.H., 2nd; Craft, S.; Danielyan, L.; Hallschmid, M.; Schioth, H.B.; Benedict, C. Intranasal treatment of central nervous system dysfunction in humans. *Pharm. Res.* **2013**, *30*, 2475–2484. [CrossRef]
6. Dhuria, S.V.; Hanson, L.R.; Frey, W.H., 2nd. Intranasal delivery to the central nervous system: Mechanisms and experimental considerations. *J. Pharm. Sci.* **2010**, *99*, 1654–1673. [CrossRef]
7. Kanazawa, T.; Akiyama, F.; Kakizaki, S.; Takashima, Y.; Seta, Y. Delivery of siRNA to the brain using a combination of nose-to-brain delivery and cell-penetrating peptide-modified nano-micelles. *Biomaterials* **2013**, *34*, 9220–9226. [CrossRef]
8. Suico, J.G.; Hövelmann, U.; Zhang, S.; Shen, T.; Bergman, B.; Sherr, J.; Zijlstra, E.; Frier, B.M.; Plum-Mörschel, L. Glucagon administration by nasal and intramuscular routes in adults with type 1 diabetes during insulin-induced hypoglycaemia: A randomised, open-label, crossover study. *Diabetes Ther.* **2020**, *11*, 1591–1603. [CrossRef] [PubMed]
9. Lee, D.; Minko, T. Nanotherapeutics for nose-to-brain drug delivery: An approach to bypass the blood brain barrier. *Pharmaceutics* **2021**, *13*, 2049. [CrossRef]
10. Kanazawa, T.; Fukuda, M.; Suzuki, N.; Suzuki, T. Novel methods for intranasal administration under inhalation anesthesia to evaluate nose-to-brain drug delivery. *J. Vis. Exp.* **2018**, *14*, 141. [CrossRef]
11. Thorne, R.G.; Pronk, G.J.; Padmanabhan, V.; Frey, W.H., 2nd. Delivery of insulin-like growth factor-I to the rat brain and spinal cord along olfactory and trigeminal pathways following intranasal administration. *Neuroscience* **2004**, *127*, 481–496. [CrossRef] [PubMed]
12. Ruigrok, M.J.; de Lange, E.C. Emerging insights for translational pharmacokinetic and pharmacokinetic-pharmacodynamic studies: Towards prediction of nose-to-brain transport in humans. *AAPS J.* **2015**, *17*, 493–505. [CrossRef]
13. Suzuki, N.; Kanazawa, T.; Suzuki, T. Intranasal administration. *Drug Deliv. Syst.* **2020**, *35*, 76–80. [CrossRef]
14. Fukuda, M.; Kanazawa, T.; Iioka, S.; Oguma, T.; Iwasa, R.; Masuoka, S.; Suzuki, N.; Kosuge, Y.; Suzuki, T. Quantitative analysis of inulin distribution in the brain focused on nose-to-brain route via olfactory epithelium by reverse esophageal cannulation. *J. Control. Release* **2021**, *332*, 493–501. [CrossRef]
15. Kurano, T.; Kanazawa, T.; Ooba, A.; Masuyama, Y.; Maruhana, N.; Yamada, M.; Iioka, S.; Ibaraki, H.; Kosuge, Y.; Kondo, H.; et al. Nose-to-brain/spinal cord delivery kinetics of liposomes with different surface properties. *J. Control. Release* **2022**, *344*, 225–234. [CrossRef]
16. Kurano, T.; Kanazawa, T.; Iioka, S.; Kondo, H.; Kosuge, Y.; Suzuki, T. Intranasal administration of N-acetyl-L-cysteine combined with cell-penetrating peptide-modified polymer nanomicelles as a potential therapeutic approach for amyotrophic lateral sclerosis. *Pharmaceutics* **2022**, *14*, 2590. [CrossRef]
17. Ullah, I.; Chung, K.; Beloor, J.; Lee, S.K.; Kumar, P. A Positioning Device for the placement of mice during intranasal siRNA delivery to the central nervous system. *J. Vis. Exp.* **2019**, *150*, e59201. [CrossRef]

18. Hanson, L.R.; Fine, J.M.; Svitak, A.L.; Faltesek, K.A. Intranasal administration of CNS therapeutics to awake mice. *J. Vis. Exp.* **2013**, *74*, 4440. [CrossRef]
19. Toray Precision, Inc. Homepage. Available online: https://www.tpc.toray/product/nozzle/noz_011.html#link_plan (accessed on 12 July 2023).
20. Kumar, N.N.; Gautam, M.; Lochhead, J.J.; Wolak, D.J.; Ithapu, V.; Singh, V.; Thorne, R.G. Relative vascular permeability and vascularity across different regions of the rat nasal mucosa: Implications for nasal physiology and drug delivery. *Sci. Rep.* **2016**, *6*, 31732. [CrossRef]
21. Rasband, W.S. *ImageJ*; U.S. National Institutes of Health: Bethesda, MD, USA, 1997. Available online: https://imagej.nih.gov/ij/ (accessed on 1 April 2023).
22. Lochhead, J.J.; Thorne, R.G. Intranasal delivery of biologics to the central nervous system. *Adv. Drug. Deliv. Rev.* **2012**, *64*, 614–628. [CrossRef]
23. Lalatsa, A.; Schatzlein, A.G.; Uchegbu, I.F. Strategies to deliver peptide drugs to the brain. *Mol. Pharm.* **2014**, *11*, 1081–1093. [CrossRef]
24. Shinde, S.C.; Mahale, N.B.; Chaudhari, S.R.; Thorat, R.S. Recent advances in brain targeted drug delivery system: A review. *World J. Pharm. Res.* **2015**, *4*, 542–549.
25. Singh, A.K.; Mishra, S.K.; Mishra, G.; Maurya, A.; Awasthi, R.; Yadav, M.K.; Atri, N.; Pandey, P.K.; Singh, S.K. Inorganic clay nanocomposite system for improved cholinesterase inhibition and brain pharmacokinetics of donepezil. *Drug Dev. Ind. Pharm.* **2020**, *46*, 8–19. [CrossRef]
26. Kamei, N.; Takeda-Morishita, M. Brain delivery of insulin boosted by intranasal coadministration with cell-penetrating peptides. *J. Control. Release* **2015**, *197*, 105–110. [CrossRef] [PubMed]
27. Kamei, N.; Shingaki, T.; Kanayama, Y.; Tanaka, M.; Zochi, R.; Hasegawa, K.; Watanabe, Y.; Takeda-Morishita, M. Visualization and quantitative assessment of the brain distribution of insulin through nose-to-brain delivery based on the cell-penetrating peptide noncovalent strategy. *Mol. Pharm.* **2016**, *13*, 1004–1011. [CrossRef] [PubMed]
28. Tanigawa, H.; Suzuki, N.; Suzuki, T. Application of ionic liquid to enhance the nose-to-brain delivery of etodolac. *Eur. J. Pharm. Sci.* **2022**, *178*, 106290. [CrossRef]
29. Thorne, R.G.; Hanson, L.R.; Ross, T.M.; Tung, D.; Frey, W.H., II. Delivery of interferon-beta to the monkey nervous system following intranasal administration. *Neuroscience* **2008**, *152*, 785–797. [CrossRef]
30. Lu, C.T.; Zhao, Y.Z.; Wong, H.L.; Cai, J.; Peng, L.; Tian, X.Q. Current approaches to enhance CNS delivery of drugs across the brain barriers. *Int. J. Nanomed.* **2014**, *9*, 2241–2257. [CrossRef]
31. Krishnan, J.K.S.; Arun, P.; Chembukave, B.; Appu, A.P.; Vijayakumar, N.; Moffett, J.R.; Puthillathu, N.; Namboodiri, A.M.A. Effect of administration method, animal weight and age on the intranasal delivery of drugs to the brain. *J. Neurosci. Methods* **2017**, *286*, 16–21. [CrossRef]
32. Flamm, J.; Hartung, S.; Gänger, S.; Maigler, F.; Pitzer, C.; Schindowski, K. Establishment of an olfactory region-specific intranasal delivery technique in mice to target the central nervous system. *Front. Pharmacol.* **2022**, *12*, 789780. [CrossRef]
33. Le Guellec, S.; Ehrmann, S.; Vecellio, L. In-vitro-in vivo correlation of intranasal drug deposition. *Adv. Drug Deliv. Rev.* **2021**, *170*, 340–352. [CrossRef]
34. Baldelli, A.; Boraey, M.A.; Oguzlu, H.; Cidem, A.; Rodriguez, A.P.; Ong, H.X.; Jiang, F.; Bacca, M.; Thamboo, A.; Traini, D.; et al. Engineered nasal dry powder for the encapsulation of bioactive compounds. *Drug Discov. Today* **2022**, *27*, 2300–2308. [CrossRef]
35. Iwasaki, S.; Yamamoto, S.; Sano, N.; Tohyama, K.; Kosugi, Y.; Furuta, A.; Hamada, T.; Igari, T.; Fujioka, Y.; Hirabayashi, H.; et al. Direct drug delivery of low-permeable compounds to the central nervous system via intranasal administration in rats and monkeys. *Pharm. Res.* **2019**, *36*, 76. [CrossRef]
36. McMartin, C.; Hutchinson, L.E.; Hyde, R.; Peters, G.E. Analysis of structural requirements for the absorption of drugs and macromolecules from the nasal cavity. *J. Pharm. Sci.* **1987**, *76*, 535–540. [CrossRef] [PubMed]
37. Parvathi, M. Intranasal drug delivery to brain: An overview. *Int. J. Res. Pharm. Chem.* **2012**, *2*, 889–895.
38. Kushwaha, S.K.; Keshari, R.K.; Rai, A.K. Advances in nasal trans-mucosal drug delivery. *J. Appl. Pharmaceut. Sci.* **2011**, *1*, 21–28.
39. Mathison, S.; Nagilla, R.; Kompella, U.B. Nasal route for direct delivery of solutes to the central nervous systems: Fact or fiction? *J. Drug Target.* **1998**, *5*, 415–441. [CrossRef] [PubMed]
40. Laddha, U.D.; Tagalpallewar, A.A. Physicochemical, biopharmaceutical, and practical considerations for efficient nose-to-brain drug delivery. In *Direct Nose-To-Brain Drug Delivery. Mechanism, Technological Advances, Applications, and Regulatory Updates*; Pardeshi, C.V., Souto, E.B., Eds.; Academic Press: Cambridge, MA, USA, 2021; pp. 39–54.
41. Merkus, P.; Ebbens, F.A.; Muller, B.; Fokkens, W.J. Influence of anatomy and head position on intranasal drug deposition. *Eur. Arch. Otorhinolaryngol.* **2006**, *263*, 827–832. [CrossRef]

pharmaceutics

Article

Improved Olfactory Deposition of Theophylline Using a Nanotech Soft Mist Nozzle Chip

Madeline X. Zhang [1,*], Frank Verhoeven [2], Pieter Ravensbergen [2], Stefan Kooij [1], Rick Geoffrion [3], Daniel Bonn [1] and Cees J. M. van Rijn [1]

[1] Van der Waals-Zeeman Institute, Institute of Physics, University of Amsterdam, 1098 XH Amsterdam, The Netherlands; s.a.kooij@uva.nl (S.K.); d.bonn@uva.nl (D.B.); c.j.m.vanrijn@uva.nl (C.J.M.v.R.)

[2] Medspray B.V., 7521 PV Enschede, The Netherlands; frank@medspray.com (F.V.); pieter@medspray.com (P.R.)

[3] Cyrano Therapeutics Inc., Delray Beach, FL 33445, USA; rick@cyranotherapeutics.com

* Correspondence: x.zhang4@uva.nl

Abstract: Currently, nasal administration of active pharmaceutical ingredients is most commonly performed using swirl-nozzle-based pump devices or pressurized syringes. However, they lead to limited deposition in the more active regions of the nasal cavity, especially the olfactory region, which is crucial for nose-to-brain drug delivery. This research proposes to improve deposition in the olfactory region by replacing the swirl nozzle with a nanoengineered nozzle chip containing micrometer-sized holes, which generates smaller droplets of 10–50 μm travelling at a lower plume velocity. Two nanotech nozzle chips with different hole sizes were tested at different inhalation flow rates to examine the deposition patterns of theophylline, a hyposmia treatment formulation, using a nasal cavity model. A user study was also conducted and showed that the patient instructions influenced the inhalation flow rate characteristics. Targeted flow rates of between 0 and 25 L/min were used for the in vitro deposition study, yielding 21.5–31.5% olfactory coverage. In contrast, the traditional swirl nozzle provided only 10.8% coverage at a similar flow rate. This work highlights the potential of the nanotech soft mist nozzle for improved intranasal drug delivery, particularly to the olfactory region.

Keywords: aerosol; nebulizer; olfactory region; intranasal delivery; soft mist; nanotechnology

1. Introduction

The nasal tract is considered an efficient pathway for the uptake of biopharmaceuticals and small molecules, as the nasal cavity is highly vascularized and has a large surface area. In the nasal mucosae, a variety of antigen-presenting cells are present, such as macrophages and dendritic cells, which continuously scan their environment for uninvited antigens [1,2]. Over the years, various nasal drug delivery devices, such as vibrating mesh nebulizers [3], propellant pressurized sprays, aqueous spray pumps, and dry powders have been used. However, aqueous spray pumps are now dominant [4,5]. This is surprising as experimental studies have shown that many spray pump devices deposit a significant amount of the drug in the nasal valve and vestibule, which are considered less active regions of the nasal cavity [6–8]. This deposition in the nasal valve and vestibule is likely due to inertial impaction since most spray pumps are designed to release a large proportion of aerosol particles substantially larger than 50 μm, which exit the devices at a high speed [9]. Several studies have suggested that nasal nebulization with much smaller droplets (<50 μm) is a more effective method of delivering topical medication beyond the nasal valve region than aqueous spray pumps [4,5,7,10]. This enhanced penetration is attributed to the fact that nebulizers are designed to generate small, slow-moving particles that traverse the nasal cavity at a resting breathing rate, thereby minimizing the inertial impact on the nasal valve and vestibule [5,7]. In addition to the delivery device, a combination of other factors can also contribute to the efficacy of the intranasal formulations. These include the drug formulation characteristics, the site of deposition, and the patient instructions for using the delivery device [11].

The olfactory region, located in the upper part of the nasal cavity, is responsible for the sense of smell, which became especially clear to patients with infection-related hyposmia during the SARS-CoV-2 pandemic. Theophylline, a natural alkaloid derivative of xanthine isolated from Camellia sinensis and Coffee arabica plants, has been shown to improve lost taste and smell when administered intranasally [12]. Theophylline appears to inhibit phosphodiesterase (PDE) and prostaglandin production, regulate calcium flux and intracellular calcium distribution, and antagonize adenosine. By inhibiting PDE, theophylline may inhibit the conversion of cAMP to AMP, increasing its concentration in the mucosal microenvironment, and thereby augmenting olfactory transduction stimulation [13]. Over time, the receptor/sensory neurons may repopulate and become stimulated, allowing the brain to process odorants. Furthermore, the olfactory region is also known to provide a pathway to deliver formulations directly to the brain through the blood–brain barrier [14], making it a unique and important region for intranasal delivery. However, normally, with current atomization techniques, only <5–10% of the formulation that is administered intranasally deposits on the olfactory mucosa [15], posing a significant challenge in achieving sufficient drug efficacy.

In this research, we performed an in vitro deposition study to investigate the extent of theophylline deposition in the olfactory region using a novel nanotech nozzle chip in combination with a simple spray pump. The nanotech nozzle chip consists of a silicon chip with micrometer-sized pores, which emits a slow-moving spray cloud upon spraying with smaller droplets and a narrower droplet size distribution than the conventional swirl nozzle [9]. It is made with semi-conductor technology, which provides several advantages for production in addition to the potential improvements in the nasal deposition investigated in this work. First, well-defined pore sizes can be maintained during the manufacturing of the nozzle chip. Compared to the effect of user instruction and user nasal dimensional variations on the deposition and efficacy, the small difference in pore size due to potential production inaccuracies is expected to have a negligible effect. Moreover, the production of the nanotech nozzle chip is scalable, as semi-conductor technology enables lower costs at larger production volumes, making the technology affordable for both pharmaceutical and OTC applications.

In addition to the deposition study, a user study was performed to measure the effect of user instructions by examining the inhalation pattern of volunteers when given different inhalation instructions. These inhalation patterns were used as inputs for the deposition study.

2. Materials and Methods

2.1. User Study

Inhalation pattern measurements were performed to identify the flow rate and the duration of inhalation. The volunteers were instructed to inhale from a nasal inhalation device consisting of a disposable nasal adaptor and a flowmeter (Sensirion SFM3019, Stäfa, Switzerland) under several different inhalation instructions. The small opening of the device was placed inside one nostril to simulate inhalation from a nasal spray pump, while the second nostril was blocked.

A total of 32 volunteers were sampled, mainly staff and students from the University of Amsterdam. The volunteers were between 21 and 67 years old, with a mean age of 35 years, and 37.5% were female (12 out of the 32). Five versions of user instructions were defined and are listed in Table 1. The instructions were given in the order described, and inhalation measurements were taken after reading each instruction to the volunteer. Volunteers were not specifically instructed to exhale before inhalation. The flow rate time series were recorded at a sampling rate of 100 Hz.

Table 1. The instructions used in the user study.

#	Instruction
1	"Inhale gently through the nose, do not sniff."
2	"Inhale normally through the nose."
3	"Inhale slowly through the nose."
4	"Inhale with the idea that you would like to smell something that is difficult to smell."
5	"Inhale firmly through the nose."

2.2. In Vitro Deposition Study

Deposition experiments were performed to determine the deposition characteristics of the nanotech nebulization chip under different conditions. The experimental procedures of the deposition study were adapted from D'Angelo et al. [9]. A transparent silicone nasal cavity model (Model LM-005 Koken Ltd., Tokyo, Japan) was used to simulate the nasal cavity. Figure 1 shows the nasal cast and corresponding intranasal regions used for analysis. During spraying, only half of the model, containing one nostril/nasal cavity with the septum attached, was used.

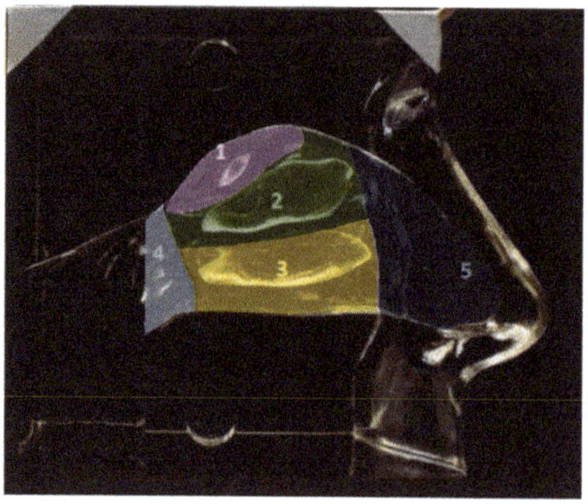

Figure 1. The image analysis mask with the intranasal regions of interest projected onto the nasal cast, showing (1) the olfactory region; (2) the middle turbinate; (3) the inferior turbinate; (4) the nasopharynx; (5) the vestibule. The mask was used for the photo analysis to determine the coverage in each region.

A 45 µL nasal spray pump in combination with two nanotech nozzle chips from Medspray (Enschede, The Netherlands) with different hole sizes, as shown in Figure 2, was used in the deposition experiments. Each nanotech nozzle had a silicon chip containing either 48 pores of 4 µm in diameter or 48 pores of 5 µm in diameter, both of which generated a slow-moving soft mist with a fixed spray plume angle of 20°. The nozzle chips with the 4 µm and the 5 µm pores created droplets with a mean diameter (Dv50) of 23.6 µm and 29.5 µm and delivered the full dose of the aerosol in approximately 2.7 s and 1.7 s, respectively. The results of the droplet size measurements and the full-dose delivery times are shown in Figure 3. The spray pump was actuated inside the nostril at an angle of 45–60°, with respect to the palate, and at an insertion depth of 10 mm, depositing a mixture of theophylline and calcein, a fluorescent dye, inside the nasal cast.

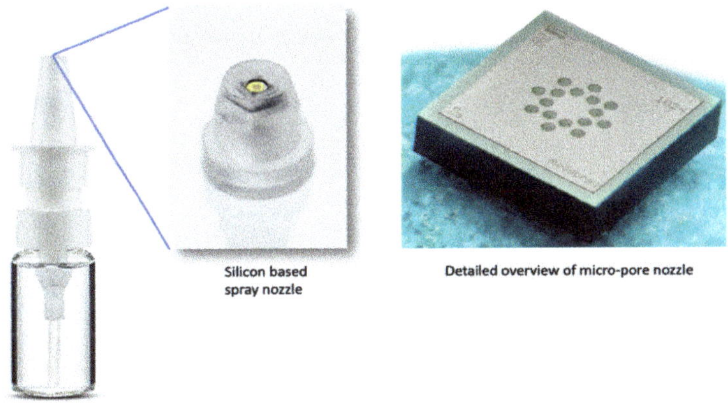

Figure 2. The nanotech nebulization device consisting of a nasal spray pump (Aero Pump GmbH, Hochheim, Germany) and an integrated silicon-based nanotech (soft mist) nozzle chip (Medspray, Enschede, The Netherlands) (image obtained from "Fluorescence-enabled evaluation of nasal tract deposition and coverage of pharmaceutical formulations in a silicone nasal cast using an innovative spray device" by D'Angelo et al. [9] licensed under CC BY-NC-ND 4.0 DEED).

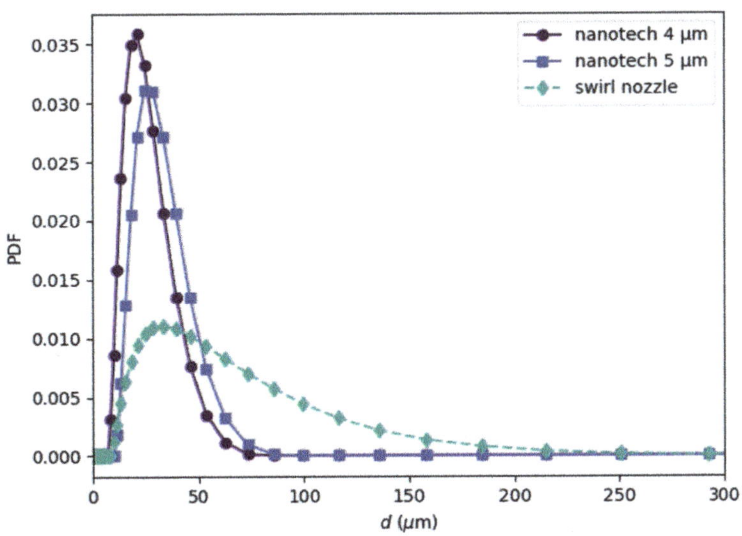

Nozzle type	Actuation time [s] at 10 bar	Dv(10) [μm]	Dv(50) [μm]	Dv(90) [μm]
4 μm nanotech chip	2.7	13.5	23.6	40.1
5 μm nanotech chip	1.7	18.0	29.5	47.6
Swirl nozzle	0.2	22.2	55.6	126.3

Figure 3. Top: the droplet size distribution (probability density function) produced by the two nanotech nozzle chips with pore sizes of 4 μm and 5 μm and a nasal swirl nozzle measured by a Malvern Spraytec laser diffraction system. Bottom: the actuation times and the droplet size volume percentiles for the three nozzles.

To prepare the theophylline–calcein mixture used for spraying, a calcein stock solution was first created. The formulation of the calcein stock solution was adapted from

D'Angelo et al. [9]. Calcein powder was solubilized in 80 µL of 1M NaOH, to which 25% (*w*/*v*) glycerol and 0.9% saline (*v*/*v*) were added to obtain a calcein concentration of 40 mg/mL. The NaOH was used to increase the pH of the stock solution to a value of 10, as calcein can only be solubilized at high pH values, and glycerol was added to increase the viscosity of the solution to prevent dripping in the nasal cast after spraying. Theophylline was then added to the stock solution as a model drug until a final calcein concentration of 1mg/mL was obtained. The formulation composition was selected to preserve fluorescence over at least 15 min, which is a sufficient time to image the nasal cast after deposition. In all the experiments, the spray pump was actuated three times, resulting in a total of 135 µL of the solution nebulized per experiment.

First, for comparing the two nanotech nozzle chips, deposition under a fixed flow was studied. To do so, a constant simulated inhalation flow of 15 L/min (as measured in the nostril) was maintained in the nasal cavity during spraying using a Copley LCP5 vacuum pump (Copley Scientific, Nottingham, UK) and a TSI 4040 flowmeter (TSI Incorporated, Shoreview United States, Shoreview, MN, USA). Measurements at the same flow rate were also performed for a nasal swirl nozzle for comparison with the nanotech nozzle chips.

Next, deposition experiments were performed at typical flow rates as found in the user study to investigate the effect of the flow rate on the deposition pattern.

Before and after spraying, images of the nasal cast were acquired using a Velleman® UV Lamp (ZLUVB, Velleman NV, Gavere, Belgium) as a source of UV rays with a wavelength of 366 nm and a digital camera (Nikon D3400, Nikon, Tokyo, Japan) set at an exposure time of 1/5 s, an f-stop of 5.6, a focal distance of 18 mm, and an ISO number of 3200. To ensure standardized photographic conditions, all images were acquired inside a black box, and the camera was fixed at a distance of 15 cm from the cast. Before each image acquisition, the septum was removed. The images were analyzed with the software ImageJ 1.53k (U.S. National Institute of Health, Bethesda, MD, USA), where a 2D mapping of the deposition in the 3D model could be determined. The cast area was divided into fixed regions of interest (ROIs) for all of the images analyzed, as shown in Figure 1. The intensity range was kept fixed between 11 and 256. Each experiment was repeated ten times.

3. Results

3.1. Effect of the User Instruction on the Inhalation Flow Characteristics

The outputs of the user study are the inhalation duration, the mean inhalation velocity, and the mean peak inhalation velocity for each of the instructions, as tabulated in Table S1. For the nanotech nasal spray to deliver the full dose, it is essential that the duration of the inhalation is sufficiently long. Using the 4 µm nanotech nebulizer as a reference, this is approximately 2 s as shown in Figure 3. Figure 4 shows the inhalation flow during the first 4 s of the inhalation maneuver averaged over all the volunteers. The percentage of the volunteers that reached a certain inhalation duration is shown in Figure 5. While all versions of the instructions achieved a sufficient inhalation time (i.e., 2 s) to deliver the entire dose for 80% of the volunteers, only instruction 3 achieved it for 100% of the volunteers. For instruction 4, the inhalation pattern consists of several short sniffs for some volunteers, resulting in a less constant flow, which is not ideal for delivering a longer-lasting soft mist nasal spray. Instruction 5 resulted in a large variation in the inhalation velocities between the volunteers. Overall, instructions 1 and 3 resulted in the most stable inhalation curve with a small variance and sufficiently long inhalation times. Based on Figure 4, we chose four flow rates: 0, 7.5, 15, and 25 L/min for the in vitro deposition studies, as the user study suggests that they are representative of in vivo conditions.

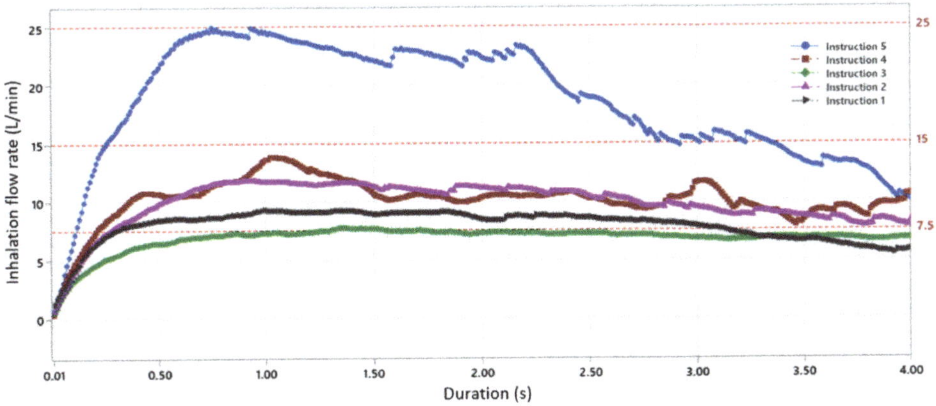

Figure 4. The average inhalation flow rate for different instructions. The flow rates used for the deposition studies are shown as red dotted lines (7.5, 15, 25 L/min). For each duration, averaging was performed over all the volunteers, excluding data from the volunteers who did not reach that duration.

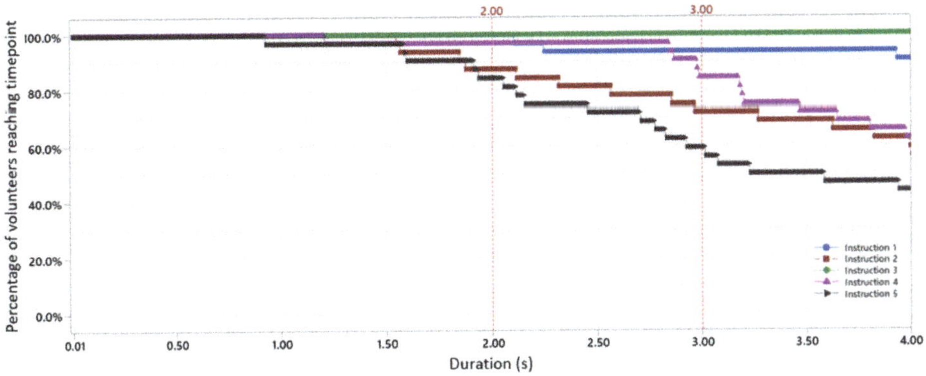

Figure 5. The percentage of the volunteers reaching a certain inhalation duration. The red dotted line at 2 s indicates the minimum time needed to deposit the complete aerosol dose.

3.2. *Effect of the Nozzle Parameters on the Deposition Pattern at a Fixed Inhalation Flow Rate*

For the deposition experiments conducted at a fixed inhalation flow rate of 15 L/min, Figure 6 shows the image comparison between the different nebulization devices in terms of the deposition pattern. It also demonstrates how an image is divided into regions, for which the covered area relative to the whole surface area of that region is calculated, as tabulated in Table S2 and summarized in Table 2. Although the deposition coverage in the nostril is similar for both types of devices, there is more coverage for the nanotech nozzle chips than for the swirl nozzle in the middle turbinate, the inferior turbinate, and especially in the olfactory region. The image also shows that the swirl nozzle leads to deposition mainly in the anterior region of the nasal cavity, and the coverage in the middle and inferior turbinate is very non-uniform. No significant difference is observed between the two nanotech nozzle chips with different size holes, reflecting the relatively small differences in the plume velocity, the spray pattern, and the droplet sizes (see Figure 3).

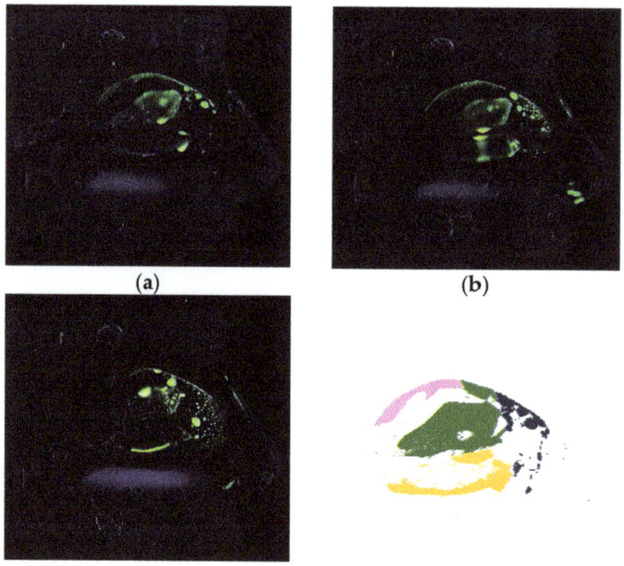

Figure 6. Fluorescence images of nasal cast coverage with calcein-stained theophylline solution deposited at a flow rate of 15 L/min: (a) 4 µm nanotech nozzle chip, (b) 5 µm nanotech nozzle chip, (c) swirl-nozzle. (d) An example photo-analysis of (a) with different regions colored (pink: olfactory region, green: middle turbinate, dark blue: nostril, yellow: inferior turbinate). Note that the nasopharynx is not visible, as this region is covered only for <0.6% in this scenario.

Table 2. An overview of the nasal coverage data for the two different nanotech nozzle chips (4 µm and 5 µm pore size) and a swirl nozzle all measured at a 15 L/min airflow. The percentages are based on the relative coverage of the region, compared to the total surface area of the region.

Device Info	Region Coverage Percentages					
Nozzle Type	Total Nasal Cast [%]	Nostril [%]	Inferior Turbinate [%]	Middle Turbinate [%]	Olfactory [%]	Nasopharynx [%]
Nanotech chip 4 µm × 48 pores	30.5% (±2.9%)	22.9% (±6.4%)	26.8% (±4.8%)	58.3% (±8.8%)	27.9% (±3.7%)	0.2% (±0.2%)
Nanotech chip 5 µm × 48 pores	29.6% (±4.9%)	23.1% (±6.5%)	27.8% (±7.9%)	54.1% (±10.6%)	24.8% (±2.6%)	0.1% (±0.1%)
Swirl nozzle	19.7% (±1.2%)	21.2% (±0.4%)	13.9% (±4.0%)	37.0% (±1.1%)	10.8% (±1.4%)	1.3% (±1.0%)

3.3. Effect of the Inhalation Flow Rate on the Deposition Pattern

For the experiments investigating the effect of the inhalation flow rates on the deposition in the nasal cavity, Figure 7a,b show the relative area coverages of each region for the four inhalation flow rates, using the 4 µm and 5 µm nanotech nozzle chips, respectively. The values are tabulated in Table S3. In two regions (in the case of the 4 µm nozzle) and all four regions (5 µm nozzle), the deposition increases slightly with increasing inhalation velocity. Overall, the deposition for the 5 µm nozzle chip has a stronger correlation with the flow rate. Deposition in the olfactory region appears least affected by the inhalation flow rate when compared to the other regions and only very slightly increases with the increasing flow rate. However, at lower inhalation velocities the variance in the olfactory coverage increases. Figure 8 compares the olfactory coverage for the two nanotech nozzle chips and the four flow rates. No significant differences are observed between the nozzles at each inhalation velocity. Both nanotech nozzle chips achieved an olfactory coverage of more than 20% when holding breath and more than 30% for a flow rate of 25 L/min.

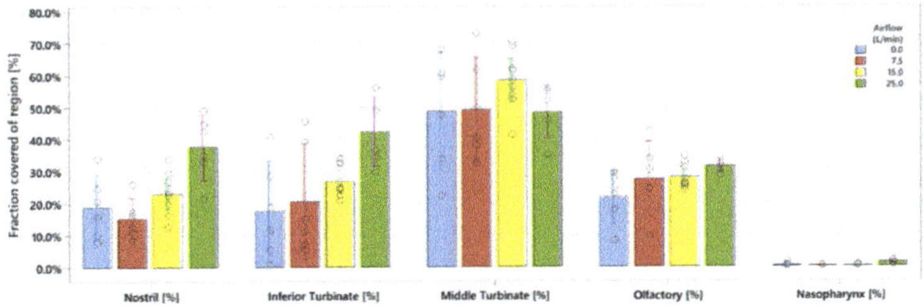

(a)

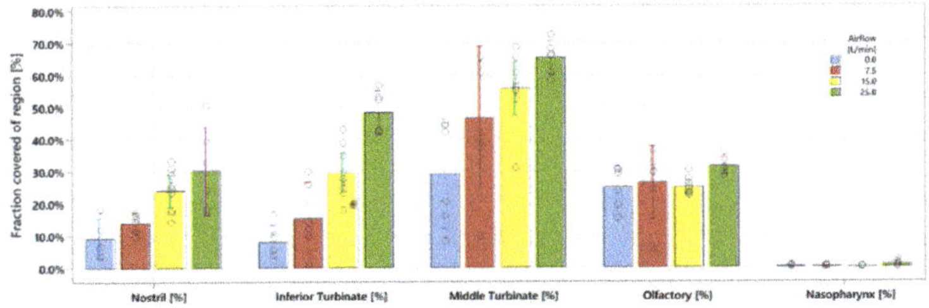

(b)

Figure 7. The deposition in different regions with the (**a**) 4 µm and (**b**) 5 µm nanotech nozzle chips at various flow rates.

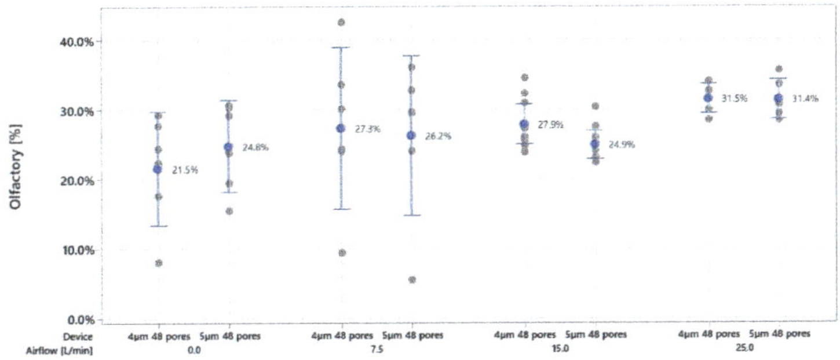

Figure 8. The olfactory region deposition for the two nanotech nozzle chips at various flow rates.

4. Discussion

The nasal cavity coverage and deposition characteristics are contingent upon the droplet size and the droplet velocity. Figure 3 shows that the swirl nozzle generates brief bursts of droplets with a wide size distribution, of which a large proportion is above 50 µm in diameter. These relatively large droplets ejected at a high velocity from the swirl nozzle follow a straight ballistic path at speeds exceeding 10 m per second [9]. Consequently, the majority of these large droplets are deposited in the front of the nasal cavity (Figure 6c), as the inertially-driven swirl nozzle droplets cannot navigate curved trajectories to reach the back of the nasal cavity. Furthermore, the interplay between the surface tension and inertial forces precludes the reduction in droplet size using a swirl nozzle. On the other hand, electric vibrating mesh nebulizers typically produce very small droplets around 5 µm [3], which are able to follow the airflow patterns more easily. However, these small droplets also more easily pass through the whole nasal cavity and continue down into the lower respiratory tract.

The nanotech nozzle device produces medium-sized droplets of around 10–50 μm (Figure 3). At this droplet size range, the droplets are likely to be in a favorable translational regime. As such, they are able to avoid ballistic impact in the anterior parts of the nasal cavity and follow the curved trajectory at a slower velocity (<1 m/s) [9], thus depositing more in the middle regions. As a result, the nanotech nozzle chip demonstrates superior deposition in the turbinate regions, including the olfactory region (Figure 8), and low passage to the nasopharyngeal region. Hence, our study showed that the slow-moving droplets of around 10–50 μm are suitable for olfactory deposition, a result that corroborates previous studies [6,16].

In the deposition study, the effect of droplet size was further tested using two different-sized nozzle chips. In both cases, the spraying duration was significantly longer than a classical swirl nozzle nasal pump (Figure 3), resulting in a lower plume velocity and a mean droplet diameter of around 25 μm and 30 μm for the 4 μm and 5 μm nanotech nozzle chips, respectively. The similar droplet sizes explain why the deposition results for the two nanotech nozzle chips are not significantly different for the same simulated inhalation flow.

Next, the user study shows that the different instructions lead to different flow rate patterns and suggests that instructions 1 and 3 provide the most constant flow rate over time, while instruction 5 gives the highest flow rate. Considering the effect of the inhalation flowrate on the deposition in the different regions inside the nasal cavity, a clear trend is visible for the 5 μm nozzle configuration (Figure 7b), which indicates that a significantly higher surface coverage can be obtained in the "nostril", "inferior turbinate", and "middle turbinate" regions at a higher inhalation velocity. This is likely because the inertial effect is stronger at higher flow rates, leading to more droplets impacting the mucosal surface in these relatively frontal regions. Therefore, in scenarios where the olfactory region is not the target delivery region, a more forceful inhalation at a higher mean inhalation flow rate between 15 and 25 L/min will give a significantly higher surface coverage in the other nasal regions. In those scenarios, provided that patients are able to inhale for long enough, higher inhalation velocities through instructions such as "inhale firmly for at least 2 s" will likely give the best results, although it is also likely to result in more variability from patient to patient.

On the other hand, deposition in the olfactory region is less affected by the inhalation flow rate. This demonstrates the robustness of the nanotech nozzle for olfactory delivery, as high area coverage (>20%) of the olfactory region can be achieved for any flow rate within the range of 0–25 L/min, making it suitable for a range of patients with different breathing patterns, provided that the inhalation time is sufficient. Since the deposition study only examined scenarios with constant flow rates, the effect of the time-varying flow rate on deposition requires future investigations but is expected to be small for realistic breathing patterns such as those obtained from the user study.

5. Conclusions

In this study, the suitability of a novel nanotech soft mist nasal spray device for the nebulization of theophylline towards the olfactory region was demonstrated. The effects of user instructions on the flow rate and subsequent deposition pattern were investigated through a user study and a deposition study. The nanotech nozzle chips achieved 21.5–31.5% coverage in the olfactory region for flow rates between 0 and 25 L/min, which is significantly higher than what is obtainable with conventional swirl nozzles. The two nanotech nozzle chips with different pore sizes did not differ significantly in terms of nasal coverage, as the droplet size distributions of the two chips are similar. The flow rate did not affect the olfactory deposition significantly within this range of flow rates tested. In future studies, the relative importance of the droplet size distribution and the spray velocity may be determined by manufacturing and testing nanotech nozzle chips with different numbers of pores, more pore sizes, and incorporating multiple pore sizes on the same chip.

In addition to hyposmia treatment with theophylline, more intranasal applications may benefit from the use of this nanotech nozzle chip technology, such as selective drug administration to the olfactory region for effective nose-to-brain drug delivery of biologics [17], oxytocin [18], polypeptides [19], and short interfering RNA for gene silencing [20], as the olfactory region can be used for crossing the blood–brain barrier. Furthermore, intranasal vaccination strategies might benefit from a more uniform formulation coverage of the mucosal tissue with the nanotech nozzle chip [21]. The pore size and the configuration of the nozzle chip may be customized for different applications to optimize the delivery.

Supplementary Materials: The following supporting information can be downloaded at: https://www.mdpi.com/article/10.3390/pharmaceutics16010002/s1, Table S1: Summary of flow measurements under the different inhalation instructions listed in Table 1; Table S2: Summary of flow measurements under the different inhalation instructions listed in Table 1; Table S3: Summarized nasal coverage data for the two nanotech nozzle chips (4 µm and 5 µm) and four airflows (0, 7.5, 15, 25 L/min).

Author Contributions: Conceptualization, M.X.Z., F.V., R.G., D.B. and C.J.M.v.R.; methodology, M.X.Z., F.V., P.R., S.K. and C.J.M.v.R.; validation, M.X.Z., F.V., P.R. and S.K.; formal analysis, M.X.Z. and F.V.; investigation, M.X.Z. and F.V.; data curation, M.X.Z. and F.V.; writing—original draft preparation, M.X.Z., F.V. and C.J.M.v.R.; writing—review and editing, M.X.Z., F.V., R.G., D.B. and C.J.M.v.R.; visualization, M.X.Z. and F.V.; supervision, D.B. and C.J.M.v.R.; funding acquisition, D.B. and C.J.M.v.R. All authors have read and agreed to the published version of the manuscript.

Funding: This research was funded by the Dutch Research Council NWO, IPP grant "Innovative Nanotech Sprays", ENPPS.IPP.019.001.

Institutional Review Board Statement: The study was conducted in accordance with the principals and rules stipulated in the Assessment framework for ethical issues of the faculty of science at the University of Amsterdam and approved by the Ethics Committee for research in the Sciences and Life sciences at the University of Amsterdam (protocol code FNWI-39_2023, date of approval 2 November 2023).

Informed Consent Statement: Informed consent was obtained from all subjects involved in the study.

Data Availability Statement: The data presented in this study are available in the main text of this article or Supplementary Materials.

Conflicts of Interest: F.V. and P.R. declare that they are employees at Medspray, B.V. and R.G. is an employee at Cyrano Therapeutics Inc. The funders had no role in the design of the study; in the collection, analyses, or interpretation of data; in the writing of the manuscript; or in the decision to publish the results.

References

1. Jahnsen, F.L.; Gran, E.; Haye, R.; Brandtzaeg, P. Human Nasal Mucosa Contains Antigen-Presenting Cells of Strikingly Different Functional Phenotypes. *Am. J. Respir. Cell Mol. Biol.* **2004**, *30*, 31–37. [CrossRef] [PubMed]
2. Fröhlich, E. Non-Cellular Layers of the Respiratory Tract: Protection against Pathogens and Target for Drug Delivery. *Pharmaceutics* **2022**, *14*, 992. [CrossRef] [PubMed]
3. Vecellio, L.; De Gersem, R.; Le Guellec, S.; Reychler, G.; Pitance, L.; Le Pennec, D.; Diot, P.; Chantrel, G.; Bonfils, P.; Jamar, F. Deposition of aerosols delivered by nasal route with jet and mesh nebulizers. *Int. J. Pharm.* **2011**, *407*, 87–94. [CrossRef] [PubMed]
4. Kundoor, V.; Dalby, R.N. Assessment of Nasal Spray Deposition Pattern in a Silicone Human Nose Model Using a Color-Based Method. *Pharm. Res.* **2010**, *27*, 30–36. [CrossRef] [PubMed]
5. Suman, J.D.; Laube, B.L.; Dalby, R. Comparison of Nasal Deposition and Clearance of Aerosol Generated by a Nebulizer and an Aqueous Spray Pump. *Pharm. Res.* **1999**, *16*, 1648–1652. [CrossRef] [PubMed]
6. Kimbell, J.S.; Segal, R.A.; Asgharian, B.; Wong, B.A.; Schroeter, J.D.; Southall, J.P.; Dickens, C.J.; Brace, G.; Miller, F.J. Characterization of Deposition from Nasal Spray Devices Using A Computational Fluid Dynamics Model of The Human Nasal Passages. *J. Aerosol. Med.* **2007**, *20*, 59–74. [CrossRef] [PubMed]
7. Suman, J.D.; Laube, B.L.; Dalby, R. Nasal nebulizers versus aqueous spray pumps: A comparison of deposition patterns in human volunteers. *Respir. Drug Deliv.* **1998**, *6*, 211–218.
8. Foo, M.Y.; Cheng, Y.-S.; Su, W.-C.; Donovan, M.D. The Influence of Spray Properties on Intranasal Deposition. *J. Aerosol Med.* **2007**, *20*, 495–508. [CrossRef] [PubMed]
9. D'Angelo, D.; Kooij, S.; Verhoeven, F.; Sonvico, F.; van Rijn, C. Fluorescence-enabled evaluation of nasal tract deposition and coverage of pharmaceutical formulations in a silicone nasal cast using an innovative spray device. *J. Adv. Res.* **2023**, *44*, 227–232. [CrossRef] [PubMed]

10. St. Martin, M.B.; Hitzman, C.J.; Wiedmann, T.S.; Rimell, F.L. Deposition of Aerosolized Particles in the Maxillary Sinuses before and after Endoscopic Sinus Surgery. *Am. J. Rhinol.* **2007**, *21*, 196–197. [CrossRef] [PubMed]
11. Merkus, P.; Ebbens, F.A.; Muller, B.; Fokkens, W.J. Influence of anatomy and head position on intranasal drug deposition. *Eur. Arch. Oto-Rhino-Laryngol. Head Neck* **2006**, *263*, 827–832. [CrossRef] [PubMed]
12. Henkin, R.I.; Schultz, M.; Minnick-Poppe, L. Intranasal Theophylline Treatment of Hyposmia and Hypogeusia: A pilot study. *Arch. Otolaryngol. Head Neck Surg.* **2012**, *138*, 1064–1070. [CrossRef] [PubMed]
13. Moon, C.; Simpson, P.J.; Tu, Y.; Cho, H.; Ronnett, G.V. Regulation of intracellular cyclic GMP levels in olfactory sensory neurons. *J. Neurochem.* **2005**, *95*, 200–209. [CrossRef] [PubMed]
14. Lochhead, J.J.; Thorne, R.G. Intranasal drug delivery to the brain. In *Drug Delivery to the Brain*; Hammarlund-Udenaes, M., de Lange, R.G.T., Eds.; Springer: New York, NY, USA, 2014; Volume 10, pp. 401–431.
15. Xi, J.; Wang, Z.; Nevorski, D.; White, T.; Zhou, Y. Nasal and Olfactory Deposition with Normal and Bidirectional Intranasal Delivery Techniques: In Vitro Tests and Numerical Simulations. *J. Aerosol. Med. Pulm. Drug Deliv.* **2017**, *30*, 118–131. [CrossRef] [PubMed]
16. Yarragudi, S.B.; Kumar, H.; Jain, R.; Tawhai, M.; Rizwan, S. Olfactory Targeting of Microparticles Through Inhalation and Bi-directional Airflow: Effect of Particle Size and Nasal Anatomy. *J. Aerosol. Med. Pulm. Drug Deliv.* **2020**, *33*, 258–270. [CrossRef] [PubMed]
17. Sasaki, K.; Fukakusa, S.; Torikai, Y.; Suzuki, C.; Sonohata, I.; Kawahata, T.; Magata, Y.; Kawai, K.; Haruta, S. Effective nose-to-brain drug delivery using a combination system targeting the olfactory region in monkeys. *J. Control. Release* **2023**, *359*, 384–399. [CrossRef] [PubMed]
18. Lochhead, J.J.; Thorne, R.G. Intranasal delivery of biologics to the central nervous system. *Adv. Drug Deliv. Rev.* **2012**, *64*, 614–628. [CrossRef]
19. Bharadwaj, V.N.; Tzabazis, A.Z.; Klukinov, M.; Manering, N.A.; Yeomans, D.C. Intranasal Administration for Pain: Oxytocin and Other Polypeptides. *Pharmaceutics* **2021**, *13*, 1088. [CrossRef]
20. Van Woensel, M.; Mathivet, T.; Wauthoz, N.; Rosière, R.; Garg, A.D.; Agostinis, P.; Mathieu, V.; Kiss, R.; Lefranc, F.; Boon, L.; et al. Sensitization of glioblastoma tumor micro-environment to chemo- and immunotherapy by Galectin-1 intranasal knock-down strategy. *Sci. Rep.* **2017**, *7*, 1217. [CrossRef] [PubMed]
21. Zhang, Y.; Almazi, J.G.; Ong, H.X.; Johansen, M.D.; Ledger, S.; Traini, D.; Hansbro, P.M.; Kelleher, A.D.; Ahlenstiel, C.L. Nanoparticle Delivery Platforms for RNAi Therapeutics Targeting COVID-19 Disease in the Respiratory Tract. *Int. J. Mol. Sci.* **2022**, *23*, 2408. [CrossRef] [PubMed]

MDPI AG
Grosspeteranlage 5
4052 Basel
Switzerland
Tel.: +41 61 683 77 34

Pharmaceutics Editorial Office
E-mail: pharmaceutics@mdpi.com
www.mdpi.com/journal/pharmaceutics

www.ingramcontent.com/pod-product-compliance
Lightning Source LLC
Chambersburg PA
CBHW061550210926
51850CB00009B/2061
9783725874002